The Electrocardiogram in Infants and Children:

A Systematic Approach

"There are comparatively few people who are not in greater danger of having their peace and happiness destroyed by an erroneous diagnosis of cardiac abnormality based on a faulty interpretation of an electrocardiogram than of being injured or killed by an atomic bomb."

FRANK WILSON
Lepeschkin's "Modern Electrocardiography" (1951)

The Electrocardiogram in Infants and Children:

A SYSTEMATIC APPROACH

Arthur Garson, Jr., M.D.

Associate Professor of Pediatrics and Medicine,
Baylor College of Medicine;
Director, Electrocardiography Laboratory,
The Lillie Frank Abercrombie Section of Cardiology,
Texas Children's Hospital,
Houston, Texas

LEA & FEBIGER   PHILADELPHIA

1983

LEA & FEBIGER, *Publishers*
600 South Washington Square
Philadelphia, Pa. 19106
U.S.A.

Library of Congress Cataloging in Publication Data

Garson, Arthur.
 The electrocardiogram in infants and children.

 Bibliography: p.
 Includes index.
 1. Electrocardiography.   2. Pediatric cardiology—Diagnosis.
I. Title. [DNLM: 1. Electrocardiography—In infancy and childhood.
WS 290 G243e]
RJ423.5.E43G37   1983   618.92′1207547   83-1039
ISBN 0-8121-0872-8

PRINTED IN THE UNITED STATES OF AMERICA
Print Number   3 2 1

DEDICATION

I would like to dedicate this book to my teachers: Beginning with my parents, Patricia and Arthur, and my sibs, Susan, Thomas and Kathleen; to Joseph Becker, Phelps Laszlo, Harold Brown, John Joseph, Alexander MacFarlane, John Bookman, Lester Barnett, Eric Rogers, Madison Spach, Samuel Katz, David Sabiston, Newland Oldham, William DeMaria, Mark Rogers, Dan McNamara, Paul Gillette, Charles Mullins, Michael Nihill, Howard Gutgesell, Thomas Vargo, Sarah Blumenschein, Jill Morriss; and, to my most recent teacher, my wife, Suzan.

Foreword

Another textbook on pediatric electrocardiography? One might ask, What makes Garson's book different from the others? Perhaps it is the author's experience with investigative intracardiac electrophysiology, which has given him the insight to understand "in depth" the surface electrocardiogram and to explain it in such a clear manner.

The book is the work of one author whose experience during the past 10 years with patients who have pediatric and congenital heart disease and with teaching the electrocardiogram to medical students, pediatric residents, and fellows as well as experienced pediatric cardiologists qualifies him for this authorship. Garson has had a receptive ear to the questions of his students, and he has used his responses to those questions in writing this book, which may be the secret to the relevance of the work.

Garson is an enthusiastic teacher who is confident that his reader can achieve success in learning the electrocardiogram. Finally, the reader who has seen the author's cleverly constructed slides will recognize his talent in many of the illustrations in this book.

DAN G. MCNAMARA, M.D.

Preface

This book was written for both the novice who is learning the fundamentals of electrocardiography as well as for the experienced clinician who seeks an update on what is becoming a science based upon electrophysiologic principles rather than an art based upon empiricism.

Our understanding of the electrocardiogram in the child has expanded even in the last five years, advancing our diagnostic capability in certain areas and defining our limitations more realistically in other aspects of the field. It has become necessary to reassess our knowledge of what we considered to be fundamental concepts as well as the application of these principles in the interpretation of the clinical electrocardiogram.

This book is entitled "A Systematic Approach" because it presents the principles of electrocardiography sequentially, in an orderly manner. It is meant to be read from cover to cover, since much of the information contained in the later chapters builds upon concepts elaborated earlier. Since most of us learn best by the Socratic method, self-assessment questions are included at the end of each chapter with a discussion of the answers.

The first half of the book is devoted to the normal electrocardiogram: electrophysiologic principles, summation of cellular events on the body surface, definition and measurement of the components of the electrocardiogram, and the variations produced solely by malposition of the heart within the thorax. The second half of the book concerns the abnormal electrocardiogram and its value in diagnosing hypertrophy, ischemia, and infarction, considering the recent advances in echocardiography and nuclear imaging. In the chapter on arrhythmias, two approaches are taken: in the electrophysiologic section, the major arrhythmias are discussed according to their site of origin and mechanism; in the morphologic section, a stepwise method of rhythm analysis is presented. Finally, a systematic approach to the recognition of artifacts is presented in the hope that the child with a normal heart will not become a victim of faulty interpretation of a normal electrocardiogram.

Houston, Texas   Arthur Garson, Jr.

Acknowledgements

I would like to thank my assistant, Candy Killebrew, in general for her support throughout this endeavor and in particular for typing and editing the manuscript several times. I would also like to thank Drs. Andre Davignon and Pentii Rautaharju for supplying their tables of the normal values for the electrocardiograms. The illustrations were expertly drawn by Bill Andrews and the other members of the Creative Arts Department, Texas Children's Hospital.

Some of the illustrations in Chapter 12 are reprinted from *A Guide to Cardiac Dysrhythmias in Children*, edited by A. Garson, P. C. Gillette, and D. G. McNamara, New York, Grune & Stratton, 1981; and *Pediatric Electrocardiography*, edited by J. Liebman, R. Plonsey, and P. C. Gillette, Baltimore, Williams & Wilkins, 1982. Permission was obtained from the publishers, the editors, and the authors.

This work was supported in part by USPH grant HL07190 from the National Institutes of Health, USPH grant RR0188 from the General Clinical Research Branch of the National Institutes of Health, a grant from the J. S. Abercrombie Foundation, and a National Institutes of Health Young Investigator Research Award HL24916.

Finally, I would like to thank the staff of the Electrocardiographic Laboratory, Texas Children's Hospital: Pat McVey, Americo Simonelli, Donalee Cushman, Sandra Jordan, Alice Mast, and Pauline Rousch. They recorded the high quality electrocardiograms displayed in these figures; they helped to find the examples that were included, and refiled the majority, which were not.

A. G., Jr.

Contents

1. Anatomy of the Conduction System   3

   —Self-Assessment Questions   6

2. Depolarization and Repolarization: Cellular Electrophysiology   9

   —The Single Cell: Cardiac Action Potential   9
   —Current Flow Within a Cell: The Dipole Concept   12
   —From the Cell to the Body Surface   16

   —Self-Assessment Questions   16

3. Recording the Sequence of Cardiac Activity   19

   —Instrumentation   19
   —Electrocardiographic Waves and Intervals   25
   —Electrocardiographic Leads   27

   —Self-Assessment Questions   33

4. Derivation of the Electrocardiogram   36

   —Atrial Depolarization and Repolarization: The P and Ta Wave   36
   —Ventricular Depolarization: The QRS Complex   39
   —Ventricular Muscle Repolarization: The T Wave   43
   —Ventricular Purkinje Repolarization: The U Wave   45

   —Self-Assessment Questions   46

5. Mean Vector ("Axis")   49
   —QRS Mean Vector   49
   —T Wave Mean Vector   55
   —P Wave Mean Vector   56

   —Self-Assessment Questions   57

6. The Normal Electrocardiogram   61
   —Normal Values   61
   —Heart Rate   62
   —P Wave   63
   —PR Interval   65
   —PR Segment   67
   —QRS Complex   67
   —ST Segment   70
   —T Wave   70
   —U Wave   71
   —QT Interval   74
   —Q-OT Interval   77
   —TP Interval   77

   —Self-Assessment Questions   79

7. The Heart Malposed in the Thorax   83
   —Atrial Situs   83
   —Ventricular Position   84
   —Pectus Excavatum and Straight Back
     Syndrome   90
   —Pneumonectomy   94
   —Pneumothorax and Pneumomediastinum   94
   —Kyphoscoliosis   95

   —Self-Assessment Questions   95

8. Chamber Enlargement and
   Hypertrophy   99
   —Right Ventricular Hypertrophy   99
   —Left Ventricular Hypertrophy   106
   —Biventricular Hypertrophy   108
   —Right Atrial Enlargement   110
   —Left Atrial Enlargement   111
   —Biatrial Enlargement   113

   —Self-Assessment Questions   113

9. **Interventricular Conduction Disturbance**   119

—Conduction Delay 119
  —Right Bundle Branch Block   119
  —Left Bundle Branch Block   126
  —Fascicular Block   130
  —Bifascicular Block   134
  —Trifascicular Block   135
  —Diffuse Interventricular Conduction Delay 135
—Preexcitation 135
  —Wolff-Parkinson-White   136
  —Lown-Ganong-Levine   137
  —Mahaim Conduction   139

—Self-Assessment Questions   143

10. **Ischemia, Injury, and Infarction**   149

—Primary and Secondary T Wave Changes   149
—Functional T Wave Changes   149
—Ischemia   151
—Injury   152
—Infarction   159
—Aneurysm   164

—Self-Assessment Questions   165

11. **Effect of Systemic Alterations on the Electrocardiogram**   170

—Action Potential Changes Reflected in the Electrocardiogram 170
—Body Chemistry   173
—Antiarrhythmic Drugs   178
—Anesthetic Agents   183
—Psychotropic Drugs   183
—Organophosphorous Insecticides   184
—Central Nervous System Effects   184
—Hypothermia   186
—Neuromuscular Disorders   186
—Connective Tissue Disease   187
—Metabolic Diseases   187
—Miscellaneous Diseases   189

—Self-Assessment Questions   189

12. Arrhythmias   195

—Ladder Diagrams   195
—The Electrophysiologic Approach   197
  —Sinus Rhythm   198
  —Escape Beats and Escape Rhythms   198
    —Sinus Arrhythmia   198
    —Atrial Escape   199
    —Junctional Escape   200
    —Ventricular Escape   201
    —Escape with Aberrancy   201
    —Wandering Pacemaker   202
    —Sinus Bradycardia   202
  —Premature Beats   205
    —Premature Atrial Contractions   208
    —Premature Junctional Contractions   210
    —Premature Ventricular Contractions   212
    —Differential Diagnosis of Premature
      Beats   214
    —Morphology of Premature Beats: Uniform
      versus Multiform   220
    —Patterns of Premature Beats: Bigeminy,
      Trigeminy, and Couplets   220
    —Coupling Interval: Parasystole   225
    —Capture Beats   229
  —Tachyarrythmias   231
    —Sinus Tachycardia   231
    —Supraventricular Tachycardia   235
    —Accelerated Atrial Rhythm and Accelerated
      Junctional Rhythm   239
    —Atrial Flutter   241
    —Atrial Fibrillation   249
    —Ventricular Tachycardia   251
    —Ventricular Fibrillation   254
    —Accelerated Ventricular Rhythm   259
    —Differential Diagnosis of
      Tachyarrhythmias   259
  —AV Block   261
    —First-Degree AV Block   263
    —Second-Degree AV Block   265
    —Third-Degree ("Complete") AV Block   269

—The Morphologic Approach   274
  —Introduction to the Systematic
    Interpretation of Cardiac Arrhythmias in
    Children   274
  —Categories of Arrythmias   301

—Self-Assessment Questions   344

13. Artifacts   376
  —Causes of Artifacts   376
  —Systematic Approach to the Recognition of
    Artifacts   385

  —Self-Assessment Questions   392

Appendix—Tables of Electrocardiographic
Normal Values   396
  —Summary Table   404

Index   405

The Electrocardiogram in Infants and Children:

A Systematic Approach

1

Anatomy of the Conduction System

The cardiac conduction system extends from the sinus node to the atrial and ventricular myocardium. The sinus node is a fusiform structure, 10 to 20 mm long in the adult, which lies in the sulcus terminalis slightly lateral to the junction of the right atrial appendage and the superior vena cava.[1] It is usually located less than 1 mm below the epicardium and extends transmurally close to the endocardium (Fig. 1-1). The sinus node surrounds the largest atrial artery, the sinus node artery, which in 55 to 65% of cases is a branch of the right coronary artery, and in the other 35 to 45%, a branch of the left circumflex coronary artery.[2]

The cellular constituents of the sinus node are supported by a collagen framework which increases in density with age. The primary cells of the sinus node are the P cells. These are round, pale-staining cells that occur in clusters close to the central artery.[3] The P cells are thought to be the true pacemaking cells. They are connected either to other P cells or to transitional cells, which are small, more fusiform cells that have some of the characteristics of P cells combined with those of atrial muscle cells. Transitional cells completely surround the borders of the sinus node and are thought to be the site of sinoatrial entrance and exit block.[4] Parasympathetic ganglia border the anterior and posterior portions of the sinus node.

The mode of conduction of impulses within the atria has been the subject of much controversy. The major question concerns the existence of the internodal tracts: Does conduction proceed preferentially through the atria by way of specialized pathways? Certain facts can be brought to bear. Electrophysiologically, the conduction velocity has been shown to be increased in three areas of the right atrium. The "anterior internodal tract" extends from the sinus node, runs anteriorly to the superior vena cava, through the anterior part of the atrial septum and to the superior part of the AV node. The "middle internodal tract" proceeds posterior to the superior vena cava and then to the limbus of the fossa ovalis where it joins the anterior internodal tract.[5] The "posterior internodal tract" runs in the crista terminalis to the inferior atrial septum adjacent to the inferior vena cava.[6] It then

3

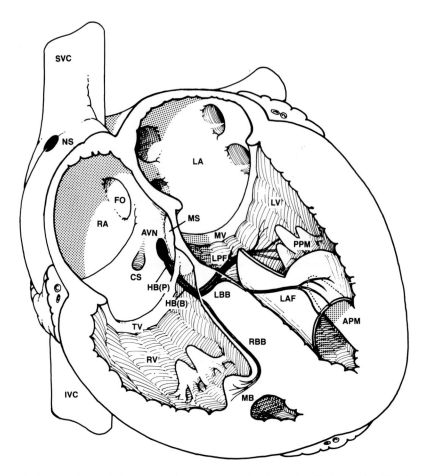

FIG. 1-1. Anatomy of the conduction system. APM, anterior papillary muscle; AVN, AV node; CS, coronary sinus; FO, foramen ovale; HB(P), His bundle, penetrating portion; HB(B), His bundle, branching portion; IVC, inferior vena cava; LA, left atrium; LAF, left anterior fascicle; LBB, left bundle branch; LV, left ventricle; LPF, left posterior fascicle; MB, moderator band; MS, membranous septum; MV, mitral valve; NS, sinus node; PPM, posterior papillary muscle; RA, right atrium; RV, right ventricle; SVC, superior vena cava.

travels superior to the coronary sinus ostium and terminates in the posterior part of the AV node. The "anterior intra-atrial tract" is a thick band of muscle that courses from the anterior part of the sinus node anteriorly to the superior vena cava, through the atrial septum to the left atrial musculature.[7]

In these areas of more rapid conduction, there is a combination of atrial muscle cells and Purkinje cells which are oriented in a parallel fashion.[8] However, these tracts are not isolated from the rest of the atrium by connective tissue.[1] These facts have been interpreted by James,[9] Waldo et al.,[10] Merideth and Titus,[11] and Liebman and Plonsey[12] as indicating the presence of true preferential conduction. On the other hand, the view that these "tracts" are the shortest anatomic distance between the sinus and AV nodes and that conduction may be facilitated only by the parallel fiber orientation (rather than the existence of true tracts) is held by Spach and Barr,[8] Lev and Bharati,[1] Durrer et el.,[13] and Janse and Anderson.[14] The finding by Gillette et al. that after the Mustard operation for transposition of the great arteries, the internodal conduction time from the high right atrium to low septal right atrium is normal, supports the view that there are no true internodal tracts.[15] If there were, these tracts should have been injured by atriotomy, suturing of the baffle, or coronary sinus cutback, and the conduction time should have been prolonged, which it was not. Our view is that conduction spreads radially and syncytially from the sinus node to the AV node by the fastest possible route. The concept of "specialized tracts" should be reserved for intraventricular conduction by way of the bundle branches and does not apply to intra-atrial conduction.

The AV node is the only normal conduction pathway from atria to ventricles. The AV node is located in the right atrium on the right side of the central fibrous body between the mouth of the coronary sinus and the annulus of the septal leaflet of the tricuspid valve (Fig. 1-1). The left surface of the AV node rests on the mitral annulus. In the adult, the AV node averages 5 to 7 mm in length, 2 to 3 mm in width, and 0.5 to 1 mm in thickness.[16,17] The blood supply to the AV node is via the artery of Haas, which arises from the right coronary artery in 90% of cases.[18] Microscopically, in the compact AV node, there are few P cells with mainly small transitional cells interweaving with collagen in all different directions in the upper and middle portions of the node. In the anterior and inferior part of the node, the fibers begin to orient longitudinally to form the AV bundle. Parasympathetic ganglia and sympathetic nerve endings are located primarily posterior to the compact node.

When the conduction tissue penetrates the central fibrous body, it is designated the penetrating portion of the AV bundle, or bundle of His. This proceeds anteriorly and medially in the central fibrous body and then inferiorly along the rim of the membranous ventricular septum immediately below the noncoronary cusp of the aortic valve. In approximately 75% of human hearts, the penetrating His bundle runs along the left side of the crest of the muscular ventricular septum; in the remainder, it courses along the right side. The penetrating bundle is made up of small oval cells which are longitudinally oriented. In this portion of the bundle, there are fibrous collagen septae. The fibers are thus thought to be "predestined" for one of the bundle branches even at this proximal level. A fibrotic lesion in part of the penetrating bundle may, therefore, simulate a more distal lesion in the bundle branches.

The "branching portion" of the AV bundle begins as fibers forming the left bundle branch exit at a right angle from the main bundle. This occurs at the level of the commissure formed by the right and noncoronary cusps. The origin of the left bundle branch is quite variable: All of the fibers may fan out together, or they may be given off in separate fascicles.[19,20] Since the AV bundle is directed in the posteroanterior direction, the first fibers of the left bundle branch to be given off form the left posterior fascicle and the last fibers form the left anterior fascicle. The left posterior fascicle in the adult is 6 mm wide and 20 mm long and extends posteroinferiorly in the inflow tract of the left ventricle to the posterior papillary muscle. The left anterior fascicle is thinner and longer, being 3 mm thick and 25 mm long in the adult. It extends obliquely, anteriorly, and superiorly across the left ventricular outflow tract to the anterior papillary muscle. Microscopically, the fascicles are made up of Purkinje cells, which are larger than ordinary myocardial cells. Each fascicle is surrounded by a connective tissue sheath and therefore makes no contact with the ventricular muscle for approximately 20 mm. Then, multiple Purkinje fibers branch throughout the endocardium of the left ventricle. The posterobasal left ventricle is virtually devoid of rapidly conducting Purkinje fibers and therefore this area of the left ventricle is the last part to be activated.

After the last fibers of the left bundle branch are given off from the branching bundle, the conduction tissue continues as the right bundle branch. The right bundle branch proceeds subendocardially in the septal band and then intramyocardially in the right side of the ventricular septum, running immediately inferior to the muscle of Lancisi (papillary muscle of the conus) until the bundle runs through the moderator band. The entire right bundle branch is insulated throughout its nonbranching course (50 to 60 mm in the adult) from the His bundle to the moderator band. When it reaches the anterior papillary muscle of the right ventricle, the right bundle separates into numerous Purkinje fibers throughout the endocardium. The conus of the right ventricle is virtually devoid of Purkinje tissue and this, added to the normally delayed right ventricular activation due to the insulated right bundle branch, makes the conus the last part of the heart to be activated.

Self-Assessment Questions

Question 1: In a patient with disease of the right atrium caused by chronic tricuspid insufficiency, which structure(s) would be affected?

A. sinus node
B. AV node
C. both
D. neither

Question 2: In the incision to divide a bundle of Kent, the surgeon may completely encircle the tricuspid annulus with his incision. Which structure(s) would necessarily be injured in this incision?

A. anterior internodal tract
B. posterior internodal tract
C. AV node
D. bundle of His
E. none of the above

Question 3: Assume an ectopic pacemaker is located in the left atrium, the same anatomic distance from the AV node as the sinus node is from the AV node. Compare the relative conduction times to the AV node.

A. the right atrium is shorter since there are tracts in the right atrium
B. the left atrium is shorter since the impulse travels via Bachmann's bundle
C. the conduction time is similar, if there is similar fiber orientation

Question 4: In patients with turbulence in the left ventricular outflow tract, which part of the conduction system is most vulnerable to injury?

A. AV node
B. bundle of His
C. right bundle branch
D. left anterior fascicle
E. left posterior fascicle

Answers to Self-Assessment Questions

Answer 1: C
The patient with right atrial disease may have both sinus node and AV node dysfunction; both structures are part of the right atrium.

Answer 2: E
All of these structures are proximal to the tricuspid annulus except the bundle of His. If the incision is superficial, the bundle of His is not necessarily injured.

Answer 3: C
In the atria, if the anatomic distance and path length are the same, and the fiber orientation is the same, the conduction time should be the same. The "tracts" most likely do not provide any preferential conduction other than parallel fiber orientation.

Answer 4: D
The left anterior fascicle is a thin structure that stretches across the left ventricular outflow tract and is therefore prone to injury with turbulence in this area.

References

1. Lev M., and Bharati S.: Anatomy of the conduction system in normal and congenitally abnormal hearts. *In* Cardiac Arrhythmias in the Neonate, Infant and Child. Edited by N. K. Roberts and H. Gelband. New York, Appleton-Century-Crofts, 1977, pp 29–50.

2. Kulbertus H., and Demoulin J.: The conduction system: anatomical and pathologic aspects. *In* Cardiac Arrhythmias, The Modern Electrophysiologic Approach. Edited by D. Krikler and S. Goodwin. London, W. B. Saunders, 1975, pp 16–38.
3. James T. N.: The sinus node. Am J Cardiol *40:*965–986, 1977.
4. Kugler J. D.: Sinoatrial node dysfunction. *In* Pediatric Cardiac Dysrhythmias. Edited by P. C. Gillette and A. Garson. New York, Grune & Stratton, 1981, pp 265–293.
5. Wenckebach K. F.: Beitrage zur kenntnis der menschlichen herztatigkeit. Arch Anat Physiol *3:*53–65, 1908.
6. Thorel C.: Ueber den aufbau des sinusknotens und seine verbindung mit der cava superior und den Wenckebachschen bundeln. MMW *57:*183–191, 1910.
7. Bachmann G.: The inter-auricular time interval. Am J Physiol *41:*309, 1916.
8. Spach M. S., and Barr R. C.: Cardiac anatomy from an electrophysiologic viewpoint. *In* The Theoretical Basis of Electrocardiography. Edited by C. V. Nelson and D. B. Geselowitz. Oxford, Clarendon Press, 1976, pp 1–23.
9. James T. N.: The connecting pathways between the sinus node and AV node and between the right and left atrium in the human heart. Am Heart J *66:*656–670, 1963.
10. Waldo A. L., Bush H. L. Jr, Gelband H., et al.: Effects on the canine P wave in discrete lesions in the specialized atrial tracts. Circ Res *29:*452–460, 1971.
11. Merideth J., and Titus J. L.: The anatomic atrial connections between sinus and AV node. Circulation *37:*566–571, 1968.
12. Liebman J., and Plonsey R.: Electrocardiography. *In* Heart Disease in Infants, Children and Adolescents. Edited by A. J. Moss, F. H. Adams, and C. G. Emmanouilides. Baltimore, Willams & Wilkins, 1977, pp 18–61.
13. Durrer D., Van Dam R., Freud G., et al.: Total excitation of the isolated human heart. Circulation *41:*899–912, 1970.
14. Janse M. J., and Anderson R. H.: Specialized internodal atrial pathways, fact or fiction. Eur J Cardiol *2:*117–136, 1974.
15. Gillette P. C., El-Said G. M., and Sivarajan N: Electrophysiologic abnormalities after Mustard's operation for transposition of the great arteries. Br Heart J *36:*186–191, 1974.
16. Widran J., and Lev M.: The dissection of the atrioventricular node, bundle and bundle branches of the human heart. Circulation *4:*863–867, 1951.
17. Massing G. K., Liebman J., and James T. N.: Cardiac conduction pathways in the infant and child. Cardiovasc Clinics *4:*27–40, 1972.
18. Haas G.: Ueber die gefassversorgung des reizleitungssystems des herzens. Anat Hefte *43:*629–635, 1911.
19. Rosenbaum M. B., Elizari M. V., and Lazzari J. O: The Hemiblocks. Oldsmar, Florida, Tampa Tracings, 1970, pp 30–60.
20. Kulbertus H. E., and Demoulin J.: Pathological findings in patients with left anterior hemiblock. *In* Vectorcardiography 3. Edited by I. Hoffman and R. I. Hamby. Amsterdam, North-Holland Publishing Company, 1976.

2

Depolarization and Repolarization: Cellular Electrophysiology

The Single Cell: Cardiac Action Potential

It is important to begin a consideration of depolarization and repolarization with a discussion of the action potential of the single cell, not only because the surface electrocardiogram is a summation of cellular potentials, but also because the effects on the electrocardiogram of alterations in the cardiac milieu (e.g., drugs, ischemia) are more easily understood at the cellular level and then applied to the intact heart. The cardiac action potential is the net result of a sequence of changes in the membrane's ionic permeabilities, with different ions carrying charges into and out of the cell. In the normal heart, two different types of action potentials are generated, depending upon the type of cell. These action potentials are the "fast response" and the "slow response,"[1] named according to the rapidity of their upstroke in the initial part of depolarization.

FAST RESPONSE
ACTION POTENTIAL

Atrial and ventricular myocardial cells and cells in the His-Purkinje system normally have fast response action potentials. The resting cell membrane is permeable to potassium and relatively impermeable to sodium ions. If a microelectrode is passed inside such a cell, the inside is negatively charged with respect to the outside, with a magnitude of approximately -90 mV (Fig. 2-1). This is the "resting membrane potential." When a cell is stimulated, sodium permeability increases

9

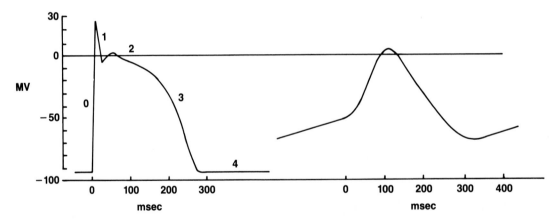

FIG. 2-1.   **Left,** Fast-response action potential similar to that found in a ventricular myocardial cell; the phases of the action potential are indicated by numbers 0 through 4. **Right,** Slow-response action potential similar to that found in a sinus node P cell.

markedly and there is a rapid inflow of sodium causing a rapid depolarization such that the inside of the cell is positive with respect to the outside.[2] This is the most rapid phase of the action potential (phase 0) and is completed within several milliseconds. The rapidity with which phase 0 occurs is defined as the change in voltage with respect to time and is called $\dot{V}max$. This correlates with the conduction velocity in a single cell. Phase 1 of "early rapid repolarization" is due primarily to an outward repolarizing chloride current. At the same time that the chloride current occurs, the inward sodium current is decreasing and the outward potassium current beginning. During phase 2, the plateau, there is a balance of currents: Slow inward currents are caused by calcium and sodium, and outward currents are caused by chloride and potassium. During repolarization (phase 3), the balance changes such that the inward currents decrease and the outward potassium current predominates.

During phase 3, it again becomes possible to stimulate the cell to depolarize. The ability to reexcite a cell depends on both the time elapsed since the last depolarization (phase 0) and the absolute voltage that the membrane has reattained during repolarization. A normal Purkinje cell cannot be reexcited unless approximately 200 msec have passed since the last depolarization, or unless the membrane potential has returned to −55 to −60 mV. In cellular electrophysiology, the time period during which the cell is inexcitable is called the absolute refractory period; in the cardiac electrophysiology catheterization laboratory, this generally corresponds to the effective refractory period. In general, a shorter action potential duration is associated with a shorter effective refractory period. In the "relative refractory period," the cell is not fully excitable but has repolarized sufficiently to generate an action potential. The resultant action potential from stimulation during the relative refractory period may be distorted with a less rapid rate of rise of phase 0 and therefore a slower conduction velocity within the cell. In some cells, rapid repolarization (phase 3) overshoots

and the membrane potential hyperpolarizes (i.e., becomes more negative than the resting membrane potential). If the cell is stimulated during this period, V̇max during phase 0 of the resultant action potential
may be increased over that of the normal action potential, resulting in
more rapid conduction. For this reason, this has been called the "supernormal period" (Fig. 2-2).[3]

When repolarization is complete, phase 4 begins. In atrial and ventricular myocardial cells, there is no net movement of charge during
phase 4, but rather a balance between slow inward sodium current
and an outward potassium current. However, in Purkinje cells, which
are distributed throughout the atria and the His-Purkinje system,
there may be spontaneous diastolic depolarization. The membrane
potential during phase 4 gradually decays to less negative values because of reduction in the outward potassium current, leaving the inward (depolarizing) sodium current. This spontaneous depolarization
during phase 4 is termed "automaticity." The automatic Purkinje cells
in the atria, His bundle, and ventricles are normally suppressed by the
sinus node, but should the sinus node fail to depolarize, these cells
will take over the pacemaker activity of the heart. The rate of diastolic
depolarization in cells of the atria is faster than that in cells of the
ventricles. The level of membrane potential at which an action potential is initiated is called the "threshold potential." The threshold can
be reached either by spontaneous diastolic depolarization of a single

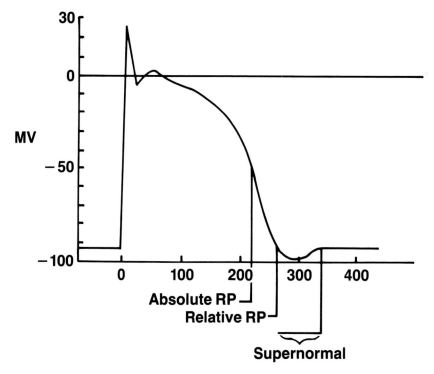

FIG. 2-2. Absolute refractory period, relative refractory period, and "supernormal period" of the ventricular muscle action potential.

cell, by spread of a depolarizing wave front from adjacent cells, or by injection of a depolarizing current from an electrode.

In summary, depolarization is caused by sodium, the plateau by calcium-potassium balance, repolarization by potassium, the level of resting membrane potential by potassium, and the automaticity in fast response fibers by sodium-potassium balance.

SLOW RESPONSE
ACTION POTENTIAL

A second type of action potential occurs in cells of the normal sinus node, AV node, coronary sinus, and AV valves.[4] In addition, other cardiac cells that are injured may display action potentials of this type.[5] Compared to the "fast" action potential, the "slow" action potential has a lower (i.e., closer to zero) maximum diastolic potential of -50 to -65 mV. The upstroke of the action potential (Vmax of phase 0) is much slower and the conduction velocity is also much slower. Depolarization of these cells depends upon a slow inward current of calcium and sodium, as opposed to the more rapid inward sodium current in the "fast" action potential (Fig. 2-1). The majority of cells with slow action potentials display automaticity with spontaneous diastolic depolarization during phase 4. In these cells, phase 4 depolarization may be due to a slow inward calcium current rather than the loss of outward potassium current found in Purkinje cells. The P cells of the sinus node have this type of action potential and normally have the most rapid diastolic depolarization, resulting in the most rapid automatic rate in the heart. It is a property of cardiac cells that stimulation from an external source suppresses their inherent automaticity.[6] Therefore, the sinus node is not only dominant because it has the fastest inherent rate, but also because the conduction of the sinus impulses to other cells naturally suppresses them. In addition, there may be selective vagal inhibition of other potentially automatic cells throughout the atrium.[7] Normally, cells in other parts of the heart with slow response action potentials do not have an opportunity to become the pacemaker of the heart, but in diseased states, these cells may be responsible for abnormal rhythms.

Current Flow Within a Cell:
The Dipole Concept

A dipole consists of a single pair of positive and negative charges lying in close proximity to each other. The cardiac cell membrane at rest can be represented as a capacitor, with negative charges on the inside and positive charges on the outside. Current flow is prevented by the high-resistance cell membrane. If an excitatory stimulus is applied to the cell surface, the resistance of the membrane is lowered and positive charge (sodium) rushes in. The flow of current also stimulates the adjacent resting membrane of the same cell and, in so doing, lowers the electrical resistance of the adjacent resting membrane. As a consequence, a new membrane current appears which initiates discharge of the next point along the cell surface.[2]

Membrane current flows *out* of the cell ahead of the depolarization wave front and back *into* the cell behind it (Fig. 2-3). The greatest amount of current flow causing a positive potential exists immediately in front of the depolarization wave front and the greatest amount of negative potential, immediately behind the wave front. Depolarization is, therefore, an advancing wave front of positive charge that extends in a plane perpendicular to the direction of propagation.

As the movement of the dipole occurs in a single cell, the potential variations at several fixed points surrounding the cell can be recorded with a galvanometer. In the "unipolar" recording configuration, one lead is close to the muscle cell while the other lead, the "indifferent lead," is relatively distant so that the indifferent lead remains at zero potential and the active lead records all local events. In Figure 2-4A, three unipolar exploring electrodes are shown surrounding a single muscle cell. These electrodes are similar to those of the chest leads in the electrocardiograph. The potential variations of the cell are recorded by the galvanometer as deflections in a moving baseline. The waveforms represent voltage plotted against time (paper speed). The size of the deflection measured from the isoelectric baseline is determined by the magnitude of the voltage, and the direction of deflection

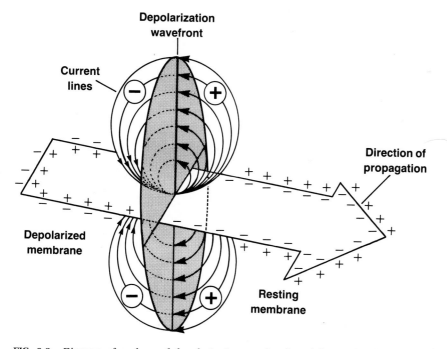

FIG. 2-3.   Diagram of a plane of depolarization moving from left to right along the surface of a membrane. The outside of the membrane is positively charged in front of the plane and negatively charged behind the plane. The plane represents a "wall" of positive charge moving from left to right.

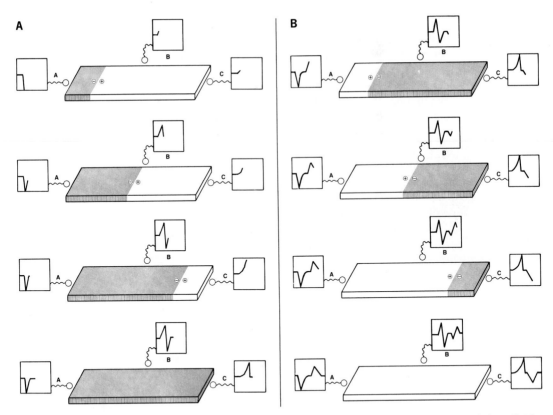

FIG. 2-4. **A,** Depolarization sequence in a hypothetical cardiac cell. Unipolar electrodes surround the cell. The potential found at these electrodes is shown in the accompanying graphs (see text). **B,** Sequence of repolarization in a hypothetical cardiac cell (see text).

by the voltage sign. Positive voltage is recorded when the wave of depolarization is moving toward the electrode and causes an up-swing of the baseline; negative voltage causes a down-swing. If the muscle cell is stimulated at its left end, electrode A facing the stimulated end of the cell is at closer proximity to the negative charge of the dipole than at any time subsequently (Fig. 2-4A, top diagram). Therefore, electrode A is at maximum negative potential, and this is evidenced graphically by a sharp downward deflection. The other two electrodes lie in the positive field of the dipole. Since electrode B, overlying the center of the cell, is closer to the positive dipole charge than is electrode C, electrode B shows a greater positive deflection. As depolarization continues and the equivalent dipole moves farther away from electrode A, the negative potential at A diminishes and the positive potential at B and C increases. The maximum positive voltage for electrode B is reached just before the dipole passes under electrode B. At the instant the dipole moves under B, the electrode is equidistant from positive and negative charges, and B is therefore at zero potential with the voltage on the isoelectric line, or zero line (Fig. 2-4A, second diagram). As the dipole continues to the right (Fig. 2-4A, third diagram), the potential at electrode B falls to a maximum negative potential because of the close proximity to the negative charge of the dipole. During the remainder of depolarization, the dipole moves steadily away from electrodes A and B (which record progressively smaller negative potentials) and approaches electrode C. The increase in positive potential at electrode C reaches its peak just before the completion of depolarization. When the fiber is completely depolarized, the dipole is extinguished and the voltage curve for each electrode returns to the isoelectric line (Fig. 2-4A, bottom diagram).

Repolarization begins at the left end of the cell and proceeds in the same direction as depolarization (Fig. 2-4B). The potential changes are similar, but of opposite polarity. Because of the long plateau of the action potential, the processes of repolarization take much longer than depolarization. In Figure 2-4B, at electrodes A and C, the different polarities can be seen. At electrode B, the deflection of repolarization is biphasic just like depolarization, except that in repolarization, the downward deflection is written before the upward deflection because the negative part of the dipole is the leading edge.

The "dipole vector" is a straight line running from the negative to the positive charges of the dipole (Fig. 2-5). In depolarization, the dipole vector parallels the direction of physiologic activity. In repolarization, the negative charge of the dipole precedes the positive charge;

DEPOLARIZATION

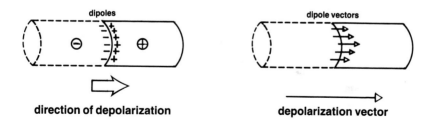

REPOLARIZATION

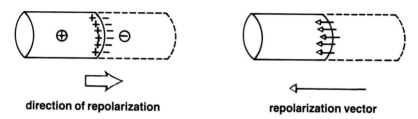

FIG. 2-5. Dipole vectors. **Top,** The dipole vector in depolarization parallels the direction of depolarization. **Bottom,** The repolarization vector occurs in the direction opposite to the direction of repolarization.

therefore, the repolarization dipole is oriented opposite to the depolarization dipole since reversed electrical processes are occurring.

From the Cell
to the Body Surface

The events of depolarization and repolarization that have been described in a single cell must be transmitted from cell to cell. The membrane surrounding each cardiac cell has a high resistance. At the ends of each cardiac cell, the opposing cellular membranes form into intercalated discs. The intercalated discs are thought to be the sites of low resistance, enabling current flow to be readily transferred from cell to cell.[8] Conduction between cells is considerably slower in a lateral direction (perpendicular to the long axis of a cell). Therefore, orientation of fiber bundles would be expected to contribute to the overall conduction velocity and sequence of electrical activity.[9]

During activation of the atria and ventricles, depolarization spreads so as to cause great cancellation of electrical force. The electrical field generated at the body surface is an "equivalent dipole," which represents the uncancelled elements. At any instant other than during the isoelectric period between ventricular repolarization and atrial depolarization, an electrical potential exists at every point on the body surface. This can be described as the summation of forces, or a vector with magnitude and direction. The magnitude is inversely proportional to the cube of the distance between the dipole and the electrode lead on the body surface. Therefore, one would expect a greater voltage in leads recorded from the chest wall than from leads recorded on the extremities. The electrocardiogram calculates the projection of the mean instantaneous vector on its lead axis by the electronic equivalent of vector addition. The changing projections of these vectors on a given lead axis, plotted against time, produce the P, QRS, and T waves.

Self-Assessment
Questions

Question 1: "Fast" response action potential refers to:

A. rapid upstroke of phase 0
B. rapid conduction velocity in a single cell
C. both
D. neither

Question 2: Slow response action potentials may be found in:

A. normal sinus node, normal atrial muscle, normal AV node
B. abnormal sinus node, normal atrial muscle, normal AV node
C. normal atrial muscle, normal ventricular muscle, normal AV node

D. normal sinus node, abnormal atrial muscle, normal AV node

E. normal sinus node, normal ventricular muscle, normal AV node

Question 3: A depolarizing wave front is:

A. positive in front and positive behind

B. positive in front and negative behind

C. negative in front and negative behind

D. negative in front and positive behind

E. none of the above

Question 4: In an electrocardiograph, if depolarization is directed towards an electrode, this causes a deflection that is:

A. negative

B. isoelectric

C. positive

D. positive or negative depending upon the distance from the electrode

E. none of the above

Answers to Self-Assessment Questions

Answer 1: C

The rapid inward sodium current is responsible for the rapid upstroke of phase 0. This, in turn, causes the rapid conduction velocity.

Answer 2: D

Slow-response action potentials that are calcium dependent are found in both the normal and abnormal sinus node and AV node. They may also be found in any other abnormal cardiac tissue.

Answer 3: B

Depolarization is an advancing wave front of positive charge, with negative charge behind the wave front.

Answer 4: C

Regardless of the distance from the electrode, if a potential is recorded moving toward the electrode, it will cause a positive deflection. If repolarization is directed toward the electrode, it causes a negative deflection.

References

1. Reder R. F., and Rosen M. R.: Basic electrophysiologic principles: application to treatment of dysrhythmias. *In* Pediatric Cardiac Dysrhythmias. Edited by P. C. Gillette and A. Garson. New York, Grune & Stratton, 1981, pp 121–143.

2. Cooksey J. D., Dunn M., and Massie E.: Clinical Vectorcardiography and Electro-cardiography. 2nd Ed. Chicago, Yearbook Medical Publishers, Inc., 1977, pp 9–112.

3. Watanabe Y., and Dreifus L. S.: Cardiac Arrhythmias. New York, Grune & Stratton, 1977, pp 208–209.

4. Cranefield P.: The Conduction of the Cardiac Impulse: The Slow Response and Cardiac Arrhythmias. Mt. Kisco, New York, Futura Publishing, 1975, pp 3–25.

5. Ten Eick R. E., and Singer D. H.: Electrophysiological properties of diseased human atrium. I. Low diastolic potential and altered cellular response to potassium. Circ Res *44:*545–557, 1979.

6. Boineau J. P., Schuessler R. B., Hackel D. B., et al.: Multicentric distribution and rate differentiation in the atrial pacemaker system. *In* Physiology of Atrial Pacemakers and Conductive Tissues. Edited by R. C. Little. Mt. Kisco, New York, Futura Publishing, 1980, pp 221–260.

7. Kang P. S., Gomes J. A. C., Kelen G., et al.: Role of autonomic regulatory mechanisms in sinoatrial conduction and sinus node automaticity in sick sinus syndrome. Circulation *64:*832–838, 1981.

8. Weidman S.: The functional significance of the intercalated discs. *In* Electrophysiology of the Heart. Edited by B. Taccardi and G. Marchetti. London, Pergamon Press, 1965, pp 43–72.

9. Spach M. S., Miller W. T., Barr R. C., et al.: Electrophysiology of the internodal pathways. *In* Physiology of Atrial Pacemakers and Conductive Tissues. Edited by R. C. Little. Mt. Kisco, New York, Futura Publishing, 1980, pp 367–380.

3

Recording
the Sequence of
Cardiac Activity

Instrumentation

THE STRING
GALVANOMETER

In 1913 Einthoven adapted the string galvanometer for recording the electrocardiogram,[1] and present-day electrocardiographs still use the concept of a galvanometer (Fig. 3-1). The string galvanometer is based on the fact that an electrical current creates a magnetic field. In the string galvanometer, electrode wires run from the patient (e.g., from the right arm and left arm in the lead I configuration—see Fig. 3-2A), to the opposite ends of a quartz string that is plated with either gold or platinum. The string is suspended under proper tension between the poles of a magnet. As the potential difference between the right arm and left arm causes current to flow in the wire, this current creates a magnetic field. This magnetic field generated by the string interacts with the magnetic field of the permanent magnet and the string moves. Displacement of the string follows Fleming's "left hand rule," which states that if the thumb, forefinger, and second finger of the left hand are held at right angles to one another, the forefinger represents the direction of magnetic field from the North to the South Pole, the second finger the direction of current flow in the string, and the thumb points in the direction in which the wire moves.[2,3] In the string galvanometer, the string interrupts a beam of light focused on it and the string projects a moving shadow onto exposed photographic paper. Appropriate timing and voltage guides are also projected onto the paper for proper calibration (Fig. 3-2A).

THE DIRECT WRITING
ELECTROCARDIOGRAPH

The direct writing electrocardiograph operates on the same principle as the string galvanometer, except that the signals are amplified several times and the amplified current passes through a coil instead

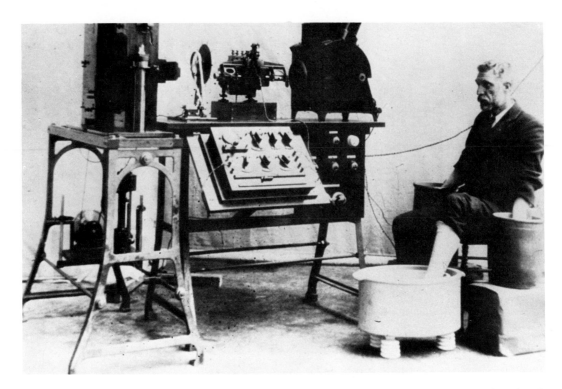

FIG. 3-1. Photograph taken in 1911 of an original electrocardiograph, using a string galvanometer. The subject's right arm, left arm, and left leg are in buckets, which were used as electrodes.

of a string. The coil is suspended between two poles of a magnet, and the stylus, which writes the electrocardiogram, is fixed to the coil. When the current passes through the coil, the coil rotates in the magnetic field, causing the stylus to move (Fig. 3-2B).[4] The stylus is usually heated, and as it moves across the wax-coated carbon paper, the wax melts, exposing the underlying carbon.

Frequency response is an important specification for direct writing electrocardiographs. Frequency response is defined in terms of faithful reproduction of a sine wave signal. For example, the Cambridge model 3803 electrocardiograph has an upper frequency response of 140 cycles/sec at 10 mm peak-to-peak deflection. This means that if a sine wave that repeats every 7 msec (1 sec divided by 140 cycles/sec) with 10 mm between the peak and the nadir of the wave is introduced into the electrocardiograph, it will be faithfully reproduced. However, in this example, there will be distortion if the sine wave repeats every 5 msec or has a greater peak-to-peak deflection. This has practical importance in the recording of an electrocardiogram. The most rapid waves (such as those generated by ventricular depolarization) may not be recorded unless there is a high enough frequency response. Also, the height and depth of a deflection can be affected by frequency response. In an electrocardiogram recorded with an inadequate frequency response, the peaks of large, narrow complexes may not be recorded and the amplitude may be falsely decreased. On the other

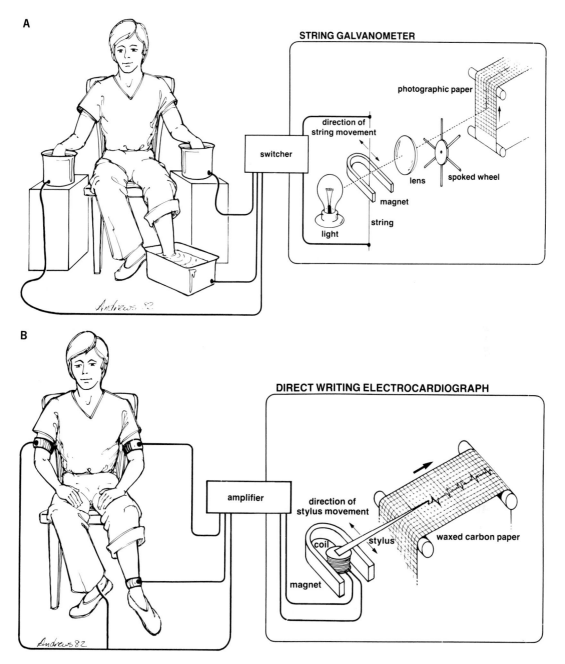

FIG. 3-2. A, Diagram of the instrumentation required for a string galvanometer. B, Diagram of the instrumentation required for a modern direct writing electrocardiograph. The basic mechanics are similar to those shown in Figure 3-2A, both relying on a galvanometer.

end of the scale, an electrocardiograph must be able to record low frequency events with a shallow slope, such as those due to ventricular repolarization. The American Heart Association recommends that all electrocardiographs have a frequency response of 0.5 to 100 cycles/sec.[5] Most direct writing electrocardiographs with waxed carbon paper can attain these standards. In models writing with an ink jet, in which there is no friction between the stylus and the paper, the frequency response is improved.[2]

*Electrocardiographic Standardization
and Measurement*

The electrocardiogram is recorded on standardized paper, with the light lines separated by 1 mm and the heavy lines separated by 5 mm (Fig. 3-3). The voltage is standardized so that 1.0 mV equals 10 mm of deflection. For large amplitude complexes, the calibration can be changed so that 1.0 mV equals either 2.5 or 5 mm; for small signals, the calibration can be changed so that 1.0 mV equals 20 mm. A calibration spike should be recorded on the electrocardiogram each time the calibration is changed (Fig. 3-4). The normal paper speed is 25 mm/sec. At this speed, the light lines are separated by .04 sec (40 msec) and the heavy lines are separated by .20 sec (200 msec) (Fig. 3-5). In order to time events more precisely, or to examine the electrocardiographic morphology during a rapid heart rate, the paper speed can be increased to 50 mm/sec. If a rapid paper speed is used, this should be indicated on the margin of the electrocardiogram for the period of 50 mm/sec recording. Since the electrocardiographic tracing drawn by the stylus has a width of its own, measurements should be

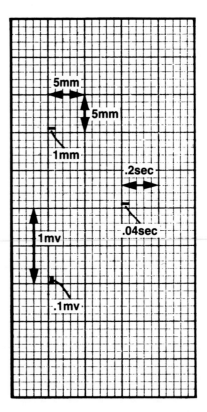

FIG. 3-3. Electrocardiographic paper with usual standardization (1.0 mV equals 10 mm) and usual timing (0.2 sec equals 5 mm).

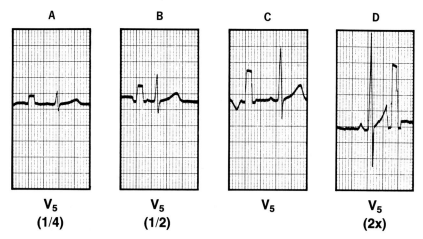

FIG. 3-4. Calibration of the electrocardiogram. A, Lead V_5 at one-quarter standardization (1.0 mV equals 2.5 mm). Since the electrocardiograph standardization output is always 1.0 mV, the height of the spike is 2.5 mm with the calibration spike at one-quarter standardization. B, Lead V_5 half standardization (1.0 mV equals 5 mm). C, Lead V_5 full (normal) standardization (1.0 mV equals 10 mm). D, Lead V_5 double standardization (1.0 mV equals 20 mm). Note: For the remainder of this book, standardization is labelled as in this diagram. Unless the standardization is different from normal calibration, the standardization is not specifically indicated.

taken consistently from the same side of the line. For example, when determining amplitude, take measurements from the bottom of one line to the bottom of the other line; and when determining intervals, take measurements from the left side of one line to the left side of the other line.

Computer Analysis
of the Electrocardiogram

In the data by Davignon et al., which are included in the Appendix as our normal values,[6] the electrocardiograms were analyzed primarily by computer. The electrocardiograms were recorded using a conven-

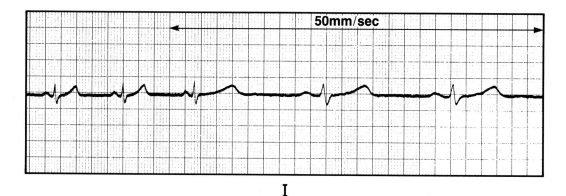

FIG. 3-5. Paper speed. The normal paper speed is 25 mm/sec. On the *right* side of this electrocardiographic tracing, the speed has been increased to 50 mm/sec and this is marked on the tracing. Note: All other electrocardiograms in this book are recorded at 25 mm/sec.

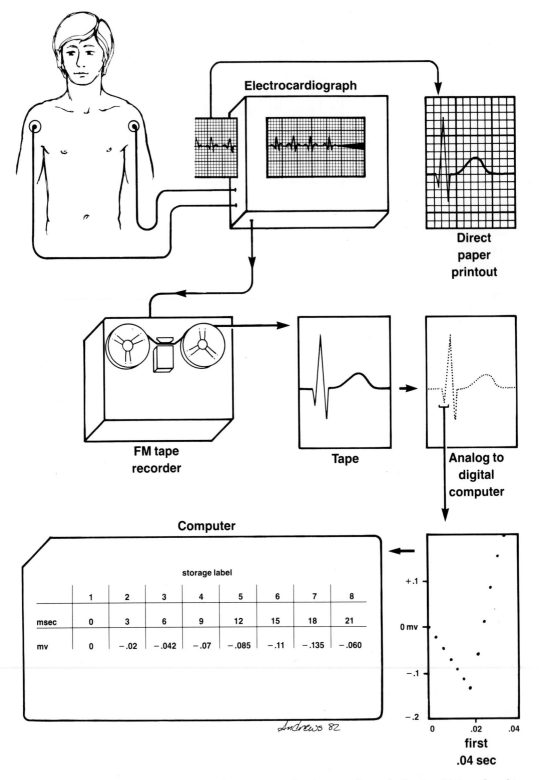

FIG. 3-6. Computer analysis of the electrocardiogram. From the electrocardiograph, the signal is transferred to a tape recorder and then to an analog to digital converter. In the diagram the first .04 sec of the electrocardiographic tracing are shown. The electrocardiogram is sampled every 3 msec and the voltages of the first .04 sec (40 msec) of the electrocardiogram are shown as they would appear in the storage registers of a computer. The storage label corresponds to the number of the sample point. For example, the seventh sample point is at the deepest point of the Q wave, 18 msec into the QRS complex, and this measures −.135 mV below the baseline.

tional electrocardiograph with a stylus, but in addition, the output was coupled to an FM tape recorder. These "analog" signals were sampled 333 times/sec (every 3 msec) for deflection from the baseline and the measured deflection was stored in a computer in "digital" form (Fig. 3-6). The analysis of these electrocardiograms using the Mayo Clinic program has been described in detail elsewhere.[6,7]

Electrocardiographic
Waves and Intervals

Cardiac activation begins in the sinus node; however, the sinus node has no expression on the surface electrocardiogram (Fig. 3-7). Atrial activation causes the P wave on the electrocardiogram. The atria begin to be activated from the high right atrium at the beginning of the

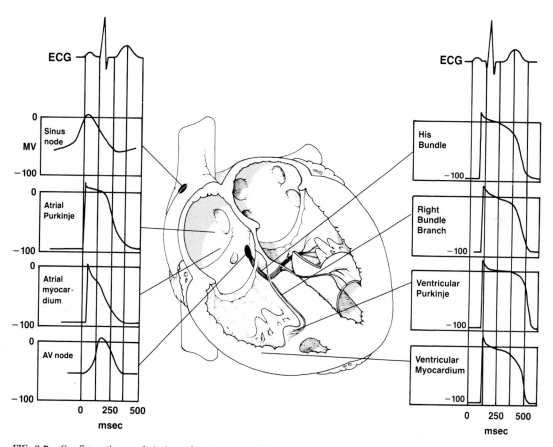

FIG. 3-7. Configuration and timing of action potentials in different parts of the heart compared to the surface electrocardiogram. Activation begins in the sinus node with a "slow" action potential. This occurs before the P wave on the surface electrocardiogram. The atrial Purkinje and atrial myocardium action potentials occur during the P wave; these are relatively short "fast" action potentials. Activation of the AV node occurs during the PR segment. The AV node has a "slow" action potential without diastolic depolarization. The remainder of the action potentials are "fast." Activation of the His bundle, right bundle branch, and ventricular Purkinje cells occurs within the PR segment. At the onset of depolarization of ventricular myocardium, the QRS complex begins.

P wave, and the distal parts of the left atrium are depolarized approximately 60 msec (1½ small boxes on the electrocardiogram) after the onset of the P wave (Fig. 3-8A). Therefore, the normal *P wave duration*, measured from the onset to the termination of the P wave, is about 60 msec. P waves are generally small (less than 2½ mm tall) "bullet shaped" waves.

It takes approximately 40 msec for the impulse to travel from the high right atrium to the low septal right atrium in the region of the AV node. Thus, the AV node may be activated before the end of the P wave. Depolarization of the AV node and His bundle do not produce visible deflections on the routine surface electrocardiogram.

The *PR interval* is caused by a relatively major delay in the AV node and usually a relatively minor delay in conduction through the His bundle and bundle branches to the ventricular myocardium. The PR interval is measured from the onset of the P wave to the onset of the QRS complex. The normal PR interval varies with age but is approximately .12 sec in children. The *PR segment* is the period between the end of the P wave and the beginning of the QRS complex. The duration of the PR segment is generally not measured. The *Ta wave*, caused by atrial repolarization, begins during the PR segment and may extend through the ST segment. In general, the Ta wave is not observed since it is obscured by other waves.

The *QRS complex* is caused by ventricular depolarization. This is usually the tallest, most rapid deflection on the electrocardiogram. If the QRS complex begins with a negative deflection, this negative de-

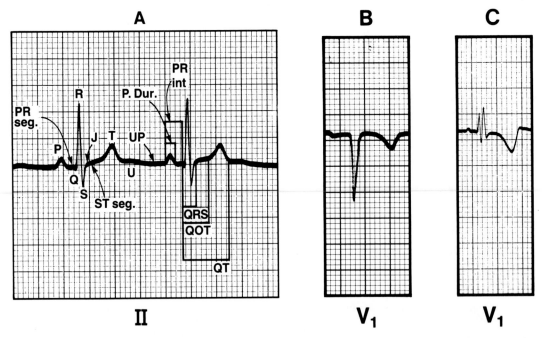

FIG. 3-8. A, Normal electrocardiographic waves and intervals, lead II. P, Q, R, S, T, and U refer to their respective waves. B, QS pattern. C, RSR′ pattern. P. Dur., P duration; PR int, PR interval; PR seg., PR segment; QRS, QRS duration; QOT, QOT interval; QT, QT interval; UP, UP interval.

flection is called a Q wave. A Q wave is not seen in all leads. The first positive deflection is the R wave. The second negative deflection is the S wave. If there is only one large negative deflection, this is called a QS wave (Fig. 3-8B). If there is a second R wave, this is called an R', and the negative deflection that follows an R' is labelled the S' (Fig. 3-8C). The *QRS duration* should be measured in leads with a Q wave. It extends from the beginning of the Q wave to the end of the QRS complex, whether the last wave is an R, S, R', or S'. The normal QRS duration varies with age but is approximately .08 sec. The *J point* occurs at the junction at the end of the QRS complex with the ST segment.

The *ST segment* extends from the end of the QRS complex to the beginning of the T wave. If there are abnormalities of ventricular repolarization, they may be marked by elevation or depression of the ST segment from the baseline. Repolarization of ventricular myocardium generates the *T wave*. The T wave is usually rounded with a shallow upstroke and a more rapid downstroke. The *QT interval* is measured from the beginning of the QRS complex to the end of the T wave and indicates the total duration for electrical depolarization and repolarization of ventricular muscle. The QT interval varies with heart rate but is usually about half the interval between QRS complexes. The *Q-OT interval* is measured from the beginning of the QRS complex to the beginning of the T wave. This measures the time to the onset of repolarization. The Q-OT is not generally measured but may be prolonged or shortened by abnormalities of serum calcium. In some leads, a *U wave* may be visible. This is thought to be due to ventricular Purkinje cell repolarization. Normally, the U wave has a lower amplitude than the T wave with an even shallower upstroke and downstroke than the T wave. The *T-P interval* (or U-P interval if there is a U wave) is the true isoelectric baseline and measurements of amplitude are usually made relative to the T-P interval.

Electrocardiographic Leads

The electrocardiograph calculates and displays the projection of the three-dimensional vector onto any single lead axis. Examination of a single bipolar lead provides much information about the timing of cardiac events, but in order to reconstruct a fuller image of the movement of the cardiac dipole in space, multiple leads are required. Three planes are used to describe the heart's electrical activity: (1) The frontal plane, which views the body from the front using the horizontal X axis (right to left) and the vertical Y axis (from head to foot); (2) the horizontal plane, which views the body from above with the horizontal X axis (right to left) and an inward Z axis (anterior to posterior); and (3) the sagittal plane, which views the body from the side with a vertical Y axis (head to foot) and an inward Z axis (anterior to posterior) (Fig. 3-9). All of the three-dimensional information can be described by two planes, and standard electrocardiography has selected the frontal

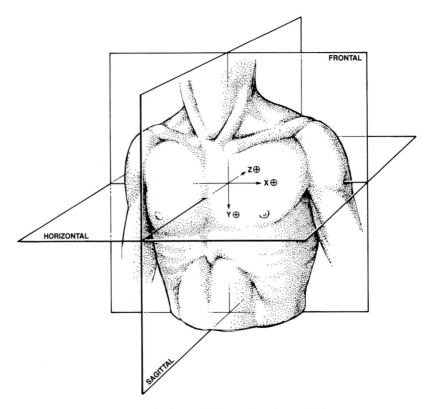

FIG. 3-9. Demonstration of the frontal, horizontal, and sagittal planes.

and horizontal planes. Six leads reflect the projection of cardiac activity on the frontal plane, and nine leads reflect the projection in the horizontal plane. In recent years, attempts have been made to simplify electrocardiography by reducing the number of leads to a total of three: an X, a Y, and a Z lead originally described by Frank.[8] This is not in general use, and at the present time 12 to 15 leads are recorded in a pediatric electrocardiogram. (Fig. 3-10).

THE FRONTAL
PLANE

Einthoven recorded activity in the frontal plane by placing recording leads on the right arm, left arm, and left leg, with a ground electrode on the right leg.[1] Because the arms and legs are relatively far from the heart, they are relatively equipotential and an electrode can be placed at any point along the extremity. Since positioning is not critical, comparison of the limb leads in serial electrocardiographic tracings is possible.

Lead I measures the potential difference between the right arm and left arm with the right arm positive. Lead II measures between the left leg and right arm with left leg positive, and lead III measures between the left leg and left arm with the left leg positive. These bipolar

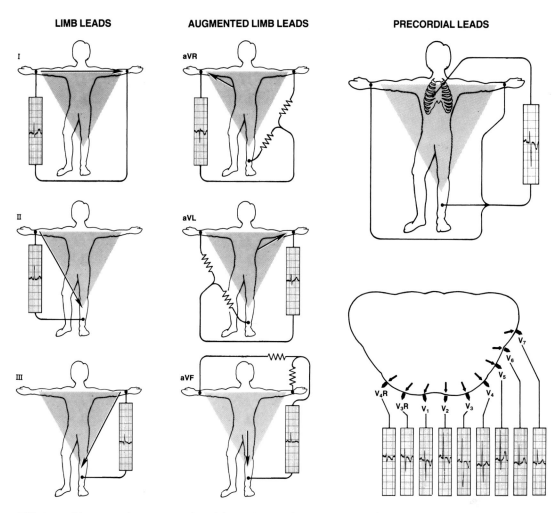

FIG. 3-10. Diagrammatic representation of the position and instrumentation for obtaining a 15-lead electrocardiogram in a child (see text). The tracings are taken from a normal 3-year-old.

leads were thought by Einthoven to represent an equilateral triangle with the heart at the center (Fig. 3-11A). From torso models, Burger and Van Milaan constructed a more accurate assessment of the lead axes and concluded that leads I, II, and III form a scalene triangle with lead I much shorter than leads II and III (Fig. 3-11B).[9] Because of the shape of the torso, the position of the heart primarily in the left chest, and the inhomogeneity of the contents of the thorax, although lead I connects the two arms, potentials recorded by this lead are slightly posterior and superior in addition to being largely left to right. Similar factors cause leads II and III to have slightly different lengths. The true direction of the lead axes is only important insofar as a depolarization that is negative in lead I may not be proceeding from left to right but may be directed slightly inferiorly or anteriorly.

Wilson et al. added three more leads to the frontal plane.[10] In the so-called "unipolar" limb leads, the right arm, left arm, and left leg

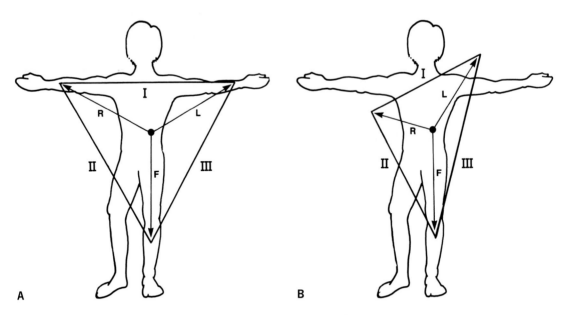

EINTHOVEN TRIANGLE
(equilateral)

BURGER TRIANGLE
(scalene)

A   B

FIG. 3-11.   A, Einthoven equilateral triangle. B, Burger scalene triangle.

electrodes are all connected to "Wilson's Central Terminal" by way of a 5000 ohm resistor. This forms the negative pole or "indifferent" electrode. Then for lead V_R, the right arm forms the positive pole; for lead V_L, the left arm; and for lead V_F, the left leg. These are called "unipolar" because the potential toward each of the three extremities is compared with an indifferent "average" electrode thought to be at zero potential. Recordings of V_L, V_R, and V_F have low amplitude, and Goldberger modified the recordings by disconnecting the central terminal connection to the extremity lead on which the exploring electrode was located.[11] For example, in recording lead V_L, the left arm connection to the central terminal is disconnected. This augments the voltage by 50%, so that the present "unipolar" limb leads are called augmented V_R, V_L, and V_F, or aV_R, aV_L, and aV_F. The frontal plane can be represented by a circle as if the patient were viewed from the front. A vector beginning at the center of the circle pointing to the left is at 0°, inferior is at +90°, superior is at −90°, and to the right is at ±180°.

Despite the minor differences in the lengths and directions of the leads, it is convenient to think of the six frontal plane leads as a hexaxial system using Einthoven's triangle. The bipolar leads (I, II, III) form the sides of the triangle, while the unipolar leads (aV_R, aV_L, aV_F) originate in the center and point toward the apices. Therefore, either the positive or negative axis of one of the leads is positioned every 30° around the circle (Fig. 3-12). The positive pole of lead I points toward

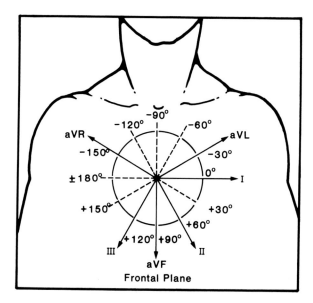

FIG. 3-12.   Frontal plane hexaxial system showing lead axes based on Einthoven's triangle.

the left arm at 0°, lead II toward the left leg at +60°, and lead III toward the right leg at +120°. The positive pole of lead aV_R points toward the right shoulder at −150°, lead aV_L toward the left shoulder at −30°, and lead aV_F toward the feet at +90°. (Fig. 3-12).

THE HORIZONTAL
PLANE

The precordial leads are also "unipolar" and are recorded by connecting the Wilson Central Terminal without augmentation to the negative pole of the electrocardiograph, with the exploring chest lead connected to the positive pole. There are six standard unipolar chest leads (V_1 to V_6) and three additional chest leads included for children: V_3R, V_4R, and V_7 (Fig. 3-13). Leads V_3R, V_4R, and V_1 are called the "right chest leads." The reason for recording two additional right chest leads in children is the usual right ventricular dominance at young ages. Also, right ventricular hypertrophy may only be manifested in these leads. Leads V_5, V_6, and V_7 are called the "left chest leads." Since rotational anomalies may accompany congenital heart defects, lead V_7 is recorded as an additional left chest lead which may be useful in determining the presence of left ventricular hypertrophy or the absence of initial "septal" forces. The leads between V_1 and V_5 are generally called the "transition" leads.

Although the chest leads do not bear the constant relationship to each other that is present in the limb leads because of the variation in torso shape, it is helpful to remember that leads V_1 and V_5 are perpendicular to each other (Fig. 3-14). Therefore, one should not necessarily

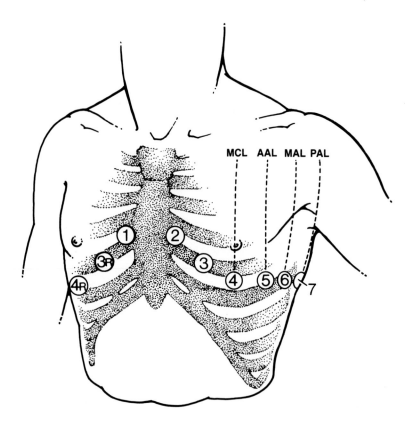

FIG. 3-13. Precordial lead positions. Lead V_1 is in the fourth intercostal space immediately to the right of the sternum; lead V_2 is in the fourth intercostal immediately to the left of the sternum; lead V_4 is in the fifth left intercostal space in the left midclavicular line; lead V_3 is midway between lead V_3 and V_4; lead V_5, V_6 and V_7 are all at the same level as V_4, but V_5 is in the anterior axillary line, V_6 is in the midaxillary line and V_7 is in the posterior axillary line; lead V_4R is in the fifth right intercostal space in the midclavicular line and lead V_3R is midway between lead V and lead V_4R.

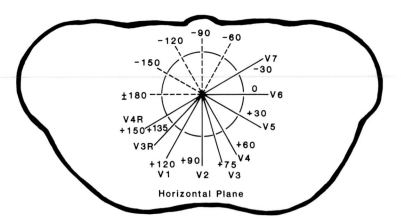

FIG. 3-14. Horizontal plane hexaxial system showing lead axes.

expect to observe opposite changes in the "right" and "left" chest leads any more than changes in lead I are opposite to those in lead aV$_F$.

The precordial leads are relatively close to the cardiac activity and therefore the proximity effect becomes important. This is stated in Poisson's formula: "The potential of a given dipole as determined at a point within its electromotive field varies inversely with the cube of the distance of the point from the center of the dipole."[2] Therefore, minor changes in the distance between the heart and the chest wall can produce marked alterations in voltage such that a thin person will have greater voltage than one with a thick chest wall. For the same reason, accurate and consistent lead placement is critical. Variation in torso shape, as well as lead placement, is reponsible for the wide range of normal values for the voltage in the precordial leads. This same variation may render comparison of the precordial leads inaccurate even in the same patient at different points in time.

Self-Assessment
Questions

Question 1: The electrocardiographic standardization that results in complexes being recorded half the normal size is:

A. 10 mV equals 5 mm
B. 1 mV equals 50 mm
C. .1 mV equals 2.5 mm
D. 10 mV equals 25 mm
E. none of the above

Question 2: At a paper speed of 50 mm/second, a PR interval measures 6 small boxes. At normal paper speed, what is the PR interval in seconds and how many small boxes would this represent?

A. .24 sec; 6 small boxes
B. .24 sec; 3 small boxes
C. .12 sec; 6 small boxes
D. .12 sec; 3 small boxes
E. none of the above

Question 3: The PR interval:

A. begins with depolarization of the sinus node and ends with depolarization of the bundle branches
B. begins with depolarization of the sinus node and ends with depolarization of the ventricles
C. begins with depolarization of the atrium and ends with depolarization of the ventricles

D. begins with depolarization of the atrium and ends with repolarization of the atrium

E. begins with depolarization of the atrium and ends with repolarization of the ventricles

Question 4: Match each frontal plane lead with its positive direction in degrees:

_____ lead I	A. +90°	G. +60°
_____ lead aV$_F$	B. −90°	H. −60°
_____ lead aV$_R$	C. +120°	I. +30°
_____ lead II	D. −120°	J. −30°
_____ lead aV$_L$	E. +0°	K. +150°
_____ lead III	F. +180°	L. −150°

Question 5: Lead V$_1$ and V$_5$ are separated by approximately _____ degrees.

A. 30
B. 60
C. 90
D. 120
E. 150

Question 6: If an electrocardiograph with an upper frequency response of 100 cycles/sec records a narrow QRS complex that is 45 mm from the top of the R wave to the bottom of the S wave, what amplitude might an electrocardiograph with an upper frequency response of 50 cycles/sec record?

A. 5 mm
B. 35 mm
C. 45 mm
D. 55 mm
E. 65 mm

Answers to Self-Assessment Questions

Answer 1: E
Normal standardization is 1 mV equals 10 mm. Therefore, half standardization is 1 mV equals 5 mm.

Answer 2: D
At 50 mm/sec, each small box (or 1 mm) is equal to .02 sec. Therefore 6 boxes equal .12 sec. At the normal paper speed of 25 mm/sec, this is 3 small boxes.

Answer 3: C

The PR interval is measured from the beginning of the P wave to the beginning of the QRS complex. The sinus node is not represented.

Answer 4: E, A, L, G, J, L

The frontal plane standard leads are equally spaced by 60°, beginning with lead I (0°), lead II (+60°), and lead III (+120°). The augmented limb leads point toward the left shoulder (aV$_L$, −30°), right shoulder (aV$_R$, −150°), and feet (aV$_F$, +90°).

Answer 5: C

V$_1$ and V$_5$ are perpendicular to each other.

Answer 6: B

An electrocardiograph with a subnormal upper frequency response is likely to clip the top and bottom of rapid QRS complexes, making smaller complexes. It will not distort them so much that a 45 mm signal is attenuated to 5 mm.

References

1. Einthoven W., Fahr G., and Dewaart A.: Über die richtung und die manifest grosse der potentialschwankungen im menschlichen herzen und über den einfluss der herzlage auf der form des electrocardiogramms. Arch Gesamte Physiol *150*:275, 1913. Hoff H., and Sekelju P. (trans.) Am Heart J *40*:163–180, 1950.
2. Cooksey J. D., Dunn M., and Massie E.: Clinical Vectorcardiography and Electrocardiography 2nd Ed. Chicago, Yearbook Medical Publishers, Inc., 1977, pp 9–112.
3. Liebman J., and Plonsey R.: Electrocardiography. *In* Heart Disease in Infants, Children and Adolescents. Edited by A. J. Moss, F. H. Adams, and C. G. Emmanouilides. Baltimore, Williams & Wilkins, 1977, pp 18–61.
4. Rogers E. M.: Physics for the Inquiring Mind. Princeton, New Jersey, Princeton University Press, 1960, p 617.
5. Pipberger H. V., Arzbaecher R. C., and Berson A. S.: Recommendations for standardization of leads and of specifications for instruments in electrocardiography and vectorcardiography. Report of the Committee on Electrocardiography, American Heart Association. Circulation *52*:11–31, 1975.
6. Davignon A., Rautaharju P., Boisselle E., et al.: Normal ECG standards for infants and children. Pediatr Cardiol *1*:123–152, 1979.
7. Smith R. E., and Hyde C. M.: Computer analysis of the electrocardiogram in clinical practice. *In* Electrical Activity of the Heart. Edited by G. W. Manning and S. P. Ahuja. Springfield, Illinois, Charles C Thomas, 1969, p 305.
8. Frank E.: Determination of the electrical center of ventricular depolarization in the human heart. Am Heart J *49*:670–676, 1955.
9. Burger H. C., and Van Milaan J. B.: Heart vector and leads. Br Heart J *10*:229, 1948.
10. Wilson F. N., Johnston F. D., Macleod A. G., et al.: Electrocardiograms that represent the potential variations of a single electrode. Am Heart J *9*:447–458, 1934.
11. Goldberger E.: Unipolar Lead Electrocardiography 2nd Ed. Philadelphia, Lea & Febiger, 1950, pp 23–35.

4

Derivation of
the Electrocardiogram

Atrial Depolarization and Repolarization:
The P Wave and Ta Wave

Atrial excitation propagates as if the atria were a two-dimensional sheet of cells.[1,2] Thus, the impulse normally begins in the sinus node and travels radially, similar to a pebble dropped in a pond, throughout the right and left atria.

Although the electrocardiogram records and summates mean vectors continually, it is often helpful to examine the vectors as if depolarization were frozen at a particular instant. In this way, the direction of depolarization can be seen closely in "stop action." In the atria of a child, approximately 60 msec are required for the impulse to conduct from the high right atrium in the region of the sinus node to the lateral left atrium. It is convenient to examine atrial depolarization in three phases: early (the first 20 msec), middle (20 to 40 msec), and late (40 to 60 msec). In the early phase, depolarization has spread approximately halfway through the right atrium and the mean vector of the dipoles points straight anteriorly, slightly to the left, and inferiorly (Fig. 4-1A). As the rest of the right atrium is depolarized in the middle period of depolarization, the mean vector points anteriorly, leftward, and inferiorly. In the terminal portion, the left atrium is activated and since the left atrium is posterior to the right atrium, the terminal vector points posteriorly, left and inferiorly (Figs. 4-1B and 4-1C). If the direction and amplitude of all the instantaneous vectors throughout atrial depolarization are averaged, the mean vector, or "axis," can be calculated. For the normal P wave, the mean vector points anteriorly, inferiorly, and to the left.

Atrial repolarization is manifested on the surface electrocardiogram by a slowly inscribed small deflection, the Ta wave, which is opposite in direction to the P wave.[3] Therefore, the mean electrical vector of the Ta wave is directed posteriorly, superiorly, and to the right. It can be seen that in the relatively simple structure of the atria, the processes of depolarization and repolarization proceed sequentially and have opposite polarities: Depolarization is a positive wave

36

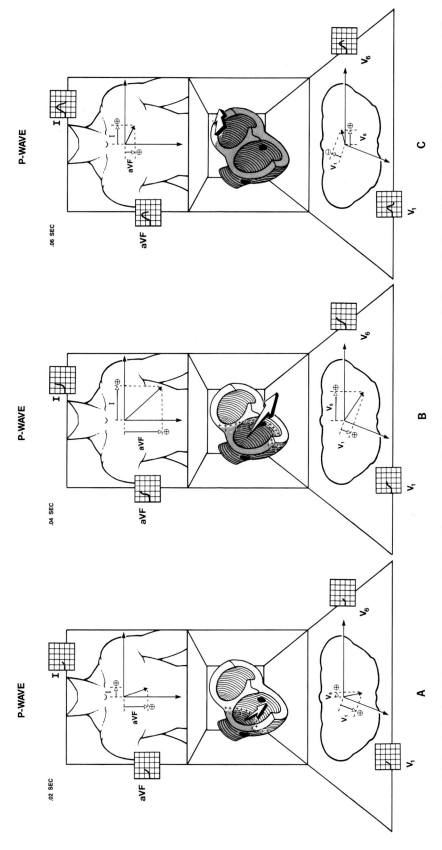

FIG. 4-1. Atrial depolarization. A, 0 to 20 msec vector. B, 20 to 40 msec vector. C, 40 to 60 msec vector. In each diagram, in the middle, a three-dimensional representation of the atria is shown with the position of the activation front at the end of each time period. The vector in three dimensions is shown as an arrow in the middle diagram. Above this, the projection of the three-dimensional vector on the frontal plane is shown on lead I and aV$_F$ axes. The horizontal component of the vector is designated by the length of the arrow in lead I and the vertical component of the vector is designated by the length of the arrow in lead aV$_F$. A diagrammatic P wave is shown on the graphs. The timing and standardization are the same as those for a standard electrocardiogram. These graphs show the position of the P wave at each of the three successive time periods. Since the P wave duration may be longer than 60 msec, the terminal portion of the P wave is indicated by dotted lines in Figure 4-1C. At the bottom of the diagrams, a similar analysis is applied to the horizontal plane.

front moving toward lead II and results in a positive deflection (Fig. 4-1); repolarization is a negative wave front moving toward lead II and results in a negative deflection (Fig. 4-2A). Because the end of the Ta wave is inscribed within 0.20 to 0.30 sec after the onset of the P wave, the Ta wave is usually superimposed upon the QRS complex and ST segment (Fig. 4-2B). The Ta wave is most easily seen when there is AV dissociation and P waves are found without following QRS complexes (Fig. 4-3). Since the Ta wave is opposite in polarity to the P wave, when the Ta wave is superimposed on the QRS complex, the Ta wave is generally negative and may result in both PR and ST depression. ST depression due to ventricular disease without atrial disease is not associated with depression of the PR segment. For this reason, when measuring ST segment changes, use the PR segment as the baseline, despite the fact that the PR segment may not be truly isoelectric.

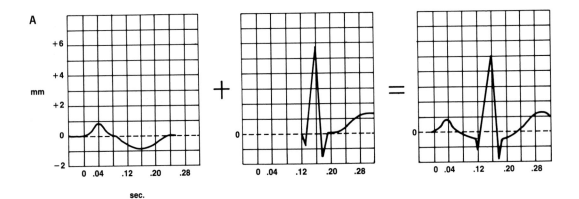

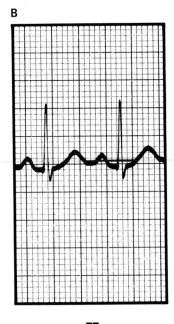

FIG. 4-2. A, Atrial repolarization. In the diagram on the *left*, a normal positive P wave is shown with a normal negative Ta wave following it. The diagram is similar to normal electrocardiographic paper. In the *middle* diagram, a normal QRS complex and T wave are shown without the preceding P or Ta wave. In the diagram on the *right*, the combination of the preceding two drawings is shown. This demonstrates how the Ta wave can result in both PR and ST depression. B, Lead II electrocardiogram from a 3-year-old child. The true isoelectric line has been drawn to extend through the PR and ST segments showing the depression produced by the Ta wave.

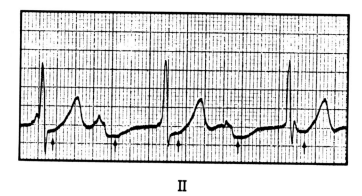

II

FIG. 4-3. Complete AV block in a 15-year-old. Arrows indicate the Ta waves that follow the P waves.

Ventricular Depolarization: The QRS Complex

The QRS complex on the body surface is much more complicated than the P wave because ventricular depolarization occurs in several different directions simultaneously. It has been estimated that only 5 to 10% of the electrical forces generated by ventricular depolarization are reflected in the QRS complex; all others cancel each other.[4] The QRS complex can best be divided into four time periods which correspond to the different major directions of activation (Fig. 4-4).

The first such time period is the .01 second initial vector (Fig. 4-4A). At the onset of the QRS, three areas on the left ventricular endocardium are activated simultaneously: (1) the central part of the interventricular septum on the left side, which results from early Purkinje fiber branches off the main left bundle branch; (2) the area high on the anterior paraseptal wall at the base of the anterior papillary muscle, from the left anterior fascicle; and (3) the posterior-inferior ventricular septum one third of the distance from the apex to the base, from the left posterior fascicle (Fig. 4-5).[5] Therefore, the initial vector is made up of three components of activation: (1) septal depolarization to the right, (2) anterior left ventricular activation proceeding radially towards the anterior chest wall, and (3) left posterior endocardial spread moving away from the anterior chest wall. In the normal heart, the anterior and posterior left ventricular forces tend to cancel, leaving the left-to-right septal vector. The base-apex axis of the ventricular septum is most often parallel to the diaphragm with the apex slightly more inferior and tilted so that the left side of the septum is caudad. Thus, left-to-right activation of the septum results in a vector that is anterior, to the right, and superior. This usually produces a Q wave in leads I, aV_F, and V_6 and an R wave in lead V_1 (Fig. 4-4A).

The second time period is the .02 sec apicoanterior vector. Approximately 0.01 sec after the endocardial surface of the left ventricle is activated, the endocardial surface of the right ventricle is activated in

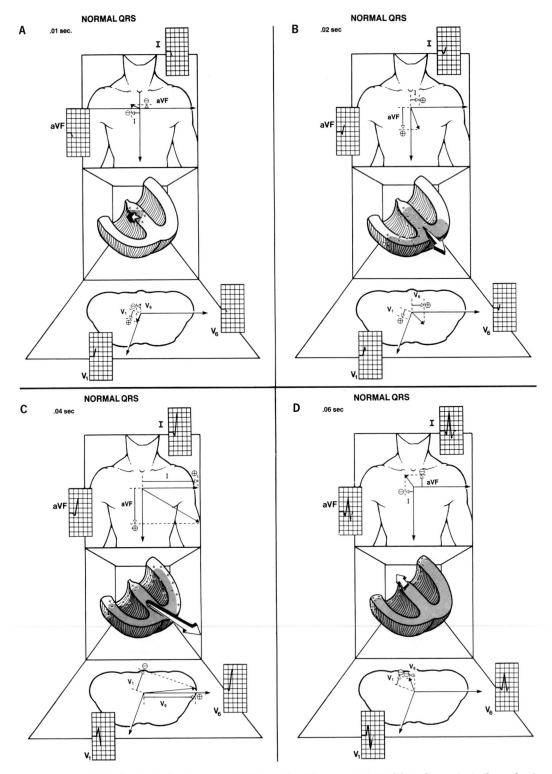

FIG. 4-4. Ventricular depolarization: the normal QRS complex. The arrangement of these figures is similar to that in Figure 4-1, except that the diagram in the middle shows the inner surfaces of the ventricles. A, .01 sec initial vector. B, .02 sec apicoanterior vector. C, .04 sec left ventricular endocardial-epicardial vector. D, .06 sec terminal vector.

ENDOCARDIAL ACTIVATION
0–5msec after QRS onset

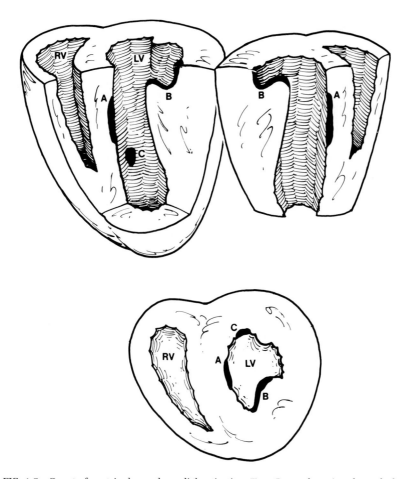

FIG. 4-5. Onset of ventricular endocardial activation. **Top,** Coronal section through the ventricles with the inner surface exposed. **Bottom,** Cross section through the ventricles midway between the base and apex. The three simultaneous areas of activation of the left ventricle are shown: left side of the interventricular septum (A), anterior paraseptal wall (B), posterior-inferior ventricular septum (C). RV, right ventricle, LV, left ventricle.

the region of the moderator band at the termination of the right bundle branch. Because the right bundle branch is longer than the left bundle branch and is insulated to this point, activation occurs later. The spread of the wave originating in the moderator band is primarily left to right as the anterior wall of the right ventricle is activated. Simultaneously, the lower two thirds of the septum have depolarized by way of the left bundle branch, with one activation front meeting the anterior right ventricular wall and the other spreading to the anteroapical left ventricle. In summary, both the right ventricular free wall and the left ventricular free wall are being activated in opposite directions. The left ventricle is thicker, so that the resultant vector is to the left, anterior, and inferior, along the long axis of the heart. Thus, the .02 sec vector is approximately +60° in the frontal plane, causing an R wave in leads I and aV$_F$. In the horizontal plane, the vector contributes to the downstroke of the R wave in lead V$_1$ as the QRS returns toward the isoelectric line (Fig. 4-4B).

Thirdly, there is the .04 sec left ventricular endocardial-epicardial vector. All of the right ventricular endocardium and most of the left ventricular endocardium have been activated. Since activation spreads from the endocardium to the epicardium, there is very little actual spread of impulses across the epicardium. Epicardial activation occurs approximately 25 msec later than the corresponding endocardial activation. There are three almost simultaneous areas of epicardial breakthrough: the anterior right ventricle, the left anterior basal left ventricle near the obtuse marginal coronary artery, and the mid-posterior paraseptal left ventricle near the posterior descending coronary artery (Fig. 4-6). Most right ventricular free wall activation is completed before left ventricular activation because the left ventricle is thicker. This leaves the activation of certain parts of the left ventricular posterior and lateral walls unopposed and the resultant vector is to the left, posterior, and slightly inferior (Fig. 4-4C). This is the peak of the R wave in leads I and V$_6$ and the bottom of the S wave in lead V$_1$.

The fourth time period is the .06 sec terminal vector. The last parts of the heart to be activated are the posterobasal left ventricle and the pulmonary outflow tract. This is because of a paucity of Purkinje cells in these areas. Terminal activation thus proceeds from apex to base. The resultant vector is directed superiorly and posteriorly, causing an S wave in leads aV$_F$ and V$_1$. Depending upon the age of the child, and

EPICARDIAL ACTIVATION
25–35 msec after QRS onset

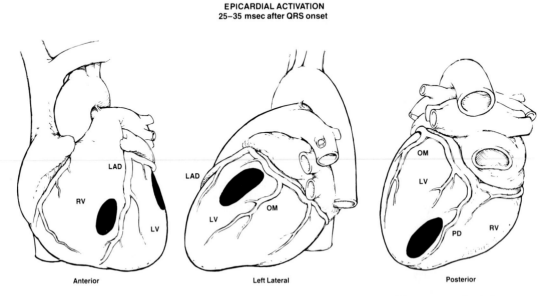

Anterior   Left Lateral   Posterior

FIG. 4-6. Onset of epicardial activation. (This begins 25 to 35 msec after the onset of the QRS complex.) Three areas are activated simultaneously: the anterior right ventricle, the left anterior basal left ventricle, and the mid-posterior paraseptal left ventricle. LAD, left anterior descending coronary artery; LV, left ventricle; OM, obtuse marginal coronary artery; PD, posterior descending coronary artery; RV, right ventricle.

therefore the degree of right ventricular dominance, this vector may be directed slightly to the right or to the left. In younger children, it is directed to the right, causing an S wave in leads I and V_6 (Fig. 4-4D). In older children, it is directed more to the left and there may be no S waves in leads I or V_6.

Ventricular Muscle Repolarization: The T Wave

Whereas ventricular depolarization relies on multiple waves of cell-to-cell conduction, ventricular repolarization appears to be an individual process of each cell and probably does not proceed as a propagated wave. Thus, although repolarization is represented by a single wave and vector on the surface electrocardiogram, it is much more complex than depolarization. The ventricular recovery properties are systematically distributed so that areas activated first have the longest refractory periods and recover last. The endocardium has a longer refractory period than the epicardium, and the apex has a longer refractory period than the base, thus tending to cause all portions of the ventricles to recover at approximately, but not exactly, the

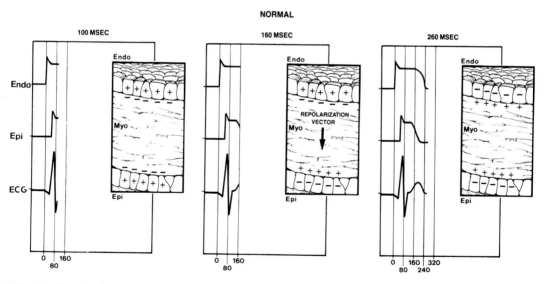

FIG. 4-7. Genesis of the normal T wave. Three phases of cardiac activity are shown. In each of the diagrams, an idealized action potential from the ventricular muscle is shown for the endocardium and the epicardium; the corresponding surface electrocardiogram is also shown. The timing in milliseconds appears at the bottom of each diagram. On the right side of each diagram, the endocardium and epicardium are diagrammed, with the relative polarities of the cells in this region. In the *left* hand diagram, 100 msec after the onset of the QRS complex, both the endocardium and the epicardium are depolarized with the inside of the cell positive relative to the outside. This generates the ST segment. In the *middle* diagram, 160 msec after the onset of the QRS complex, the epicardium has begun to repolarize and the endocardium is still depolarized during the plateau phase. The epicardium is therefore relatively negative compared to the endocardium, and the repolarization vector extends from endocardium to epicardium. This generates the onset of the T wave. In the *right* hand diagram, repolarization of both the endocardium and epicardium is complete and the T wave has ended.

same time. Nevertheless, net repolarization appears to proceed from epicardium to endocardium. This may be due to the shorter epicardial action potentials. Since the epicardium recovers slightly before the endocardium, the extracellular potential in the epicardium is positive with respect to the unrecovered endocardium. The vector of repolarization (T wave) points toward the positive, or already recovered, areas with short action potential duration (Fig. 4-7). This has been shown experimentally. It is known that warming a cell decreases its action potential duration and refractory period. If the epicardium is warmed, the action potentials shorten further and the T wave amplitude increases.[6,7]

Repolarization is electrically the opposite process of depolarization. In the atrium, since depolarization and repolarization follow the same sequence, the polarity of the P and Ta waves are opposite, re-

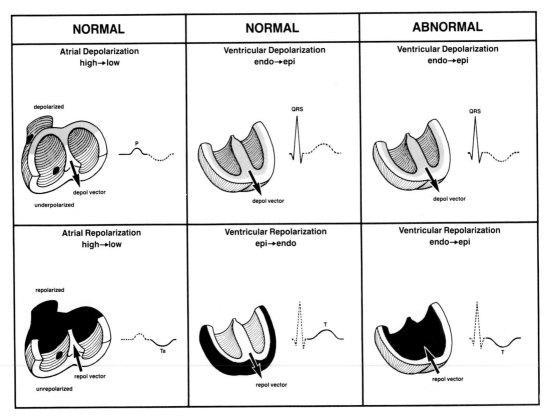

FIG. 4-8. Comparison of atrial and ventricular depolarization and repolarization. In the *left* hand diagram, atrial depolarization begins in the high right atrium and is directed inferiorly, causing a positive P wave in lead II. Atrial repolarization extends in the same direction but has an opposite polarity, causing a negative Ta wave in lead II. In the *middle* diagram, normal ventricular depolarization is shown to occur from endocardium to epicardium. This results in a positive depolarization vector directed towards lead II. Since ventricular repolarization occurs in the opposite direction and also has the opposite sign, the repolarization vector has the same direction as the depolarization vector and the QRS and T waves are both positive in lead II. In the *right* hand diagram, in an abnormal repolarization sequence of the ventricles, the endocardium is depolarized before the epicardium and the directions of depolarization and repolarization are the same. The situation in the abnormal ventricle is analogous to that in the normal atrium in which the depolarization vector and repolarization vector have the same direction but opposite polarities. In the normal atrium, the P and Ta waves have different polarities; in the abnormal ventricle, the QRS and T waves have different polarities.

flecting the different electrical properties (Fig. 4-8, left diagram). In the ventricles, however, the sequence of depolarization and repolarization is reversed: Depolarization proceeds from endocardium to epicardium and repolarization from epicardium to endocardium (Fig. 4-8, middle diagram). Thus, the opposing electrical properties of depolarization and repolarization occur in opposite directions in the ventricles and the net effect is QRS-T concordance: The mean QRS vector and T vector have a similar direction. In abnormal ventricular repolarization, there is QRS-T discordance (Fig. 4-8, right diagram).

Ventricular Purkinje Repolarization: The U Wave

The U wave is apparently due to normal repolarization of ventricular Purkinje cells. Watanabe measured the action potential duration in ventricular muscle and Purkinje cells and found that the U wave corresponds to repolarization in those parts of the ventricle with the longest action potential duration.[8] In the normal heart, the Purkinje cells have the longest action potential duration; the end of the T wave corresponds to the end of ventricular muscle repolarization and the end of the U wave corresponds to the end of Purkinje repolarization. In the abnormal heart, an increased amplitude of the U wave implies that certain portions of the ventricular muscle or Purkinje cells are repolarizing later than normal. Therefore, if the onset of the T wave occurs at the normal time and there is a large U wave, this implies that parts of ventricular muscle are repolarizing on time and other parts are delayed, and this increased "dispersion of refractoriness" may lead to arrhythmias. Factors that prolong phase 3 of the action potential are associated with increased U waves: hypokalemia, bradycardia, hypothermia, and quinidine. In the Jervell-Lange-Nielsen syndrome of congenitally prolonged "QT interval," the original description stated, "It can be discussed as to whether the end deflections in these cases should be interpreted as T waves, U waves, or perhaps T-U waves. The electrocardiograms in our cases did not give any possibility to decide this question. The abnormal complexes were, in our opinion, caused by delayed repolarization of the heart. The nomenclature, therefore, seems to be of less importance."[9] We, and others,[10,11] agree that if the terminal vector of repolarization has an increased magnitude, whether this is called a "long T wave" or an "enlarged U wave," the significance is the same, namely, a vulnerability to ventricular arrhythmias.

The normal U wave has the same polarity as the preceding T wave. This may be accounted for by the observation that the action potential duration in Purkinje cells is longest at the left ventricular cavity and gets shorter toward the subendocardium. Thus, the cells closest to the cavity are repolarized last, producing a negative vector of repolarization directed toward the cavity or a positive vector of the U wave directed away from the cavity toward the chest wall. An inverted U wave may have the same implications as an inverted T wave (see Chapter 10 on Ischemia). In adults, inverted U waves are most often associated with conditions causing stretch in either ventricles, such as chronic volume overload, acute hypertension, or acute pulmonary embolism.[12,13]

Self-Assessment Questions

Question 1: If atrial depolarization originates high in the left atrium, the Ta wave of atrial repolarization will be _____ in lead III.

A. isoelectric
B. positive
C. negative
D. biphasic
E. none of the above

Question 2: If the ST segment in lead II is depressed 2 mm below the TP segment, this can be due to:

A. abnormal ventricular repolarization
B. normal atrial repolarization
C. abnormal atrial repolarization
D. A and B
E. A and C

Question 3: The .01 second initial vector of the QRS complex can potentially be due to:

A. septal depolarization to the right
B. anterior left ventricular activation toward the chest wall
C. posterior left ventricular activation away from the chest wall
D. all of the above
E. none of the above

Question 4: In the normal left ventricle, which of the following is true?

A. endocardium depolarizes first, repolarizes first
B. epicardium depolarizes first, repolarizes first
C. endocardium depolarizes first, repolarizes last
D. epicardium depolarizes first, repolarizes last

Question 5: If the ventricles were thin-walled like the atria, with a positive QRS complex in lead II, the T wave in lead II would be:

A. isoelectric
B. positive
C. negative
D. biphasic

Question 6: Increased amplitude of the U wave implies:

A. delayed repolarization of ventricular muscle or Purkinje cells
B. early repolarization of ventricular muscle or Purkinje cells
C. increased vulnerability to ventricular arrhythmias
D. decreased vulnerability to ventricular arrhythmias
E. A and C
F. B and D

Answers to Self-Assessment Questions

Answer 1: C
In this case, atrial depolarization is directed toward lead III and the P wave is positive in this lead. Atrial repolarization is also, therefore, directed toward lead III, but since this is an advancing wave front of negative charge, the Ta wave is negative in lead III.

Answer 2: D
Because both abnormal ventricular repolarization and normal atrial repolarization (Ta wave) can cause ST segment depression when compared to the TP segment in lead II, it is best to compare the ST segment to the PR segment when trying to distinguish the cause of an ST segment shift. If the PR segment is also depressed (compared to the TP segment), then the ST depression is due to normal atrial repolarization. If the PR segment is at the same level as the TP segment but the ST segment is depressed, then this is due to abnormal ventricular repolarization. Usually abnormal atrial repolarization causes PR segment and ST segment elevation in lead II.

Answer 3: D
The .01 second vector is due to a summation of all of these forces. Usually, the anterior and posterior activation cancel, leaving the septal depolarization uncancelled to predominate. However, in abnormal states, one of the other forces may become predominant.

Answer 4: C
Depolarization spreads from endocardium to epicardium and repolarization spreads from epicardium to endocardium. Thus, the endocardium has the longest action potential duration and the epicardium the shortest, tending to make all repolarization occur at approximately the same time.

Answer 5: C
If the ventricles acted similar to a sheet of cells in which repolarization followed depolarization in the same direction, the T wave caused by an advancing negative wave would be negative in lead II. However, in the normal thick-walled ventricle, the negative wave of repolarization

occurs in the opposite direction to the positive wave of depolarization, causing the QRS and T wave to be concordant.

Answer 6: E

The delayed repolarization of some parts of the ventricles or Purkinje cells compared to other parts generates U waves. If a large proportion of repolarization is delayed, the U waves have increased amplitude. The difference in potential between the normally repolarized cells and those with delayed repolarization may contribute to ventricular arrhythmias.

References

1. Spach M. S., Miller W. T., Barr R. C., et al.: Electrophysiology of the internodal pathways. *In* Physiology of Atrial Pacemakers and Conductive Tissues. Edited by R. C. Little. Mt. Kisco, New York, Futura Publishing, 1980, pp 367–380.
2. Weidman S.: The functional significance of the intercalated discs. *In* Electrophysiology of the Heart. Edited by B. Taccardi and G. Marchetti. London, Pergamon Press, 1965, pp 43–72.
3. Burch G. E., and DePasquale N. P.: Electrocardiography in the Diagnosis of Congenital Heart Disease. Philadelphia, Lea & Febiger, 1967, pp 30–105.
4. Scher A. M.: Excitation of the heart. *In* The Theoretical Basis of Electrocardiography. Edited by C. V. Nelson and D. B. Geselowitz. Oxford, Clarendon Press, 1976, pp 44–95.
5. Durrer D., Van Dam R., Freud G., et al.: Total excitation of the isolated human heart. Circulation *41*:899–912, 1970.
6. Surawicz B.: The pathogenesis and clinical significance of primary T wave abnormalities. *In* Advances in Electrocardiography. Edited by R. C. Schlant and J. W. Hurt. New York, Grune & Stratton, 1972, pp 377–421.
7. Burgess M. J.: Physiologic basis of the T wave. *In* Advances in Electrocardiography. Edited by R. C. Schlant and J. W. Hurt. New York, Grune & Stratton, 1972, pp 367–375.
8. Watanabe Y.: Purkinje repolarization as a possible cause of the U wave in the electrocardiogram. Circulation *51*:1030–1037, 1975.
9. Jervell A., and Lange-Nielsen F.: Congenital deafmutism, functional heart disease with prolongation of the Q-T interval and sudden death. Am Heart J *54*:59–68, 1957.
10. Karhunen P., Ludmanmaki K., Heikkila J., et al.: Syncope and QT prolongation without deafness: the Romano-Ward syndrome. Am Heart J *80*:820–823, 1970.
11. James T. N.: The sinus node. Am J Cardiol *40*:965–986, 1977.
12. Lepeschkin E.: The U wave of the electrocardiogram. Mod Concepts Cardiovasc Dis *38*:39–45, 1969.
13. Lepeschkin E., and Surawicz B.: The measurement of the QT interval of the electrocardiogram. Circulation *6*:378–388, 1952.

5

Mean Vector ("Axis")

The vector of cardiac forces changes in direction and magnitude from instant to instant as different regions of the heart activate and recover. For each of the four processes of atrial and ventricular depolarization and repolarization, a *mean* vector can be calculated which is the average direction and magnitude of all instantaneous vectors during that interval. In standard electrocardiography, we are concerned with the direction of the mean vector as it projects onto the frontal and horizontal planes. The three mean vectors most often considered are for the QRS complex, T wave, and P wave.

QRS Mean Vector

FRONTAL PLANE

The most commonly calculated mean vector is for the QRS complex in the frontal plane. The term "QRS axis" has become a popular substitute phrase for this term. The frontal plane QRS mean vector can be calculated in three ways.[1]

The most accurate and most tedious method of determining the QRS mean vector is to determine the area subtended by each wave of the QRS deflection (Figs. 5-1 and 5-2). Each component is measured as if it were a triangle. The formula used is for the area of a triangle (one-half times the base in seconds times the height in millimeters). The area of the deflections below the baseline are subtracted from the area of the deflections above the baseline, yielding the algebraic sum of the areas. The algebraic sums in leads I and aV$_F$ can be plotted and the angle calculated.[2]

The second most accurate method for determining mean vector is to use the algebraic sum of the *amplitudes* of the components rather than the areas (Fig. 5-3).

The most practical method for estimating the mean vector is to determine the most isoelectric complex (Fig. 5-4). This is defined as the lead in which the sum of positive and negative deflections equals

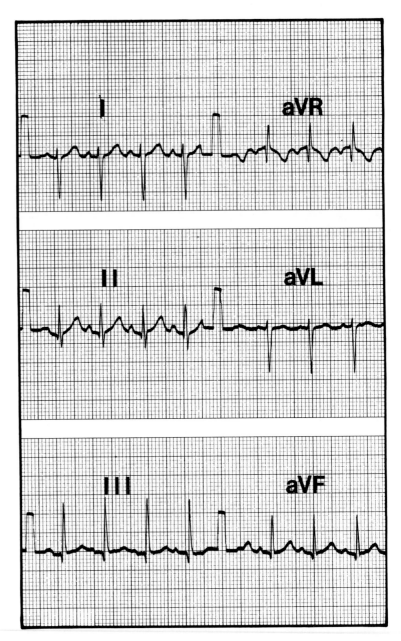

FIG. 5-1. Limb leads from a 4-year-old child. These tracings are used in the calculation of mean vector in Figures 5-2 through 5-4.

zero. The QRS mean vector is directed perpendicular to this lead. However, there are two possible perpendiculars. For example, if lead II is isoelectric, this implies that the mean vector is directed 90° away from (perpendicular to) lead II. Since lead II points toward +60°, the mean vector would be directed toward either −30 or +150°. To determine which of the two perpendiculars is the true mean vector, the lead with the maximum net positive deflection is examined. If lead III

QRS FRONTAL PLANE
MEAN VECTOR—AREA METHOD

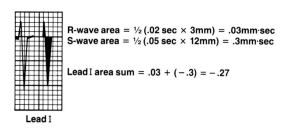

R-wave area = ½ (.02 sec × 3mm) = .03mm·sec
S-wave area = ½ (.05 sec × 12mm) = .3mm·sec

Lead I area sum = .03 + (−.3) = −.27

Lead I

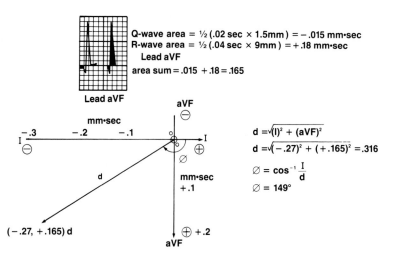

Q-wave area = ½ (.02 sec × 1.5mm) = −.015 mm·sec
R-wave area = ½ (.04 sec × 9mm) = +.18 mm·sec
Lead aVF
area sum = .015 + .18 = .165

Lead aVF

$d = \sqrt{(I)^2 + (aVF)^2}$

$d = \sqrt{(-.27)^2 + (+.165)^2} = .316$

$\varnothing = \cos^{-1} \dfrac{I}{d}$

$\varnothing = 149°$

FIG. 5-2. Calculation of QRS frontal plane mean vector by the area method. The area of each wave of the QRS complex is calculated as if it were a triangle (½ × base × height). The algebraic sum of the areas is calculated for lead I and lead aV$_F$. Then each area is plotted. For lead I the area is −.27 and for lead aV$_F$ it is +.165. To calculate the mean vector or angle (ϕ), first calculate the hypotenuse of the triangle (d). This is done by the Pythagorean theorem. Once d has been calculated, the angle ϕ can be calculated as shown.

has the maximum net positive deflection, the frontal plane mean QRS vector is +150°. It is more accurate to base the calculation on the perpendicular to the isoelectric lead rather than simply on the direction of the largest deflection, because of the true difference in lengths of the lead axes. If all the QRS complexes in the frontal plane are equiphasic, the mean vector is termed "indeterminate" and no calculation can be made.

The calculation of mean vector based upon each of these three methods may differ by as much as 35° because the three standard leads do not truly form an equilateral triangle and the adjacent axes

QRS FRONTAL PLANE
MEAN VECTOR—AMPLITUDE METHOD

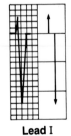

R-wave amplitude = 3mm
S-wave amplitude = 12mm
Lead I
amplitude sum = 3 + (− 12) = −9mm

Lead I

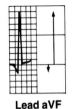

Q-wave amplitude = 1.5mm
R-wave amplitude = 9mm
Lead aVF
amplitude sum = − 1.5 + 9 = +7.5mm

Lead aVF

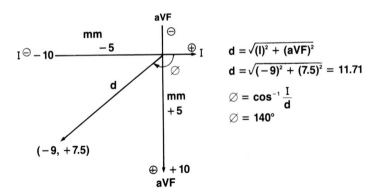

$$d = \sqrt{(I)^2 + (aVF)^2}$$
$$d = \sqrt{(-9)^2 + (7.5)^2} = 11.71$$
$$\varnothing = \cos^{-1}\frac{I}{d}$$
$$\varnothing = 140°$$

FIG. 5-3. Calculation of QRS frontal plane mean vector by the amplitude method. See Figure 5-2.

are not separated by exactly 30°. The normal values for the QRS frontal plane mean vector given in Table A-1 (see Appendix) were based upon the area method.

*"Axis
Deviation"*

If the value for the QRS mean vector falls outside the range of normal values for age (see Appendix, Table A-1), "axis deviation" is diagnosed. In the first month of life, "right axis deviation" occurs when the

QRS FRONTAL PLANE
MEAN VECTOR — PERPENDICULAR METHOD

1. **Inspection: Isoelectric to leads II and aVR**
   maximum positive : lead III
2. **Deduction:**

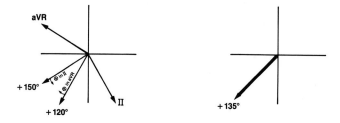

   a. isoelectric to II:
   either −30° or +150°

   b. maximum in III:
   +150°

   a. isoelectric to aVR:
   either −60° or 120°

   b. maximum in III:
   +120°

3. **Fine Tuning:**
   a. II slightly positive (Q (−2mm) + R (+8mm) + S (−4mm) = +2mm)
   ∴ slightly towards II from +150°
   b. aVR slightly positive (R (+1mm) + S (−4mm) + R' (+6mm) = +3mm)
   ∴ slightly towards aVR from + 120°

4. **Conclusion = Mean vector between +120° and +150° = +135°**

FIG. 5-4. Calculation of QRS frontal plane mean vector by the perpendicular method. In Figure 5-1, leads II and aV$_R$ are the most isoelectric and lead III has the maximum positive voltage. Therefore, the mean vector is between +90 and 180° (see text). However, II is not completely isoelectric—it is slightly positive (amplitude sum = +2 mm). This implies that the mean vector is toward II (+60°) from 150°. aV$_R$, however, is also slightly positive, implying that the mean vector is toward aV$_R$ (−150°) from +120°. Therefore, the mean vector is between +120 and +150°, or approximately +135°.

mean vector is between the upper limit for age and −90° (see discussion of northwest axis below). In older children, right axis deviation occurs when the mean vector is between the upper limit for age and ±180°. For a 3-month-old, right axis deviation is between +105 and +180°. In a 10-year-old, right axis deviation is between +120 and +180° (Fig. 5-5). Using logic from the "method of perpendiculars," if the QRS complex is isoelectric or positive in lead aV$_R$ (and isoelectric and positive in aV$_F$) in a 10-year-old, right axis deviation is diagnosed. The most common cause of right axis deviation in children is right ventricular hypertrophy.

"Left axis deviation" occurs when the mean vector is between the lower limit for age and −90°. Above the age of 2 months, left axis deviation is between 0 and −90° (Fig. 5-5). Using logic from the method of

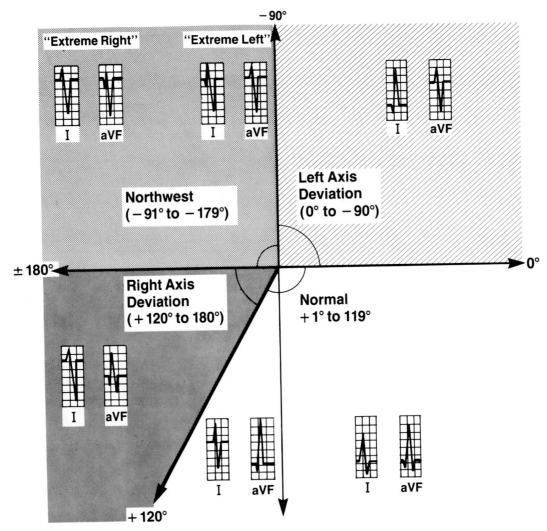

FIG. 5-5. "Axis deviation." Limits for normal and abnormal frontal plane mean vector in a 10-year-old child. The electrocardiograms have been drawn to reflect the mean vector in each of the quadrants.

perpendiculars, if the QRS complex is isoelectric or negative in lead aV$_F$ (and isoelectric or positive in lead I) in a child older than 2 months, left axis deviation is diagnosed. The most common causes of left axis deviation in childhood are those due to abnormal intraventricular conduction associated with congenital heart disease, namely complete AV canal, ostium primum atrial septal defect, tricuspid atresia, and single ventricle (see Chapter 9, "Left Anterior Hemiblock"). Concentric left ventricular hypertrophy generally does not cause left axis deviation.

If the frontal plane QRS mean vector is between −90 and ±180°, "northwest axis" is diagnosed (Fig. 5-5). This may be either an extreme form of right axis deviation or left axis deviation. In general, in *northwest axis only*, if the initial QRS forces are directed at +120° (Q wave in lead I or aV$_L$), left anterior hemiblock coexists with the northwest axis and this is a form of extreme *left* axis deviation. On the other hand, if the initial forces are directed at $-60°$ (Q waves or QS pattern in leads II, III, and aV$_F$) this is extreme right axis deviation.

HORIZONTAL
PLANE

The QRS mean vector in the horizontal plane is not routinely calculated.

T Wave
Mean Vector

FRONTAL
PLANE

The T wave mean vector in the frontal plane can be calculated using the same methods as for the QRS complex. Generally, the T wave mean vector and QRS mean vector point in the same direction: positive QRS complexes have positive T waves. The amount of deviation between these mean vectors is called the QRS-T angle and the maximum allowable QRS-T angle varies with age. In early infancy, the QRS-T angle in the frontal plane is quite variable, but by 3 to 6 months, an angle greater than 75° is abnormal; after 6 months, the upper limit of normal is 60°.[3] If the QRS-T angle is abnormally large, this is called "QRS-T discordance" and indicates either a primary or secondary T wave change (see Chapter 10, "Ischemia"). In practice, rather than calculating the QRS-T angle, remember that in normal children, the T waves should be upright in leads I and II (above 48 hours of age), upright in lead aV$_F$ (above 5 days of age), and inverted in lead aV$_R$ (at all ages) (Fig. 5-6).

HORIZONTAL
PLANE

The QRS-T angle in the horizontal plane can be calculated. In practice, however, this is not done and the far right and far left chest leads are examined. Between approximately 5 days of age and adolescence, the T waves should be inverted in leads V$_1$ and V$_3$R.[4] If they are positive, this is usually a sign of right ventricular hypertrophy. In infants less than approximately 5 days of age or in adolescents, the T waves in lead V$_1$ or V$_3$R are variable. The T waves in lead V$_6$ should be positive at all ages. T wave inversion in lead V$_6$ may be a primary or secondary T wave change (see Chapter 10, "Ischemia").

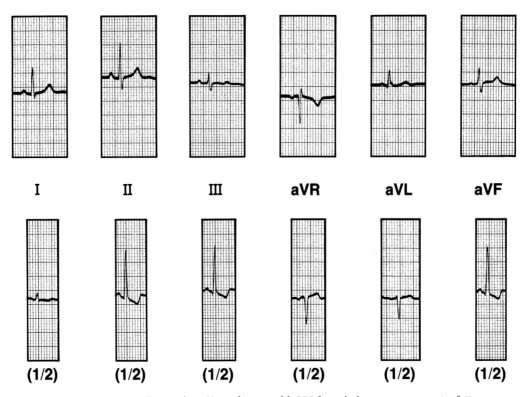

FIG. 5-6.   T wave mean vector. **Top** tracings; Normal 7-year-old; QRS frontal plane mean vector +17°, T wave mean vector +34°; the QRS-T angle is 17°. **Bottom** tracings; 7-year-old with severe aortic stenosis; QRS frontal plane mean vector +85°, T wave mean vector −90°; the QRS-T angle is 175°.

P Wave
Mean Vector

FRONTAL
PLANE

The P wave mean vector is directed away from the site of origin of atrial depolarization. Although it is possible to calculate the exact P wave mean vector, in practice only the quadrant of the vector in the frontal plane is determined. If the P wave is isoelectric or positive in lead I and isoelectric or positive in lead aV_F (P wave mean vector between 0 and +90°), we infer that the atria begin depolarization from the high right atrium, in other words, from the sinus node (Fig. 5-7). If the P wave is negative in lead aV_F and isoelectric or positive in lead I (P wave mean vector between −1 and −90°), the atria begin depolarization from the low right atrium. If the P wave is negative in lead I (P wave mean vector between +91 and −91°), the atria begin depolarization from the left atrium (see Chapter 7).

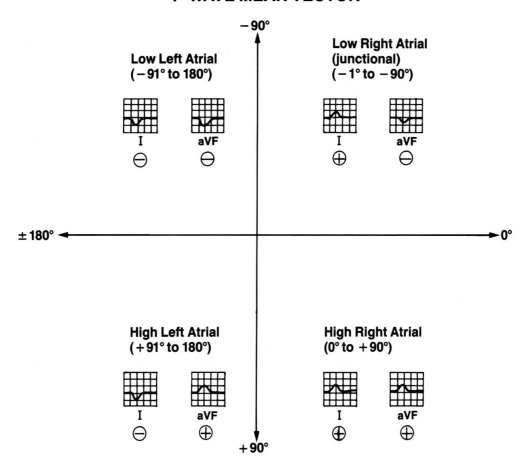

FIG. 5-7. Frontal plane P wave mean vector.

HORIZONTAL
PLANE

The P wave mean vector in the horizontal plane is variable and is not helpful in determining the site of origin of atrial depolarization.

Self-Assessment
Questions

Question 1: Calculate the frontal plane QRS mean vector in the tracing on next page (Fig. 5-8), using the perpendicular method.

A. +120°   C. −30°   E. −90°
B. +60°   D. −60°

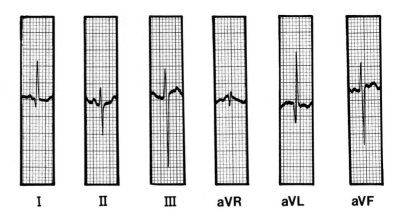

FIG. 5-8.   Questions 1 and 2.

Question 2: Which of the following is commonly associated with the frontal plane QRS mean vector as shown in Question 1 (Fig. 5-8):

A. normal heart
B. ostium primum atrial septal defect
C. tetralogy of Fallot
D. aortic stenosis
E. none of the above

Question 3: Calculate the approximate QRS-T angle for this 9-year-old child (Fig. 5-9).

A.   0°
B. 25°
C. 50°
D. 75°
E. 90°

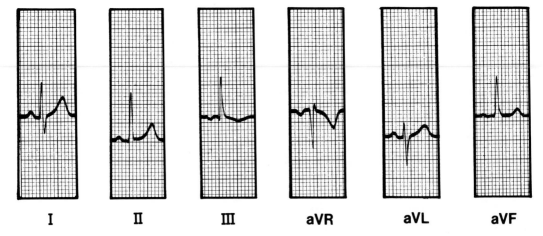

FIG. 5-9.   Questions 3 and 4.

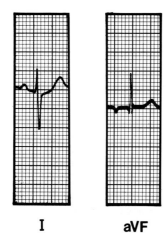

I   aVF

FIG. 5-10. Question 5.

Question 4: In a 9-year-old child, the diagnosis in the electrocardiogram in Figure 5-9 is:

A. normal (QRS-T concordance)
B. abnormal (QRS-T discordance)

Question 5: The P wave mean vector in the frontal plane is approximately _____, indicating a site of origin of atrial depolarization in the _____ (Fig. 5-10).

A. 0 to +90°; HRA
B. 0 to +90°; HLA
C. −1 to −90°; LRA
D. −1 to −90°; LLA
E. none of the above

Answers to Self-Assessment Questions

Answer 1: D
The most isoelectric lead is aV_R. The lead with the largest voltage is III, which is negative. Therefore, the mean vector is perpendicular to aV_R, away from III, or −60°.

Answer 2: B
The common causes of left axis deviation are complete AV canal, ostium primum atrial septal defect, tricuspid atresia, and single ventricle.

Answer 3: C

The QRS frontal plane mean vector is approximately $+75°$ and the T wave mean vector is approximately $+25°$, giving a QRS-T angle of approximately $50°$.

Answer 4: A

After the age of 6 months, a QRS-T angle of $60°$ or less is normal.

Answer 5: C

A P wave that is positive in lead I and negative in lead aV_F has a mean vector between -1 and $-90°$, indicating the low right atrium as the site of origin. Answers B and D are internally incorrect since a high left atrial pacemaker has a mean vector of $+91$ to $+180°$; a low left atrial pacemaker has a mean vector of -91 to $-179°$.

References

1. Cooksey J. D., Dunn M., and Massie E.: Clinical Vectorcardiography and Electrocardiography. 2nd Ed. Chicago, Yearbook Medical Publishers, 1977, pp 9–112.
2. Dubin S., and Staib J.: Numerical calculation of the mean electrical axis of electrocardiographic deflections. J Electrocardiol *10:*77–78, 1977.
3. Liebman J., and Plonsey R.: Electrocardiography. *In* Heart Disease in Infants, Children and Adolescents. Edited by A. J. Moss, F. H. Adams, and C. G. Emmanouilides. Baltimore, Williams & Wilkins, 1977, pp 18–61.
4. Hait G., and Gasul B. M.: The evaluation and significance of T wave changes in the normal newborn during the first several days of life. Am J Cardiol *28:*494–504, 1963.

6

The Normal Electrocardiogram

As the transition is made from the fetus to the neonate, infant, child, and adult, changes in the physiology, changes in the size and position of the cardiac chambers relative to each other, changes in the size and position of the heart relative to the body, and changes in the overall body habitus contribute to the different patterns of normal in the pediatric electrocardiogram. The major changes in amplitudes and direction of depolarization and repolarization occur in the first year of life; thereafter, changes slowly occur in the timing of cardiac events as reflected in the electrocardiographic intervals. Because most of the measurements made on a neonate's electrocardiogram would be abnormal in an adult (Fig. 6-1), it is important to refer to the Tables of Normal Values in the Appendix, which are given by age. In the following discussion, we will consider the normal electrocardiogram from the term newborn through the adolescent. Discussion of the normal premature[1] and adult[2] electrocardiograms can be found elsewhere.

Normal Values

The normal values included in Tables A-1 through A-17 (see Appendix) are those collected and published by Davignon et al.[3] The population in this study consisted of 2141 white children. Each child had a normal physical examination. The total population was divided into 12 age groups, with 7 age groups in the first year of life to reflect the greater changes in the electrocardiogram during this time. There were at least 100 children in each age group. The data were analyzed by computer (see Chapter 3, "Instrumentation"). In addition, the electrocardiograms that fell in the upper or lower tenth percentile were displayed with an electrocardiograph and were verified visually by a physician. If the computer and physician disagreed, the visually determined value by the physician was substituted in the data file.

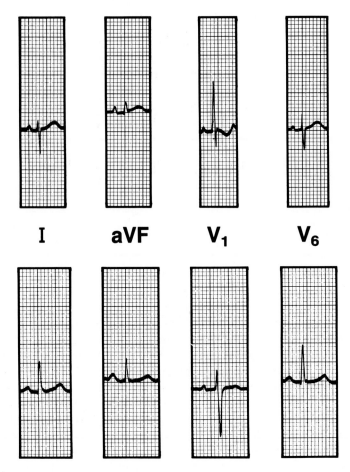

FIG. 6-1. Comparison of the normal neonatal and adolescent electrocardiogram. The neonate is shown in the *top* row and the adolescent is shown in the *bottom* row.

These normal values are therefore applicable to all tracings recorded from an electrocardiograph that meets the American Heart Association's standards (see Chapter 3, "Instrumentation"). The limits of "normal" include the 2nd and 98th percentiles in each age range. A Summary Table of Normal Values is presented in Table A-17 (see Appendix).

Heart
Rate

In sinus rhythm, the heart rate is measured by determining the interval between successive P waves or R waves on the electrocardiogram. The onset of each deflection rather than the peak should be used for timing, since a change in the shape of a complex may result in a faulty measurement if the peak occurs at a different time relative to the beginning of the complex (Fig. 6-2). The exact heart rate can be calculated by dividing the RR intervals (in seconds) into 60. For exam-

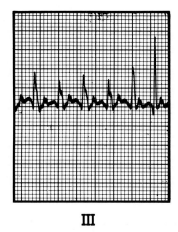

III

FIG. 6-2. Measurement of heart rate. In this patient with supraventricular tachycardia with varying intraventricular conduction, the QRS morphology changes sufficiently that the peak of each complex does not occur at the same time relative to the onset of each beat. Therefore, in measuring heart rate, rather than measuring from peak to peak, use the onset of the QRS complex at all times.

ple, assume an RR of .46 sec; the heart rate is 60/.46 or 130/min. An approximation can be made by counting the number of .2 sec blocks (large boxes on the electrocardiographic paper) that are contained in the RR interval. If the RR interval is approximately one box (.2 sec), the heart rate is 300/min; for two boxes, it is 150/min, and so on: 300, 150, 100, 75, 60, 50, 43, 38. For a more exact heart rate, it is helpful to remember that the small boxes (.04 sec) between 100 and 150 represent 10 beats/min and those between 150 and 300 represent 30 beats/min (Fig. 6-3). This can be committed to memory.

The normal heart rate increases from the first day of life to a maximum between 1 and 2 months of age and then slowly declines (see Appendix, Table A-2). The reason for this has not been demonstrated but probably is related to the relative immaturity of the sympathetic nervous system at birth.

P
Wave

The *configuration* of the P wave is generally symmetric in leads I and II. The normal shape is of a bullet and not of a steeple (right atrial enlargement) or a bent staple (left atrial enlargement) (Fig. 6-4). With the improved frequency response of most electrocardiographic machines, over 25% of normal children will have a notch in the middle of the P wave. Therefore, notching by itself must be considered normal. In lead V_1, the P wave may normally be biphasic, but the terminal negative portion should be less than .04 sec in duration and less than 1 mm deep (less than one small box by one small box). The overall *duration* of the P wave in lead II should be between .03 and .09 sec in

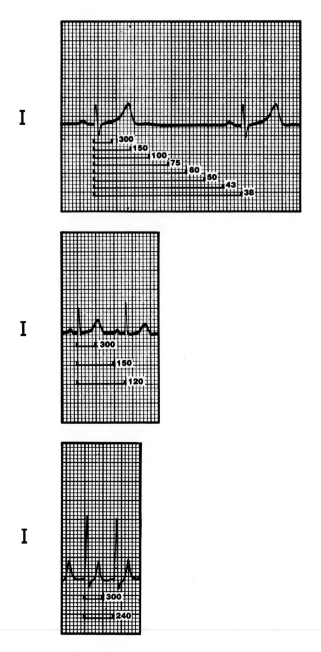

FIG. 6-3.   Calculation of heart rate. **Top** tracing, A heart rate of 38/min. This is exactly nine large boxes on the electrocardiogram. The method of counting large boxes is illustrated. **Middle** tracing, Sinus rhythm at a rate of 120/min. The QRS complexes are separated by two large boxes and three small boxes. **Bottom** tracing, Supraventricular tachycardia at 240/min. The QRS complexes are separated by one large and three small boxes.

children 3 years old and younger; over the age of 3 years, the normal duration is between .05 and .10 sec. The normal P wave *amplitude* is less than 2.5 mm at all ages. The P wave *mean vector* normally is directed between 0 and +90° in sinus rhythm with situs solitus atria (see Chapter 5, "P Wave Mean Vector").

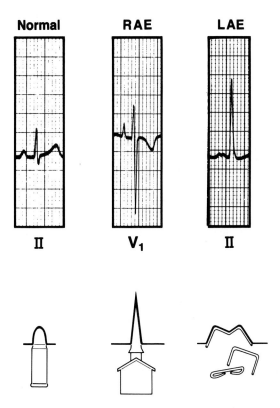

FIG. 6-4. P wave shape. **Left,** Normal P wave shape, which is similar to that of a bullet. **Middle,** P wave of right atrial enlargement (RAE). This is similar to a church steeple. **Right,** P wave of left atrial enlargement (LAE). This is similar to a bent staple.

PR
Interval

The PR interval is measured from the beginning of the P wave to the beginning of the QRS complex. The true onset of atrial or ventricular depolarization may not be recorded in a lead because the initial forces are directed perpendicular to the lead and the initial portion of the P wave or QRS complex may therefore be isoelectric in that lead. Thus, the PR intervals measured in different leads may vary by as much as .04 sec (Fig. 6-5), but usually vary only by .02 sec or less.[2] It has been the practice to measure either the longest PR interval or the PR interval in lead II. Standards are available in children only for lead II (see Appendix, Table A-3). If a "delta wave" is present (see Chapter 9, "Preexcitation"), the shortest "PR interval" (actually a P-delta interval) should be sought in the diagnosis of the Wolff-Parkinson-White syndrome. With an isoelectric delta wave, the PR interval may be normal, and only in certain leads will the truly short PR interval be observed (Fig. 6-6). (See the section in Chapter 9 on Preexcitation for other causes of a short PR interval.) A more common cause for a short PR interval in a normal

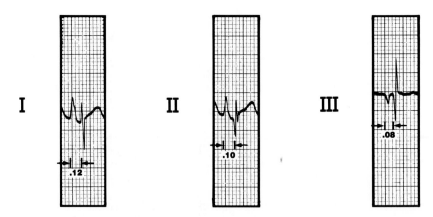

FIG. 6-5. PR interval. Simultaneous leads I, II, and III. The PR interval in lead I is .12 sec, in lead II .10 sec, and in lead III .08 sec. The reason for the seemingly short PR interval in lead III is that the early part of the P wave is isoelectric in that lead.

heart is a low right atrial pacemaker. In this instance, the P wave is negative in lead aV_F and positive or isoelectric in lead I. When the impulse originates low in the atrium, the normal high to low right atrial conduction time (which accounts for up to .04 sec of the PR interval) is eliminated and therefore low right atrial pacemakers may have a PR interval up to .04 sec less than normal.

The PR interval normally increases with age and decreases with heart rate. The increase in PR interval with increased heart rate can be accounted for by the fact that heart rate decreases normally with age. Therefore, in Table A-3 (see Appendix), the PR interval is correlated with age and not heart rate.

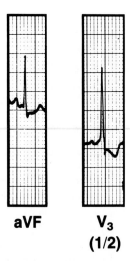

aVF   **V₃**
(1/2)

FIG. 6-6. PR interval in Wolff-Parkinson-White syndrome. In lead aV_F, the PR interval is normal and there is no delta wave. The short PR interval and delta wave are only apparent in lead V_3, taken from the same patient.

PR
Segment

The PR segment is measured from the end of the P wave to the beginning of the QRS complex. The length of this segment is variable and depends upon the duration of the P wave. Normal values for the duration of the PR segment in children are not available. A short PR segment is most often due to a long P wave with a normal PR interval, rather than to the Wolff-Parkinson-White syndrome.

The importance of the PR segment in pediatrics is that it may provide the only estimation of the *isoelectric line* on the electrocardiogram. The true isoelectric line is the TP segment but in children at rapid heart rates, the T and P waves may merge, without the electrocardiogram returning to the baseline between waves. In this case, the PR segment can be used as the isoelectric line. However, the PR segment may be depressed from the true baseline by as much as .8 mm (or elevated in aV_R by .5 mm) by a normal Ta wave of atrial repolarization. When the Ta wave depresses the PR segment, the ST segment may be depressed to the same extent (see Chapter 4). Therefore, it has been argued that although the PR segment is not the true isoelectric line, when diagnosing ST segment shifts, one should compare the ST segment to the PR segment.[4]

QRS
Complex

QRS
DURATION

The QRS duration is measured from the beginning to the end of the ventricular depolarization complex. It should be measured in a lead with a Q wave. The precordial leads may have a QRS duration that is .01 to .02 sec longer than that measured in the limb leads.[2] For the normal values included in Table A-4 (see Appendix), lead V_5 was chosen to measure the duration because there usually is a Q wave and a defined termination to the QRS complex. As ventricular muscle mass increases, the QRS duration increases. Because the muscle mass increases with age, the QRS duration tends to increase with age.

QRS
MEAN VECTOR

The measurement of the QRS mean vector in the frontal plane is considered in Chapter 5. The QRS frontal mean vector moves to the left with age, as shown in Table A-1 (see Appendix).

QRS
MORPHOLOGY

Depending upon the lead and orientation of the initial forces, a Q wave may or may not be present. The remainder of ventricular depolarization is written as an R wave followed by an S wave. This is true in all normal precordial leads and limb leads other than lead aV_R with the following exception: An R wave without an S wave may be present normally in lead V_1 up to 5 months of age and in lead V_6 at any age. In approximately 7% of normal children, in the right chest leads, a second R wave or R' may follow the S wave, giving an RSR' pattern.[5] In these normal children, the overall QRS duration may be prolonged by .01 sec above the normal children given in Table A-4 (see Appendix), but the R' wave has a rapid deflection and has the same duration as the preceding R and S waves. In normal children, with an RSR' pattern, the S wave usually has a greater amplitude than either the R or R' wave. The RSR' pattern can be found in complete right bundle branch block and right ventricular hypertrophy. In complete right bundle branch block, the total QRS duration is increased and there is a true terminal conduction delay with an increase in the duration of the slurred R' compared to the normal duration of the initial R and S waves (see Chapter 9). In mild to moderate right ventricular hypertrophy, the R and especially the R' waves have a greater amplitude than the S wave. With a normal duration QRS complex, right ventricular hypertrophy can be diagnosed by an R' amplitude greater than 15 mm in an infant under a year of age or one greater than 10 mm in a child over a year of age. In children with a normal duration QRS complex and an RSR' pattern with a small R' wave, since the distinction between mild to moderate right ventricular hypertrophy, incomplete right bundle branch block, and normal is difficult, we prefer the designation "RSR' pattern in right chest leads" without a further attempt at diagnosis.

QRS
AMPLITUDE

Q
Wave

A normal Q wave may be present in almost any lead. A QS pattern (or initial S wave) may be normal in lead aV_R at any age and in V_3R and V_4R in older children. A QR pattern (Q wave followed by an R wave) is not normal in lead aV_R or the right chest leads, and if present, usually indicates right ventricular hypertrophy (see Chapter 8, "Right Ventricular Hypertrophy"). If Q waves are present in the midprecordial leads, this generally implies counterclockwise rotation of the heart (see Chapter 7).

The distinguishing points between normal and abnormal Q waves are the duration and the amplitude of the Q wave. A normal duration Q wave is less than .015 sec. Any Q wave greater than .03 sec is definitely abnormal.[5,6] The normal amplitude of Q waves varies with the lead and with age:[3] At all ages, lead aV_L normal is less than 2 mm; lead I, less than 3 mm; leads II and aV_F, less than 4 mm; leads III and V_6 are the most variable with age (see Appendix, Tables A-5 and A-6).[7] The implications of abnormal Q waves are further discussed in the section on infarction in Chapter 10.

R and S
Waves

Since the ventricles overlie each other to a great extent in the frontal plane, the attempt to separate right ventricular from left ventricular forces is best made in the horizontal plane. Therefore, R wave and S wave amplitudes will only be considered in the horizontal plane. In the normal heart with normally related ventricles, the right ventricular forces are directed anteriorly and to the right. The anterior forces are reflected by the height of the R wave in lead V_1 and the rightward forces by the depth of the S wave in lead V_6. Conversely, the posterior forces generated by the left ventricle are reflected by the depth of the S wave in lead V_1 and the leftward forces generated by the left ventricle are reflected by the height of the R wave in lead V_6. Left ventricular forces can also be represented by the sum of the posterior and leftward forces, or the sum of the depth of the S wave in lead V_1 and the height of the R wave in lead V_6. The normal values by age for the amplitudes and ratios of R waves and S waves in leads V_1 and V_6 are given in Tables A-7 through A-13 (see Appendix).

The transition leads are the precordial leads in which the QRS complexes are approximately equiphasic (R and S waves have equal amplitude). The transition leads record activity from both ventricles, and if the total amplitude of the R wave plus the S wave in the transition leads is increased, this represents biventricular hypertrophy. The normal total amplitude of R plus S in lead V_4 is given in Table A-14 in the Appendix.

The mean amplitudes of the waves reflecting the right ventricle decrease with age while those reflecting the left ventricle increase with age. The variability of these amplitudes also decreases with age. With adolescence, in the 12-to-16-year-old age group, sex differences in the electrocardiogram become manifest (see Appendix, Table A-15). R waves, especially in the left chest leads, are smaller in girls. This may represent breast development or the smaller cardiac size in women. In adolescence, changes in race and body habitus become more manifest. Larger midprecordial voltages are found in blacks and in those with thin chests.[4]

Lower Limit
of QRS Amplitude

Heretofore, we have been concerned with the upper limts for QRS amplitude. The lower limit is important because low-voltage QRS complexes are usually a sign of myocardial edema (in myocarditis, myxedema, or generalized edema), loss of functioning myocardium (in congestive heart failure, tumor, or amyloid), or increased distance between the heart and chest wall (in obesity, pneumothorax, constrictive pericarditis, pericardial, or pleural effusion) (see Chapter 10, "Injury Due to Myocarditis"). The criterion for abnormally low voltage of QRS complexes is a total amplitude of R plus S of 5 mm or less in each of the limb leads or 8 mm or less in each of the chest leads.[6]

ST
Segment

The ST segment is that portion of the electrocardiogram between the end of the S wave and the beginning of the T wave. Normally the ST segment gently curves into the proximal limb of the T wave and is not perfectly horizontal. To determine ST segment deviation above or below the baseline, it is best to consider the PR segment as the baseline (see "PR Segment" in this chapter). The ST segments should not be elevated more than 1 mm or depressed more than ½ mm in any lead in children. The exception is the "early repolarization" syndrome of adolescence, in which the ST segment can be elevated to 4 mm in the midprecordial leads (see Chapter 10, "Functional T Wave Changes").

T
Wave

The T wave is normally asymmetric in *shape*, with the upstroke having a more gradual slope than the downstroke (Fig. 6-7A). The T wave usually has a smooth, curved form but it may have a notch near its summit (Fig. 6-7B).

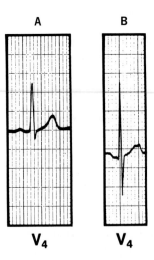

FIG. 6-7. T waves. A, Normal smooth T wave. B, Normal notched T wave.

The T wave *amplitude* is generally not measured in specific leads, since it is so variable in normal children. However, low-voltage or "flattened" T waves in several leads may indicate an abnormality (see Chapter 10). The T waves in leads I, II, and V_6 should be greater than 2 mm in all children over 48 hours old. An abnormally tall T wave is generally defined at any age as greater than 7 mm in a limb lead or 10 mm in a precordial lead.

The T wave *mean vector* generally parallels the QRS mean vector, resulting in positive T waves in leads I, II, and V_6 in children over 48 hours old (see Chapter 5).

U

Wave

The normal U wave has the same polarity as the preceding T wave but the normal U wave has only 2 to 24% of the T wave's amplitude. There is a wide variation of normal; however, the normal U wave should not be more than 50% of the amplitude of the T wave (Fig. 6-8). The U waves with the largest amplitudes are recorded in leads V_2 through V_4. The shape of a normal U wave is different from the normal T wave: In the U wave, the upstroke is steeper than the downstroke.[6,8]

DIFFERENTIATING
T, U AND P WAVES

It is important to differentiate between T waves and normal U waves so that the U wave can be discounted in the measurement of the QT interval. A normal U wave is one with an amplitude no more than 50% of the preceding T wave. At slow heart rates, the T and U waves are usually separated by a distinct isoelectric line, but at rates over

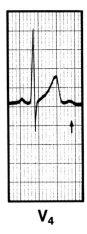

V₄

FIG. 6-8. U wave (arrow).

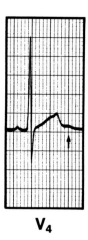

V₄

FIG. 6-9. Notched T wave followed by a U wave. (Arrow indicates U wave.)

90/min, there may be no intervening isoelectric line and it may be difficult to determine whether the terminal portion of the deflection is a U wave or the second half of a notched T wave. If, in the same or a different lead, another wave is seen later in timing than the questionable wave, then the questionable wave is a notched T wave (Fig. 6-9). It may be possible to bring out a U wave by recording the electrocardiogram in the sitting position. This tends to decrease the T wave and increase the U wave amplitude in the left precordial leads.[9]

If there is a single wave in all leads, it is not possible to determine whether this represents a T wave or fusion of a T wave and U wave. If there is not a notch in any lead, but this wave is smooth throughout, this should be considered a T wave (Fig. 6-10). If there is a notch in the terminal part of the wave and the amplitude is 50% or less of the peak, then the downstroke of the early portion of the wave should be extrapolated as the T wave (see Fig. 6-11). If the terminal portion of the wave in any lead (usually V₄ is the clearest) is more than 50% of the ampli-

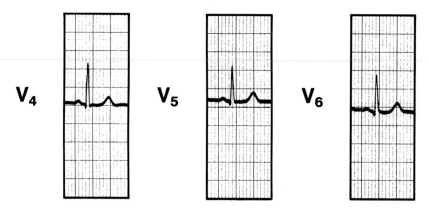

V₄   **V₅**   **V₆**

FIG. 6-10. There is no notch in any of the waves following the QRS complex, so these should all be considered T waves. Simultaneous leads V₄, V₅, and V₆.

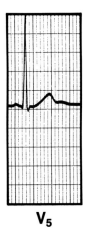

V₅

FIG. 6-11.   T wave followed by a notch with an amplitude less than 50% of the peak of the T wave. In this case, the T wave is considered to have merged with the U wave and the T wave ends at the extrapolated downslope of the larger wave.

tude of the peak, the terminal portion of the wave should be included as part of the T wave (Fig. 6-12). Whether this terminal portion should be called a T wave is a semantic question.[10] The important electrocardiographic question to be answered is whether there is a significant increase in the amount of late repolarization. This can be indicated either by a separate U wave with an amplitude more than 50% of the T wave, *or* by a single fusion wave whose terminal portion is more than 50% of the amplitude of the peak. The causes and consequences of increased late repolarization are the same. Therefore, the same consideration should be given to long T waves and to excessively large U waves.

The distinction of P waves from T or U waves in sinus rhythm is simplified by examining multiple leads. P waves are most obvious in

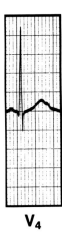

V₄

FIG. 6-12.   T wave with a notch, and the peak of the terminal segment is greater than 50% of the peak of the T wave. In this case, both these waves should be considerd part of the T wave.

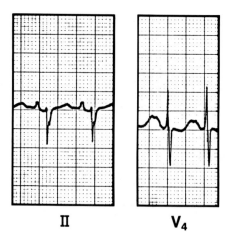

II   **V₄**

FIG. 6-13.   Distinction of P waves from T waves. In lead V₄, it is not possible to tell whether these waves are merged P waves with T waves or T and U waves. It is apparent from examination of lead II in the same patient that the second notch in lead V₄ is caused by the P wave.

lead II and least obvious in leads V_4 through V_7. T and U waves are most obvious in leads V_4 through V_7. Therefore, a synthesis can be made of the different waves by using the timing from different leads (Fig. 6-13). In sinus tachycardia, the P wave may begin before the T wave has been completed. At rapid rates, P waves become much more pointed than T waves. Again, in leads V_6 or V_7 almost all of the wave is likely to be a T wave, while in lead II the maximum P wave is likely to be visible. In supraventricular tachycardia, the most pointed of the waves are P waves. P waves can also be identified as discrete deflections usually lasting .06 sec or less which occur with an improper timing for a QRS complex or a T wave (Fig. 6-14). Using this type of analysis, we have found it possible to distinguish P waves in 55% of children during supraventricular tachycardia.[11]

QT
Interval

The QT interval begins at the onset of the QRS complex and terminates at the end of the T wave. The longest interval in any lead should be used. As noted in the previous section, in certain conditions, it may be difficult to choose the proper end of the T wave. We agree with Dr. James that "in electrocardiography, there is no more nebulous measurement than the QT interval,"[12] but the following rules may be helpful (Fig. 6-15). (1) If a separate T and U wave are visible and the U wave amplitude is 50% or less than the T wave amplitude, the QT interval ends at the end of the T wave. (2) If a single wave is visible and there is no notch in any lead, the entire wave is included in the QT interval. (3) If a single wave is visible but a notch is present in the wave and the terminal portion of the wave has an amplitude 50% or less than the

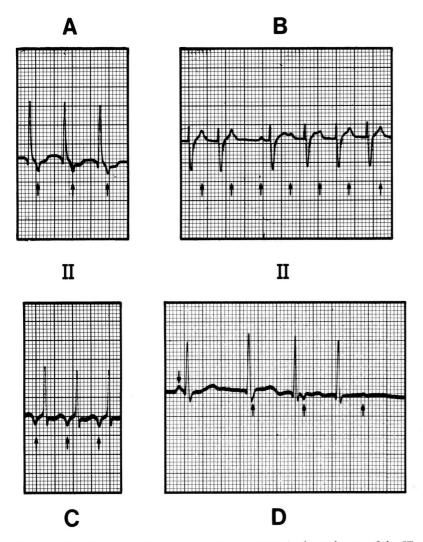

FIG. 6-14. Identification of P waves (arrows). A, P waves in the early part of the ST segment. B, P waves directly on top of T waves. The only way of distinguishing these waves was to observe an episode of spontaneous type I second-degree AV block in which the P wave was not followed by a QRS complex. This allowed observation of the P wave preceding the next QRS complex with a lengthening PR interval in subsequent beats. C, P waves on the downslope of the wave. D, P waves with differing relation to the QRS and T wave. In the second QRS complex, the widened S wave is caused by a superimposed P wave. The first P wave is upright and comes from the sinus node. The last three are inverted and due to retrograde conduction through the AV node.

peak, then the initial downslope should be extrapolated and the extrapolation used for the QT interval. (4) If a single wave is visible with a notch and the terminal portion has an amplitude more than 50% of the peak, then the entire wave is included as the T wave. (5) If a P wave is superimposed, extrapolate the T wave back to the baseline from the initial downstroke (Fig. 6-15).

The QT interval varies with heart rate. The QT interval can be corrected for heart rate by using Bazett's formula: corrected QT interval is

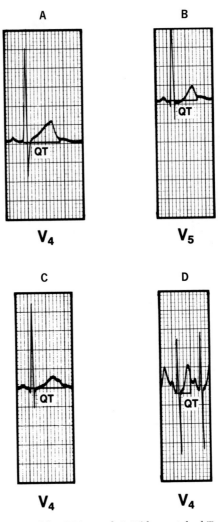

FIG. 6-15.   Measurement of the QT interval. **A,** With a notched T wave followed by a U wave, the downslope of the T wave is extrapolated to the baseline. **B,** With a notch less than 50% of the peak of the T wave, the early segment is extrapolated to the baseline. **C,** With a notch greater than 50% of the peak of the T wave, the second portion of the wave is extrapolated to the baseline. **D,** With superimposed P waves, the downslope of the T wave is extrapolated to the baseline.

equal to the QT interval (in seconds) divided by the square root of the RR interval (in seconds).[13] In the data of Davignon et al.,[3] the mean corrected QT (QTc) is .40 in children; the upper limit of normal (98th percentile) is .45 up to 6 months of age, and .44 in older children. While these limits generally apply throughout childhood, the QTc begins to decrease during early adolescence such that in adults,[2] the upper limit of normal QTc is .425. Alternatively, a patient's data can be compared with the normal QT interval derived from a plot of Bazett's data (Fig. 6-16). The actual measured QT interval in lead V_5 in children as it varies with heart rate is shown in Table A-16 (see Appendix).

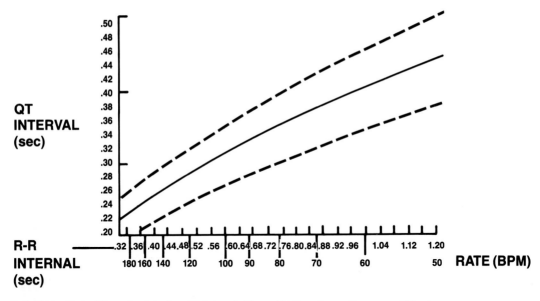

FIG. 6-16. Plot of Bazett's data for QT interval. The solid line shows the mean QT interval for each heart rate and cycle length. The dotted lines mark the upper and lower limits of normal calculated as ±2 standard deviations from the mean.

Q-OT Interval

The interval from the onset of the QRS complex to the onset of the T wave is the Q-OT interval. This interval may be corrected for heart rate in a similar way to the QT interval, thus determining the Q-OTc interval. In hypocalcemia, the entire T wave is shifted later in the cardiac cycle (due to a prolonged ST segment) and the Q-OTc interval provides a measure of this prolongation (Fig. 6-17). In premature infants, the normal corrected Q-OTc is .20 or less and in full term infants, it is .19 or less.[14]

TP Interval

The TP interval is that segment between the end of the T wave (or U wave) and the beginning of the P wave. This is the true isoelectric segment of the electrocardiogram between the last ventricular repolarization and the onset of atrial depolarization (Fig. 6-18). In cases with both PR and ST segment depression, it is best to use the PR segment as the isoelectric reference for the ST segment (see "PR Segment" in this chapter).

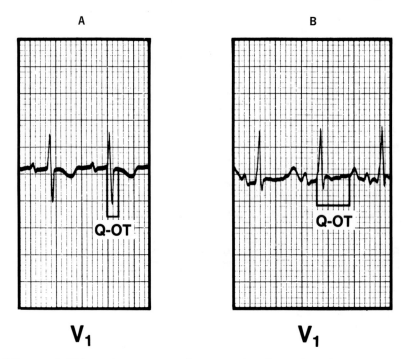

FIG. 6-17.   Q-OT interval. A, Q-OT interval in a normal newborn infant. The Q-OT interval is .10 sec and the PR interval is .45 sec. Therefore, the Q-OTc interval is .15. A normal Q-OT interval is .20 or less. B, Q-OT interval in an infant with hypocalcemia. The Q-OT interval is .27 sec and the RR interval is .47 sec. The Q-OTc interval of .39 is prolonged.

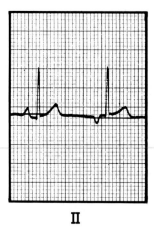

FIG. 6-18.   Importance of using the TP segment as the baseline. In the beat on the left, in sinus rhythm, using the TP segment as the baseline, there is PR segment depression of approximately 1 mm due to an inverted Ta wave. In the beat on the right with a low atrial rhythm, there is PR segment and ST segment elevation due to an upright Ta wave. In this tracing, the TP segment remains constant while the PR segment and ST segments change.

Self-Assessment Questions

Question 1: The heart rates (based on RR intervals) in Figure 6-19 vary between _____ and _____.

A. 33–69
B. 33–110
C. 69–110
D. 85–130
E. 98–150

Question 2: The PR interval _____ with increasing age.

A. increases
B. decreases
C. does not change
D. increases to age 8 and then is constant
E. none of the above

Question 3: The following QRS complex in lead V_1 in a 7-month-old should be interpreted as (Fig. 6-20):

A. normal
B. right ventricular hypertrophy
C. incomplete right bundle branch block
D. complete right bundle branch block
E. cannot distinguish between A, B, or C

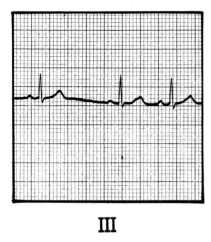

III

FIG. 6-19. Question 1.

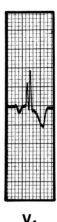

V₁

FIG. 6-20. Question 3.

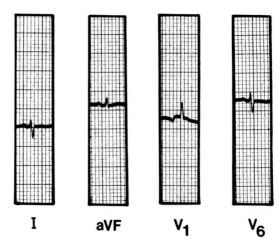

FIG. 6-21.   Question 4.

Question 4: Which of the following should be considered as the cause of the above electrocardiogram (Fig. 6-21):

A. myocarditis
B. pneumothorax
C. pleural effusion
D. improper standardization
E. all of the above

Question 5: In the measurement of the QT interval which *one* of the following is *false?*

A. If the U wave amplitude is 50% or less of the T wave amplitude, the QT interval ends at the end of the T wave.
B. If the terminal portion of a notched wave is 50% or less than the peak, the initial downstroke should be extrapolated for the QT interval.

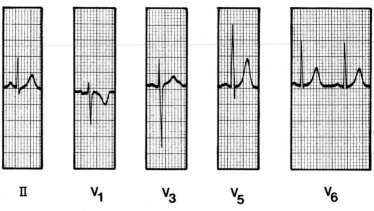

FIG. 6-22.   Question 6.

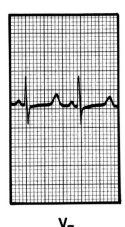

V₅

FIG. 6-23. Question 7.

C. If the terminal portion of a notched wave is more than 50% of the peak, the entire wave should be included in the QT interval.
D. If a P wave is superimposed, the QT interval cannot be measured in that lead.

Question 6: Measure the following on the electrocardiogram of this 4-year-old (Fig. 6-22). Refer to the tables in the Appendix and note any abnormalities. PR interval _____ seconds, QRS duration _____ seconds, Q-OT interval _____ seconds, Q-OTc interval _____ seconds, QT interval _____ seconds, QTc interval _____ seconds, R wave in V₁ _____ mm, S wave in V₁ _____ mm, R wave in V₆ _____ mm, S wave in V₆ _____ mm.

Question 7: Measure the Q-OT interval, the Q-OTc interval, the QT interval, and the QTc interval (Fig. 6-23). Note any abnormalities.

Answers to Self-Assessment Questions

Answer 1: C
This first interval contains 4 large and 2 small boxes. The exact heart rate is 69. The second interval contains 2 large and 4 small boxes. The heart rate is 110.

Answer 2: A
The PR interval lengthens with increasing age and shortens with increasing heart rate. Age is the more important factor.

Answer 3: E
The QRS duration is normal, and therefore complete right bundle branch block is incorrect. Otherwise, this QRS complex is compatible

with normal, mild right ventricular hypertrophy, or incomplete right bundle branch block and should be designated "RSR' complex in V_1."

Answer 4: E

Low voltage QRS complexes are seen in myocardial edema, loss of functioning myocardium, or increased distance between the heart and chest wall. If the standardization is improper, this also can result in "low-voltage" QRS complexes.

Answer 5: D

If a P wave is superimposed, extrapolate the T wave back to the baseline from the initial downstroke.

Answer 6:

The PR interval is .12 sec (measure in lead II); QRS duration (lead V_5) is .05 sec; Q-OT (V_5) is .12; Q-OTc is .12/square root (.56) = .16; QT (V_5) is .29; QTc is .29/square root (.56 = .39; RV_1 is 9 mm; SV_1 is 19 mm; RV_6 is 14 mm; SV_6 is 0.5 mm.

Answer 7:

Q-OT is .30; Q-OTc is .30/square root (.57) = .40; QT is .40; QTc is .53. All these intervals are prolonged.

References

1. Sreenivasan V., Fisher B. J., Liebman J., et al.: Longitudinal study of the standard electrocardiogram in the healthy premature infant during the first year of life. Am J Cardiol *31*:57–71, 1973.
2. Cooksey J. D., Dunn M., and Massie E.: Clinical Vectorcardiography and Electrocardiography. 2nd Ed. Chicago, Yearbook Medical Publishers, 1977, pp 9–112.
3. Davignon A., Rautaharju P., Boisselle E., et al.: Normal ECG standards for infants and children. Pediatr Cardiol *1*:123–152, 1979.
4. Chou T.: Electrocardiography in Clinical Practice. New York, Grune & Stratton, 1979, pp 114–150.
5. Burch G. E., and DePasquale N. P.: Electrocardiography in the Diagnosis of Congenital Heart Disease. Philadelphia, Lea & Febiger, 1967, pp 30–105.
6. Marriott H. J. L.: Practical Electrocardiography. 5th Ed. Baltimore, Williams & Wilkins, 1972, pp 16–50.
7. Gerard R., Seichter J., Lasry F., et al.: Les critères de surcharge ventriculaire gauche distonique chez l'enfant dans le canal arteriel et la communication interventriculaire. Arch Mal Coeur *64*:1590–1612, 1971.
8. Lepeschkin E.: The U wave of the electrocardiogram. Mod Concepts Cardiovasc Dis *38*:39–45, 1969.
9. Lepeschkin E., and Surawicz B.: The measurement of the QT interval of the electrocardiogram. Circulation 6:378–388, 1952.
10. Jervell A., and Lange-Nielsen F.: Congenital deafmutism, functional heart disease with prolongation of the Q-T interval and sudden death. Am Heart J *54*:59–68, 1957.
11. Garson A., Gillette P. C., and McNamara D. G.: Supraventricular tachycardia in children: clinical features, response to treatment, and long-term follow-up in 217 patients. J Pediatr *98*:875–882, 1981.
12. James T. N.: The sinus node. Am J Cardiol *40*:965–986, 1977.
13. Bazett H. C.: An analysis of the time relations of electrocardiograms. Heart 7:353–370, 1918.
14. Colletti R. B., Pan M. W., Smith E. W. P., et al.: Detection of hypocalcemia in susceptible neonates: the Q-OTc interval. N Eng J Med *290*:931–935, 1974.

7

The Heart Malposed
in the Thorax

Atrial
Situs

In the majority of cases, the atrial situs may be determined from the electrocardiogram. In situs solitus of the atria and viscera, the P wave mean vector in the frontal plane is approximately $+60°$, pointing away from its site of origin in the high right atrium or away from the right shoulder. This results in a positive P wave in leads I and aV_F (Fig. 7-1). In atrial situs inversus, a normal sinus impulse still originates high in the anatomic right atrium but because the anatomic right atrium is on the patient's left, the P wave appears to originate from the left shoulder and the P wave mean vector in the frontal plane, pointing away from the site of origin, is $+120°$ resulting in a P wave that is negative in lead I and positive in aV_F. The P wave mean vector in the horizontal plane is generally not helpful, because activation proceeds posteroanteriorly in this plane.

It may be impossible to determine atrial situs in the presence of an ectopic atrial rhythm.[1] However, in patients with normal situs and left atrial ectopic rhythm, despite the negative P wave in lead I, there may be a "dome-and-dart" P wave (a slow, rounded wave followed by a rapid, spiked wave) in lead V_1 (Fig. 7-1), indicating that the anatomic left atrium is activated before the anatomic right atrium.[2] In the rare case of a patient with atrial situs inversus and an ectopic rhythm originating from the right-sided anatomic left atrium, this patient would have a normal frontal plane P wave axis $(+60°)$ but with a dome-and-dart configuration in lead V_1 (Fig. 7-1).

In cases of situs ambiguous associated with splenic malformations, the P waves may be characteristic. In asplenia, there may be two anatomic right atria, one on either side, and there may be two sinus nodes.[3] In such cases, competition between the sinus nodes may occur with two P waves (one positive in lead I and one negative in lead I), each having a slightly different rate (Fig. 7-2). In polysplenia, there

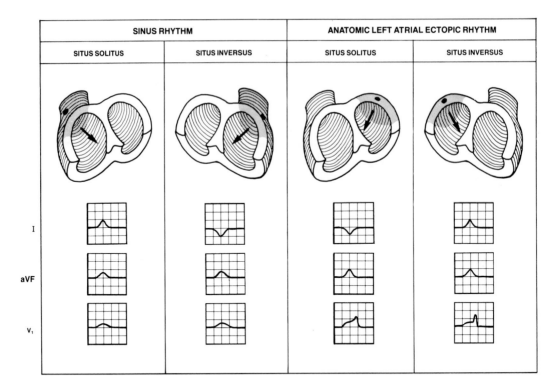

FIG. 7-1.   P wave morphology in sinus rhythm and anatomic left atrial ectopic rhythm with different atrial position. In sinus rhythm, the P wave is positive in lead I with situs solitus and negative in lead I with situs inversus. If the anatomic right atrium is depolarized before the anatomic left atrium, there is a normal P wave in lead V_1. If the anatomic left atrium is activated before the anatomic right atrium, a "dome and dart" P wave is found in lead V_1. Therefore, in situs solitus with anatomic left atrial ectopic rhythm, there is a negative P wave in lead I and a dome and dart P wave in lead V_1. With atrial situs inversus and anatomic left atrial ectopic rhythm, there is a positive P wave in lead I and a dome and dart P wave in lead V_1.

may be no sinus node and the pacemaker characteristically is located in the low atrium, giving a frontal plane P wave mean vector that is directly superior (−90°) (Fig. 7-3).

Ventricular Position

Since atrial situs is independent of ventricular position, the P waves and QRS complexes should be interpreted independently (i.e., a negative P wave in lead I suggests atrial situs inversus but not necessarily dextrocardia). There are four major electrocardiographic patterns that describe ventricular position: normal, mirror-image dextrocardia, dextrorotation, and ventricular inversion (Fig. 7-4). In the normally positioned heart, the maximal biphasic QRS voltage in the chest leads (transition) is at the left midclavicular line at lead V_3 or V_4. In the frontal plane, the initial forces are directed superiorly and to the right (Q wave in leads I, aV_F, and V_6), the major forces are directed

R Atrial

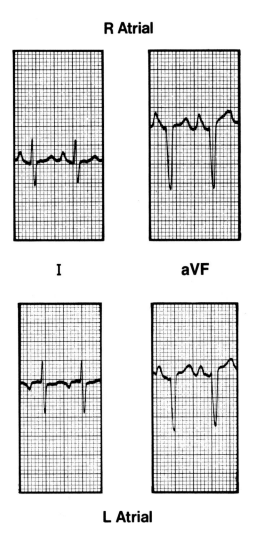

I   aVF

L Atrial

FIG. 7-2. P waves in asplenia. In the *top* two tracings, the patient has positive P waves in leads I and aV_F, indicating the site of origin of the P waves high in the atrium on the right side. In the *bottom* two tracings, taken several minutes later, the P waves have changed so that they are negative in lead I and positive in aV_F, indicating the origin of the P wave high and on the left side. The QRS complexes are identical.

inferiorly and to the left (tall R wave in leads I, aV_F, and V_6), and the terminal forces are directed superiorly and to the left (small S wave in lead aV_F; R wave in leads I and V_6) (Fig. 7-5).

MIRROR-IMAGE
DEXTROCARDIA

"Dextrocardia" implies only that the ventricular mass is in the right chest. In mirror-image dextrocardia, however, there is a reversal of the anatomic left-right relationship, but with anteroposterior relationships maintained—in other words, the anatomic right ventricle is to

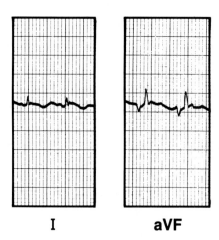

I   **aVF**

FIG. 7-3.   P waves in polysplenia. The P wave mean vector is −90°.

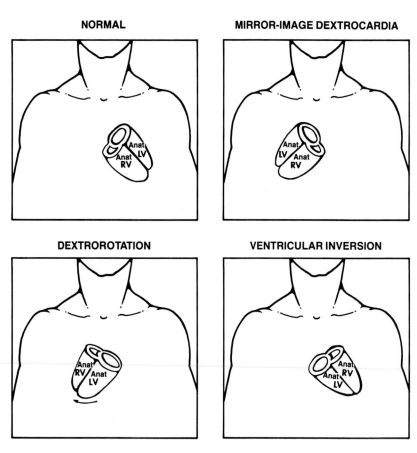

FIG. 7-4.   Ventricular position. In the normally positioned heart, the anatomic right ventricle is to the right and anterior to the anatomic left ventricle. The cardiac mass is in the left chest. In mirror-image dextrocardia, the anatomic right ventricle is to the left and anterior to the anatomic left ventricle. The ventricular mass is in the right chest. In dextrorotation, the anatomic right ventricle is to the right and posterior to the anatomic left ventricle. The ventricular mass is in the right chest to a varying degree. In ventricular inversion, the anatomic right ventricle is to the left and usually side-by-side to the anatomic left ventricle. In ventricular inversion without dextrocardia, the ventricular mass is in the left chest.

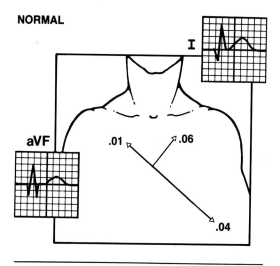

NORMAL

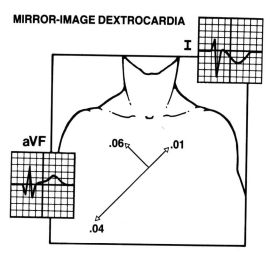

MIRROR-IMAGE DEXTROCARDIA

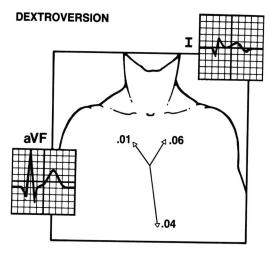

DEXTROVERSION

FIG. 7-5. Frontal plane QRS vectors in different ventricular positions. Top tracing, The directions and amplitudes of the early (.01 sec), middle (.04 sec), and terminal (.06 sec) vectors. In the normally positioned heart, the early vector is to the right and superior, the middle vector is to the left and inferior, and the terminal vector is to the left and superior. In mirror-image dextrocardia, the initial vector is to the left and superior, the middle vector is to the right and inferior, and the terminal vector is to the right and superior. In dextroversion, the initial vector is to the right and superior, the middle vector is inferior, and the terminal vector is to the left and superior.

the left and anterior. Whenever the ventricles are in the right chest, the maximal biphasic voltage is recorded in one of the *right* chest leads. *If the total voltage (top of the R wave to bottom of the S wave) in leads V_3R or V_4R is larger than the total voltage in lead V_3 or V_4, the patient has dextrocardia.* In *mirror-image* dextrocardia, if all the right chest leads are recorded (V_1, V_3R through V_7R), the QRS morphologies in these leads should be the same as those found recording the left chest leads in a normally situated heart. In the frontal plane, in a patient with mirror-image dextrocardia, the initial forces are directed superiorly and to the left (initial deep Q wave in leads I, aV_F, and V_6), the major forces are directed inferiorly and to the right (small R, deep S in leads I and V_6, tall R in aV_F) and the terminal forces are directed superiorly and to the right (S wave in leads I, aV_F, and V_6) (Figs. 7-5 and 7-6).

In summary, mirror-image dextrocardia should be suspected: (1) If the magnitude of the total QRS deflection is greater in leads V_3R or V_4R than in lead V_3 or V_4; (2) if lead I has a deep Q wave and a small R wave; or (3) if in leads V_3 through V_7, the QRS complexes become progressively smaller with a small R deep S, or QS, configuration.[4]

In assessing ventricular hypertrophy in mirror-image dextrocardia, one can apply the same criteria as with normally situated ventricles except that instead of lead V_6, lead V_6R should be substituted and instead of lead V_1, lead V_2 should be substituted (Fig. 7-7). Therefore, even in the absence of a tracing with all the right chest leads, ventricular hypertrophy can be assessed by interpreting lead V_2 as if it were lead V_1 in a normally situated heart.

DEXTROROTATION

In dextrorotation, the anatomic relationships between the ventricles are preserved (i.e., the right ventricle is on the right and the left ventricle is on the left), but the heart is *shifted* to a varying degree into the right chest. This shift is usually accompanied by a counterclockwise rotation of the heart (viewed from the apex) making the left ventricle anterior to the right ventricle (Fig. 7-4). Since the amount of rightward shift is variable, the classic signs of dextrocardia with greater voltage in the right chest leads than the left may be missing. In the frontal plane, the direction of the initial, major, and terminal deflections may be similar to that in normally situated ventricles. The mean frontal plane QRS vector is inferior and slightly to the left or right (Fig. 7-5). The major effect is on the precordial leads in which the transition is found in leads more to the right than normal, namely, in lead V_3R or V_4R (Fig. 7-6). The far right chest leads (lead V_6R) appear similar to the normal V_1, and the anterior leads (V_3) appear similar to the normal V_6. This can be suspected in a routine electrocardiogram when the anterior chest leads (V_2 through V_4) have small Q waves and tall R waves (similar to the normal V_6) and the transition is just beginning in lead V_1 or V_3R (Fig. 7-8).

Ventricular hypertrophy is less accurately assessed in dextrorotation since the degree of rotation is unknown, but similar criteria to those used for mirror-image dextrocardia may be applied with caution.

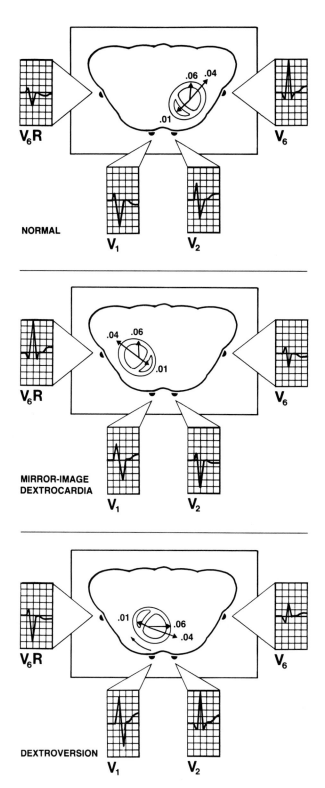

FIG. 7-6. Horizontal plane vectors in different cardiac positions. In the normally positioned heart, the middle (.04 sec) vector points left and posterior. In mirror-image dextrocardia, the middle (.04 sec) vector points right and posterior. In dextroversion, the middle (.04 sec) vector points left and slightly anterior.

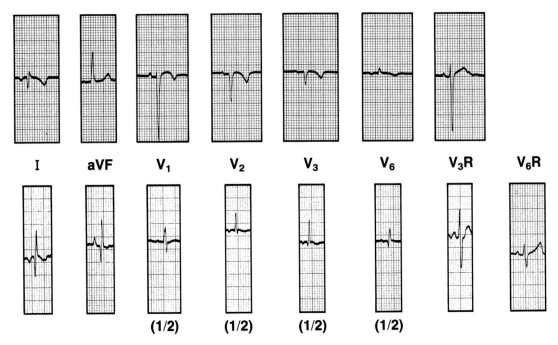

| I | aVF | V₁ | V₂ | V₃ | V₆ | V₃R | V₆R |

| | (1/2) | (1/2) | (1/2) | (1/2) | |

FIG. 7-7. Top tracing, 7-year-old with dextrocardia and situs inversus with an otherwise normal heart. Bottom tracing, 6-month-old with dextrocardia, situs inversus, and anterior ventricular hypertrophy. There is a QR pattern in lead V₂ and a deep S wave in lead V₆R.

VENTRICULAR INVERSION

One other condition in which the ventricles are malposed is ventricular inversion. In ventricular inversion with otherwise normal cardiac position (i.e., with the ventricles in the left chest), such as in atrial situs solitus and levocardia, the ventricular septum is oriented straight anteroposteriorly and parallel to the diaphragm with the ventricles side by side and the anatomic right ventricle to the left of the anatomic left ventricle (Fig. 7-4). Since the anatomic left bundle branch is on the right, this results in reversed septal depolarization with a Q wave in lead V₁ and an absent Q wave in lead V₆ (Fig. 7-9). The other characteristics of ventricular inversion and an otherwise normal heart are left axis deviation in the frontal plane and AV block—first, second, or third degree. Usually ventricular inversion is accompanied by additional anatomic abnormalities.

Pectus Excavatum and Straight Back Syndrome

In both of these conditions, the mediastinum is shortened in the anteroposterior dimension, causing the heart to shift to the left and rotate clockwise viewed from the apex. This brings the right atrium

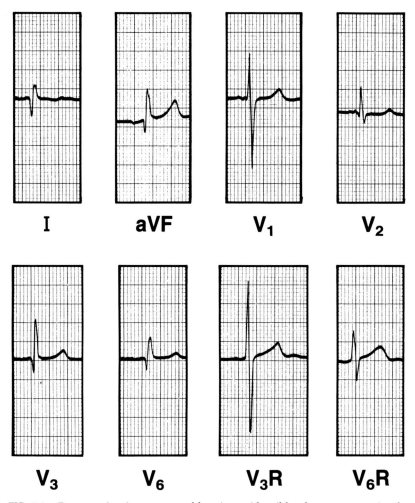

FIG. 7-8. Dextroversion in a 12-year-old patient with mild pulmonary stenosis. The transition occurs in lead V_3R, and there are Q waves in leads V_2 through V_6. Lead V_6R in this patient appears similar to lead V_1 in a patient with normally positioned ventricles and mild pulmonary stenosis.

more anteriorly relative to the left atrium and so the mean vector of atrial depolarization is oriented straight posteriorly. Therefore, in lead V_1, the P wave may be entirely negative (Figs. 7-10 and 7-11).[5]

Clockwise rotation moves the left side of the heart posteriorly and superiorly, causing some patients to have left axis deviation of the QRS in the frontal plane.[6] The right side of the heart is rotated anteriorly and inferiorly such that the vector of depolarization in the pulmonary outflow tract is shifted from its normal superior and rightward position to a straight anterior position. This is responsible for the normal duration RSR′ pattern in V_1 often found in these patients.[7] The transition is shifted to the left and there may be a persistent S wave in lead V_7. Abnormally deep QS waves followed by a normal duration R wave and inverted T wave in the anterior and midprecordial leads may occur instead of the RSR′ and simulate anterior myocardial infarction.

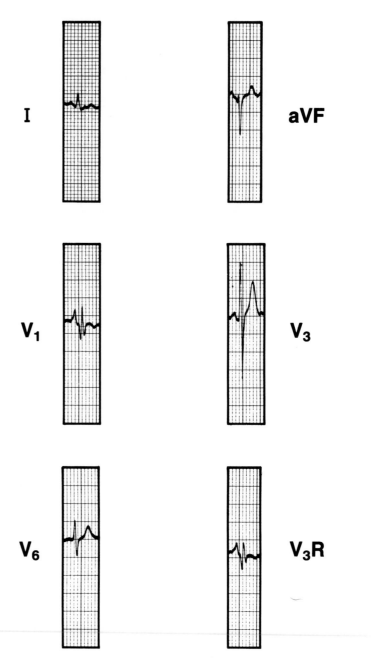

FIG. 7-9. Ventricular inversion. Note the deep Q waves in lead V_1 with a relatively small R wave. There are no Q waves in lead V_6.

These changes can be explained by the clockwise rotation shifting the major QRS forces even more posteriorly, causing the deep QS and concordantly inverted T wave. The terminal R wave has the same genesis as the R' that may be found in this condition: normal terminal depolarization of the right ventricular outflow tract.

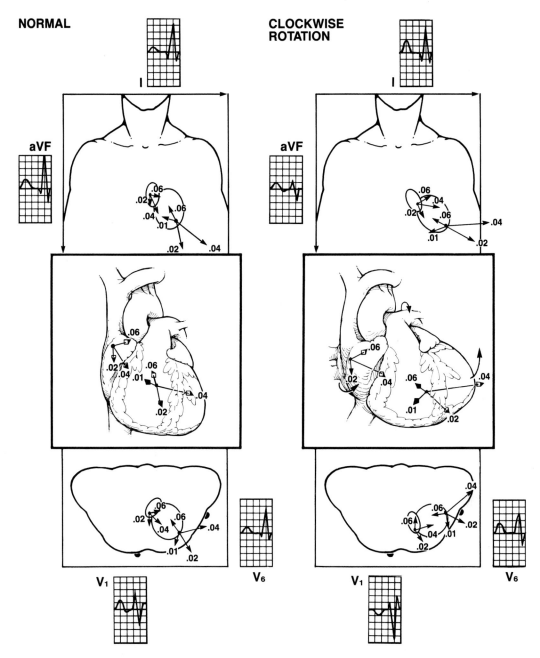

FIG. 7-10. Comparison of normal with clockwise rotation. The three-dimensional vectors for the different timings of the P wave are shown overlying the atrium; for the QRS complex they are shown overlying the ventricles. In the *top* part of the diagrams, the projections of the vectors on the frontal plane are shown. The small circle denotes the atria and the larger circle denotes the ventricles. In the frontal plane with clockwise rotation, both the P wave and QRS vectors are shifted to the left and superiorly. In the *bottom* parts of the diagrams the horizontal plane vectors are shown. In the horizontal plane, the vectors are shifted to the left and posteriorly.

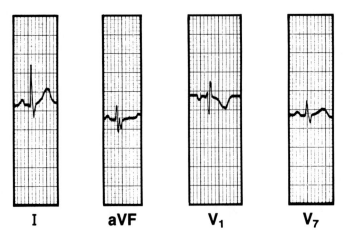

I   aVF   V₁   V₇

FIG. 7-11.   Electrocardiogram from a 4-year-old patient with pectus excavatum. The frontal plane QRS mean vector is −45°. There is an RSR′ pattern in lead V₁ and a persistent S wave in lead V₇.

Pneumonectomy

The chronic electrocardiographic changes following pneumonectomy result from shift and rotation of the heart. Following a right pneumonectomy, the findings are similar to those of congenital dextrorotation with the transition moved to the right in the chest leads.[8] In over 90% of children who underwent a left pneumonectomy, the heart was rotated clockwise with findings similar to those reported in pectus excavatum.

Pneumothorax and Pneumomediastinum

Because air is a poor conductor of electrical activity, if there is air between the heart on the recording electrode, the voltage of the P, QRS, and T waves will be decreased. In pneumomediastinum, the voltage may be decreased in all leads. In pneumothorax, the voltage may be decreased only in certain leads corresponding to the location of the air. Depending upon the amount of air, a pneumothorax may cause shift or rotation of the heart similar to that found following pneumonectomy on the opposite side. Finally, depending upon the amount of hemodynamic compromise caused by the condition, nonspecific ST and T wave changes as well as arrhythmias may occur. In pneumothorax, if the patient is placed in a sitting position, the electrocardiogram may normalize as the air moves superiorly away from the heart.

Kyphoscoliosis

There may be virtually any positional abnormality with kyphoscoliosis.[5] In severe cases, both rotation and shift occur, thus making it even more difficult to interpret the electrocardiogram. Since respiratory insufficiency and cor pulmonale may occur in these children and cause right atrial enlargement, right axis deviation, and right ventricular hypertrophy, an electrocardiographic diagnosis may be helpful in the management of the patient. As a general rule, a P wave amplitude of more than 2.5 mm in any lead constitutes right atrial enlargement. Right ventricular hypertrophy should be considered if a complex is found in any precordial lead to the right of the transitional leads with a tall R wave and a small S wave, and the height of the R wave is greater than the normal value for age given for lead V_1.

Self-Assessment
Questions

Question 1: In dextrocardia,

A. the atria begin depolarization high on the left side of the body
B. the total voltage in lead V_3R or V_4R exceeds the total voltage in lead V_3 or V_4
C. there is rarely a Q wave in lead I
D. the QRS complexes become progressively smaller in leads V_3R through V_7R
E. none of the above

Question 2: In mirror-image dextrocardia, the lead that should be substituted for V_1 in assessing anterior ventricular hypertrophy is:

A. V_3R
B. V_4R
C. V_2
D. V_3
E. V_4

Question 3: Match the correct term with the most common electrocardiographic finding:

_____ dextrorotation	A. RSR' in V_1
_____ ventricular inversion	B. Q waves in V_1
_____ pectus excavatum	C. Q waves in V_2 through V_4
_____ pneumonectomy	D. A or C
	E. none of the above

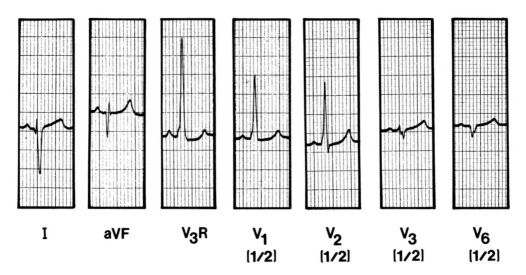

FIG. 7-12. Question 4.

Question 4: Diagnose the disorder in this 4-year-old on the basis of the electrocardiogram (Fig. 7-12).

A. Wolff-Parkinson-White   D. A and C
B. situs inversus   E. B and C
C. dextrocardia

Question 5: Diagnose the disorder in this 5-month-old on the basis of the electrocardiogram (Fig. 7-13).

A. dextrocardia   D. A and C
B. situs inversus   E. A and D
C. reversed limb leads

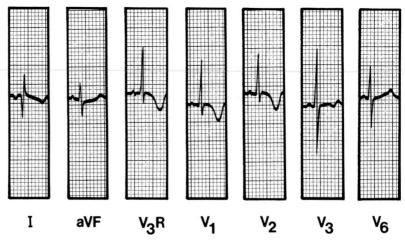

FIG. 7-13. Question 5.

Answers to Self-Assessment Questions

Answer 1: B

The cardiac mass is in the right chest and therefore the voltage in the right chest leads is greater than in the left chest leads. Answer A is false because dextrocardia does not necessarily imply atrial situs inversus. Answers C and D are false. Usually there is a deep Q wave in lead I and the QRS complexes become progressively smaller in the left chest leads, V_3 through V_7.

Answer 2: C

Lead V_2 is located immediately to the left of the sternum and lead V_1 is located immediately to the right of the sternum. Therefore, V_2 in mirror-image dextrocardia is in the same relative location as V_1 in the normally situated heart.

Answer 3: C, B, A, D

In dextrorotation, the transition is shifted to the right so that the anterior leads, V_2 through V_4, have small Q waves and tall R waves similar to the normal V_6 (answer C). In ventricular inversion, there is reversed septal depolarization, usually causing a QR pattern in lead V_1 (answer B). In pectus excavatum, there is anterior and inferior movement of the right side of the heart causing an RSR′ pattern in lead V_1 (answer A). In pneumonectomy, the heart may rotate either clockwise (left pneumonectomy) simulating pectus excavatum or counterclockwise (right pneumonectomy) simulating dextrorotation (answer D).

Answer 4: C

The voltage in V_3R is much greater than the voltage in V_3, so the patient has dextrocardia. In addition, she has left axis deviation and anterior ventricular hypertrophy (read in V_2). There is not atrial situs inversus. The PR interval is normal.

Answer 5: C

The P wave is negative in lead I but positive in lead V_6. This is the best sign for reversed limb leads (see Chapter 13).

References

1. Hoffman J. I. E.: The place of electrocardiography in pediatric cardiology. Praxis 64:816–822, 1975.
2. Mirowski M., Neill C. A., and Taussig H. B.: Left atrial ectopic rhythm in mirror image dextrocardia and in normally placed malformed hearts. Report of 12 cases with "dome and dart" P waves. Circulation 27:864–877, 1963.
3. Momma K., and Linde L. M.: Abnormal P wave axis in congenital heart disease associated with asplenia and polysplenia. J Electrocardiol 2:395–405, 1969.
4. Burch G. E., and DePasquale N. P.: Electrocardiography in the Diagnosis of Congenital Heart Disease. Philadelphia, Lea & Febiger, 1967, pp. 30–105.

5. Chou T.: Electrocardiography in Clinical Practice. New York, Grune & Stratton, 1979, pp 114–150.
6. De Leon A. C., Perloff J. K., and Twigg H.: The straight back syndrome. Clinical cardiovascular manifestations. Circulation *32:*193–200, 1965.
7. De Oliveira J. M., Sambi M. P., and Zinnerman H. A.: The electrocardiogram in pectus excavatum. Br Heart J *20:*495–499, 1958.
8. Calleja H. B.: Diagnostic value of electrocardiographic changes in pneumonectomies. Cardiologia *49:*228–238, 1966.

8

Chamber Enlargement and Hypertrophy

The electrocardiogram can be helpful in the diagnosis of enlargement or hypertrophy of the cardiac chambers. Although the electrocardiogram correlates with chamber size better in pediatric patients than in adults, it nevertheless has only about a 60 to 70% predictive value in children.[1,2] Therefore, if either the presence or absence of an abnormality on an electrocardiogram does not agree with the clinical or echocardiographic findings, the electrocardiogram should be viewed quite critically. In the following discussion, criteria are listed for chamber enlargement or hypertrophy with the most reliable signs presented first.

Right Ventricular Hypertrophy

The electrocardiogram can provide important data on right ventricular hypertrophy or elevated right ventricular systolic pressure that are not currently available by noninvasive means. The criteria for right ventricular hypertrophy follow.

1. QR PATTERN IN THE RIGHT CHEST LEADS (Fig. 8-1). The Q wave is due to a dominant early wave of excitation moving posteriorly. This may be due to the hypertrophied and dilated right side of the septum providing a larger surface area for a normally insignificant posterior vector. In this case, left-to-right septal activation occurs normally but is overshadowed by a stronger posterior vector. Alternatively, in right ventricular hypertrophy, the inferior wall of the right ventricle directly contiguous to the septum may bulge posteriorly and to the left of the septum. Therefore, instead of the earliest activation continuing left to right, the initial septal depolarization may begin normally towards the right for a few milliseconds but then change orientation and move to the left as those parts of the inferior wall of the right ventricle that are situated to the left of the septum depolarize.[3]

99

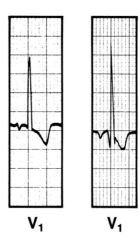

V_1 V_1

FIG. 8-1.   Left, Typical QR pattern in lead V_1 with a small Q wave. This is from a 9-month-old patient with unoperated transposition of the great arteries. Right, Deep Q wave with a tall R wave and ST depression in a 4-year-old after Mustard operation for transposition of the great arteries.

The Q wave in the QR pattern of right ventricular hypertrophy is generally only 0.5 to 1 mm deep in infants but may become 3 to 5 mm deep in older children. The QR pattern is quite reliable and implies a right ventricular systolic pressure of 70 mmHg or more at any age.[4] A QR pattern may also be seen in ventricular inversion with reversed septal depolarization. In general, in the QR pattern of right ventricular hypertrophy in lead V_1 or V_4R, the R wave is tall (15 to 20 mm). In ventricular inversion, the Q wave may be slightly deeper than the usual Q wave seen in right ventricular hypertrophy and the R wave may not be as tall (Fig. 7-9). This distinction may not be possible in an individual patient. A final cause of a QR pattern in lead V_1 or V_3R is the rare case of an anterior myocardial infarction involving either the right ventricle or the anterior ventricular septum. Before making the diagnosis of a QR pattern, make sure to ascertain that the QRS complex does not begin with a tiny R wave, which would make the complex an RSR' pattern rather than a QR pattern.

2. T WAVE CHANGES. Between one week of age and the onset of adolescence, the T waves in the right chest leads should be negative. In mildly increased right ventricular systolic pressure, the electrocardiogram is normal with a small R wave and a symmetrically inverted T wave in lead V_1 (Fig. 8-2A). With increasing severity of pulmonary stenosis, usually before the R wave height is abnormal, the T wave becomes isoelectric or upright (Fig. 8-2B). The upright T wave is due to elevated right ventricular systolic pressure and not necessarily right ventricular hypertrophy, since in a patient with increased right ventricular systolic pressure due to upper airway obstruction and hypoxia, the upright T waves may invert immediately with intubation and ventilation. In general, if the height of the R wave in lead V_1 is less than 10 mm, an inverted T wave is associated with less severe disease than an isoelectric or upright T wave (Fig. 8-2C). When the R wave

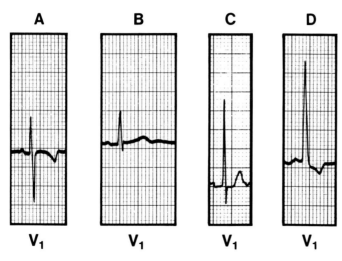

FIG. 8-2. Progression of T wave changes in lead V_1 in right ventricular hypertrophy. A, Normal T wave in a 4-year-old child. B, Upright T wave in a 7-year-old child with mild pulmonary stenosis. The R wave is 9 mm tall. C, Tall R wave with upright T wave in a 2-year-old with severe pulmonary stenosis. D, Tall R wave with asymmetrically inverted T wave ("right ventricular strain") in a 3-year-old patient with critical pulmonary stenosis.

height increases above 10 mm, the upright T wave may become asymmetrically inverted with a concave upward terminal portion (Fig. 8-2D). Therefore, the progression and severity are as follows: normal R with symmetrically inverted T; normal or slightly increased R with upright T; tall R with upright T; and tall R with asymmetrically inverted T. The asymmetrically inverted T wave in lead V_1 is called the "right ventricular strain" pattern and may be associated with ST depression in the same lead. This is thought to be a primary T wave change due to the reversed direction of repolarization that occurs from endocardium to epicardium in hypertrophy.[5] The right ventricular strain pattern generally indicates a right ventricular systolic pressure equal to or greater than systemic pressure.[4,6] The deeply asymmetrically inverted T waves in the right ventricular strain pattern may extend as far to the left as lead V_4, and rarely V_5, but usually not to V_6.[3] Conversely, the T wave inversion found in leads V_5 and V_6 indicating "left ventricular strain" may cause reciprocally *upright* T waves in the right chest leads (Fig. 8-3). Therefore, before the diagnosis of right ventricular hypertrophy is made on the basis of an upright T wave in lead V_1, leads V_5 and V_6 should be examined for left ventricular strain.

One other T wave change of severe right ventricular hypertrophy is T wave inversion in lead aV_F.[4] This is a nonspecific sign since it may also be indicative of left ventricular strain or other conditions (see Chapter 10). However, in the presence of other signs of right ventricular hypertrophy, T wave inversion in lead aV_F indicates severe right ventricular hypertrophy.

3. R WAVE AMPLITUDE IN LEAD V_1. If the amplitude of the R wave in lead V_1 exceeds the 98th percentile for age (see Appendix, Table A-7),

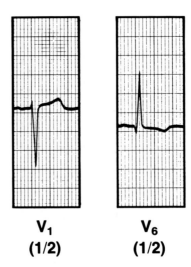

V₁
(1/2)

V₆
(1/2)

FIG. 8-3. Left ventricular strain with T wave inversion in lead V_6 causing upright T waves in lead V_1.

right ventricular hypertrophy is suspected. This sign is more specific but less sensitive; in other words, there may be children with right ventricular hypertrophy with a normal R wave in lead V_1.[7] The magnitude of the R wave in lead V_1 is directly proportional to the right ventricular systolic pressure. Two correlative formulas have been devised from children with pulmonary stenosis. Right ventricular systolic pressure equals 3 times the R wave in V_1 plus 47, or right ventricular systolic pressure equals 5 times the R wave in V_1.[3,4] If the R wave in V_1 is 20 mmHg or more at any age, the right ventricular systolic pressure is equal to or more than systemic pressure.

One other reason for an abnormally tall R wave in lead V_1 in a patient without right ventricular hypertrophy is ventricular septal hypertrophy. This may cause deep Q waves in leads V_5 and V_6 with reciprocally tall R waves in lead V_1. Since septal depolarization is completed relatively early in the QRS complex, the tall R wave in lead V_1 due to septal hypertrophy is "narrow" and usually lasts .03 sec or less. Conversely, in right ventricular hypertrophy, ventricular activation is slightly prolonged and the R wave of right ventricular hypertrophy in lead V_1 generally lasts .04 sec or longer[7] (Fig. 8-4). Finally, in patients with muscular dystrophy, a similar pattern of a tall narrow R wave in V_1 may occur with Q waves in the left chest leads. This is thought to be due to posterobasal left ventricular fibrosis (Fig. 8-4).

4. S WAVE AMPLITUDE IN LEAD V_6. If the depth of the S wave in lead V_6 exceeds the 98th percentile for age (see Appendix, Table A-10), right ventricular hypertrophy is suspected. This is more sensitive and less specific (i.e., a deep S wave in lead V_6 may be associated with conditions other than right ventricular hypertrophy). One of these conditions is left ventricular hypertrophy localized to the superior septum.

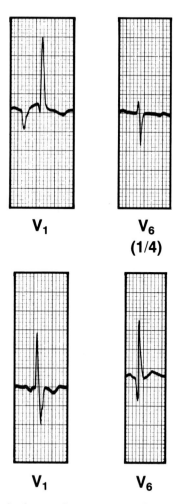

FIG. 8-4. Tall R wave in lead V_1. In the *top* tracings, the patient has right ventricular hypertrophy due to pulmonary atresia. In the *bottom* tracings, the tall R wave in lead V_1 is caused by the deep Q wave in lead V_6 in a patient with muscular dystrophy. The duration of the R wave in lead V_1 in the *top* tracing is .07 sec and in the *bottom* tracing is .04 sec.

This part of the left ventricle is the last to be activated and since it is usually in the anterior part of the left ventricle, this may cause a delayed vector directed anteriorly, causing an S wave in lead V_6 or even a normal duration RSR' in lead V_1. This has been termed the "incomplete right bundle branch block of coarctation of the aorta or aortic stenosis."[3] One other cause of a deep S wave in lead V_6 is left anterior hemiblock caused by delayed activation of the anterior left ventricle (Fig. 8-5) (see Chapter 9 on conduction abnormalities).

5. R/S RATIO IN LEAD V_1. This ratio suffers the inaccuracies of each of the single measurements. Nonetheless, an abnormally large RS ratio does correlate with right ventricular hypertrophy (see Appendix, Table A-11).

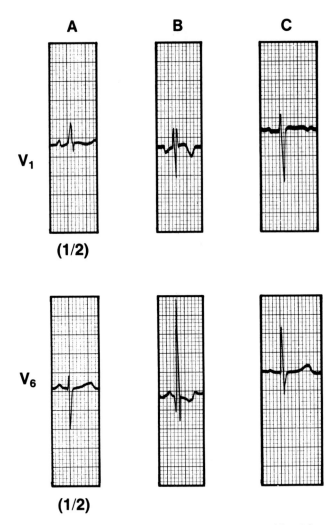

FIG. 8-5. Deep S wave in lead V$_6$. A, The deep S wave is caused by right ventricular hypertrophy in a 2-year-old. B, The deep S wave is caused by hypertrophy of the anterior part of the left ventricle in a 1-year-old patient with coarctation of the aorta. C, The deep S wave is caused by left anterior hemiblock in an 8-year-old patient.

6. RSR′ IN V$_1$. In over 90% of children with a secundum atrial septal defect, there is a normal duration RSR′ pattern in lead V$_1$. This correlates well with the mild right ventricular hypertrophy found in these children.[6] Thus, the RSR′ pattern is quite sensitive for mild right ventricular hypertrophy but also quite nonspecific since it may be found in normal children and those with incomplete right bundle branch block (see Chapters 6 and 9). In right ventricular hypertrophy, the S wave tends to be smaller and the R′ wave larger than in normal children. With a normal duration QRS complex, right ventricular hypertrophy is usually the cause of an R′ wave greater than 15 mm in an infant under a year of age or an R′ greater than 10 mm in a child over a year of age (Fig. 8-6). If the R′ is small with a normal duration RSR′ complex, the diagnosis could be normal, incomplete right bundle branch block

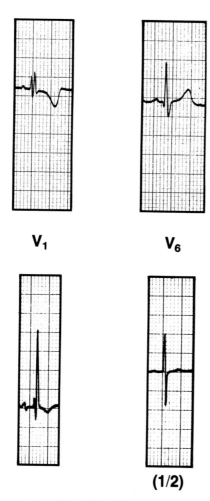

V₁ **V₆**

(1/2)

FIG. 8-6. The RSR'. **Top** tracings, Normal duration QRS complex with RSR' pattern in V₁ in a 6-year-old child. The R' is not tall. No specific diagnosis can be applied. **Bottom** tracings, Normal duration QRS complex with an RSR' pattern in lead V₁. The R' wave is tall. This is a 6-month-old child with right ventricular hypertrophy.

pattern, or right ventricular hypertrophy and we would prefer the description "RSR' pattern in right chest leads" rather than attempt to make a specific diagnosis.

7. RIGHT AXIS DEVIATION. Over the age of 3 months, right axis deviation correlates with right ventricular hypertrophy.[8] In adults, one of the common causes of right axis deviation is left posterior hemiblock (see Chapter 9 on conduction abnormalities). Left posterior hemiblock is rare in children and therefore right ventricular hypertrophy is by far the leading cause of right axis deviation in children. Nonetheless, right axis deviation should be considered as supporting evidence, and the electrocardiogram should meet one of the other criteria for right ventricular hypertrophy. The diagnosis of right axis deviation may be stronger supporting evidence for right ventricular hypertrophy in the patient with an RSR' pattern in lead V₁.[9]

Left Ventricular Hypertrophy

Recent echocardiographic and autopsy studies have shown that the electrocardiographic diagnosis of left ventricular hypertrophy is only accurate approximately 50% of the time. The greater the number of the following criteria met by an electrocardiogram, the more certain is the diagnosis of left ventricular hypertrophy.[5]

1. T WAVE CHANGES. The T waves are normally upright in leads V_5 and V_6 after 48 hours of age. The most reliable sign of left ventricular hypertrophy is asymmetric T wave inversion with an upward convexity in the terminal portion of the T wave in lead V_5 or V_6: the so-called "left ventricular strain" pattern (Figs. 5-6, 8-3, and 8-7). This may coexist with ST depression in the same leads. These changes become more prominent with increasing left ventricular to aortic gradient in aortic stenosis in children. In all children with a gradient less than 50 mmHg, the T waves in lead V_6 were upright, whereas 50% of those with gradients of 80 mmHg or more had inverted T waves in lead V_6. The T waves

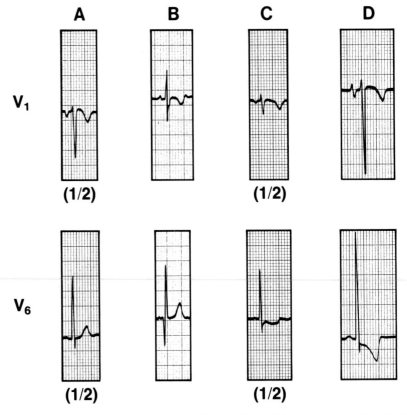

FIG. 8-7.   Left ventricular hypertrophy. A, Voltage criteria with deep S wave in V_1 and tall R wave in V_6. B, Deep Q waves in lead V_6. C, Absent Q wave in lead V_6. D, T wave inversion in lead V_6 with ST depression ("left ventricular strain").

in lead aV_F also became inverted with increasing gradient in aortic stenosis, but the findings in leads V_5 and V_6 were more reliable.[2]

The ST-T wave changes of "left ventricular strain" are the opposite of what would be expected in hypertrophy. In mild hypertrophy, the R wave in lead V_6 is increased in amplitude and the positive T waves are also increased in amplitude. In severe left ventricular hypertrophy, there is a variable amount of conduction delay and endocardial repolarization begins before epicardial depolarization has ended, causing T wave inversion and ST depression (Fig. 8-7). Left ventricular strain is therefore a primary change unrelated to the height of the R wave.[5]

T wave inversion in the inferior and lateral leads is found in conditions other than severe left ventricular hypertrophy (see Chapter 10). However, if no other cause is found for the T wave inversion, even in the absence of other criteria, the diagnosis of severe left ventricular hypertrophy should be suspected on the basis of the T waves.

2. R WAVE AMPLITUDE IN LEAD V_6 OR S WAVE AMPLITUDE IN LEAD V_1. An R wave in lead V_6 or an S wave in lead V_1 that is greater than the 98th percentile for age (see Appendix, Tables A-8 and A-9) should be designated as "left ventricular hypertrophy by voltage criteria" (Fig. 8-7A). Morganroth et al. reported 11 teenagers with either an abnormally deep S wave in lead V_1 or an abnormally tall R wave in lead V_6, all of whom had a normal echocardiogram and no other evidence of cardiac disease.[10] All of these children had normal T waves. Therefore, an individual adolescent may have prominent voltage without an increased left ventricular mass. In the absence of T wave changes, the diagnosis of left ventricular hypertrophy based entirely on voltage criteria must be viewed critically.

3. AMPLITUDE OF R WAVE IN LEAD V_6 PLUS AMPLITUDE OF S WAVE IN LEAD V_1. This measurement suffers from the same problem as the individual measurements, but does correlate with left ventricular hypertrophy. This should also be considered "left ventricular hypertrophy by voltage criteria" if greater than the 98th percentile for age (see Appendix, Table A-13). The R/S ratio in the precordial leads is less helpful in left ventricular hypertrophy than in right ventricular hypertrophy.

4. Q WAVE ABNORMALITIES. The .01 sec vector consists of the net result of almost simultaneous activation of the anterior left ventricle, posterior left ventricle, and left side of the septum. Therefore, if any of these areas is hypertrophied, the normal balance of forces may be upset and the initial portion of the QRS may change. The Q waves may vary independently from the R and S waves.

In left ventricular hypertrophy due either to a dilated left ventricle (aortic insufficiency or ventricular septal defect), septal hypertrophy (hypertrophic cardiomyopathy), or mild aortic stenosis, the initial forces may be increased in the right anterior-superior direction causing abnormally deep Q waves in the inferior and lateral leads—leads

II, III, aV$_F$, V$_5$, and V$_6$[11] (Fig. 8-7B) (see Chapter 6). The other causes for abnormally deep Q waves are discussed in Chapter 10.

In advanced concentric left ventricular hypertrophy with increased thickness of the posterior wall and septum, the QRS vector shifts to the left and posteriorly causing the initial forces to be directed more to the left. This may cause the absence of a Q wave in lead V$_6$ (Fig. 8-7C). In children with aortic stenosis, an absent Q wave in lead V$_6$ was more than twice as common in those with a severe gradient than in those with a gradient less than 50 mmHg.[2] Nonetheless, 53% of those with a gradient of at least 80 mmHg had a 1- or 2-mm Q wave in lead V$_6$. The terms "volume overload" and "pressure overload" type of left ventricular hypertrophy have been associated with deep Q waves and absent Q waves respectively.[11] Because there is so much overlap, we prefer not to use this terminology. Nonetheless, the absence of a Q wave or the presence of an abnormally deep Q wave may be supportive evidence of left ventricular hypertrophy.

Biventricular Hypertrophy

1. ABNORMAL VOLTAGE IN BOTH THE RIGHT AND LEFT CHEST LEADS. In the presence of isolated hypertrophy of one ventricle, the forces reflecting the other normal ventricle usually appear diminished on the electrocardiogram. For example, in isolated right ventricular hypertrophy with a tall R wave in lead V$_1$ and a deep S wave in lead V$_6$, the forces reflecting the left ventricle (S wave in lead V$_1$ or R wave in lead V$_6$) are usually diminished because of the dominance of the other ventricle. Therefore, biventricular hypertrophy can be diagnosed if, in the presence of voltage criteria for hypertrophy of one ventricle, the other ventricle generates at least normal forces. We have formalized this idea into the following criteria for biventricular hypertrophy: (a) right ventricular hypertrophy (abnormally tall R wave in lead V$_1$ or deep S wave in lead V$_6$) and either an S wave in lead V$_1$ or an R wave in lead V$_6$ exceeding the *mean* for age; or (b) left ventricular hypertrophy (abnormally tall R wave in lead V$_6$ or deep S wave in lead V$_1$) and either an S wave in lead V$_6$ or an R wave in lead V$_1$ exceeding the *mean* for age (Figs. 8-8A and 8-8B). Biventricular hypertrophy should not be diagnosed based upon Q wave or T wave morphology.

2. ABNORMAL VOLTAGE IN THE MIDPRECORDIAL LEADS. Prominent midprecordial voltage is a sign of biventricular hypertrophy. Katz and Wachtel originally described large biphasic QRS complexes in the limb leads of patients with congenital heart disease.[12] The "Katz-Wachtel" criterion has become broadened to refer to increased midprecordial voltage in patients with biventricular hypertrophy (Fig. 8-8C). In lead V$_4$, the voltage from the top of the R wave to the bottom of the S wave varies with age (see Appendix, Table A-14). Biventricular hypertrophy

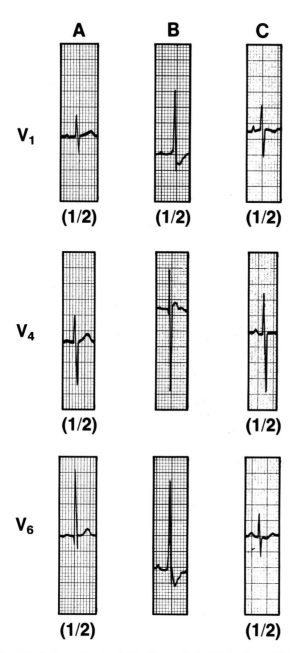

FIG. 8-8. Biventricular hypertrophy. **A,** The R wave in lead V$_6$ is 42 mm high. This meets the criterion for left ventricular hypertrophy. The R wave in lead V$_1$ is 15 mm high. This exceeds the mean voltage for the R wave in lead V$_1$ for this 1½-year-old child, and therefore the diagnosis of biventricular hypertrophy is made. **B,** The R wave in lead V$_1$ is 40 mm high. This meets the voltage criteria for right ventricular hypertrophy. The R wave in lead V$_6$ is 12 mm high. This exceeds the mean for the R wave in lead V$_6$ at 1 week of age, and so the diagnosis of biventricular hypertrophy is made. **C,** The voltages in V$_1$ and V$_6$ are not distinctly abnormal for a 1-week-old baby; however, the voltage in lead V$_4$ constitutes abnormally prominent midprecordial voltage, and the diagnosis of biventricular hypertrophy is made on this basis. This is the "Katz-Wachtel" criterion.

can be diagnosed if the total R plus S wave exceeds the 98th percentile. The "Katz-Wachtel" criterion of increased midprecordial voltage may be inaccurate because of proximity effects enlarging the midprecordial QRS voltage or cancellation effects reducing the voltage.

Right Atrial Enlargement

Right atrial depolarization is responsible for the early part of the P wave and therefore when right atrial enlargement occurs, this is manifest in the first .04 to .06 sec of the P wave. The following criteria may be used.

1. INCREASED AMPLITUDE OF THE P WAVE. The right atrium enlarges anteriorly and inferiorly causing an enlarged P wave of normal duration. The increased early vector causes the P wave to appear peaked. If the P wave in any lead is greater than 2.5 mm in amplitude at any age, right atrial enlargement is diagnosed (Fig. 8-9A).[3,13] The right atrium may occasionally enlarge and wrap around the superior vena cava and inferior vena cava posteriorly as well as anteriorly. In this case, there is an early negative deflection in the first .04 to .06 sec which is usually pointed (Fig. 8-9B). This negative deflection, by itself, is not a criterion for right atrial enlargement but needs to be distinguished from the more rounded late terminal negative deflection, which is a criterion of left atrial enlargement. If the mean vector of the P wave is such that atrial depolarization is thought to originate from an area other than the sinus node, the electrocardiogram should not be interpreted for atrial enlargement.

The electrocardiographic criteria of right atrial enlargement are related both to high right atrial pressure and to high right atrial volume

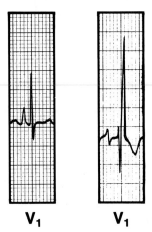

V_1 V_1

FIG. 8-9. Right atrial enlargement. Left, Tall peaked P wave. Right, Early (first .04 sec) pointed, negative deflection in lead V_1.

in children.[14] The presence of these changes immediately after an episode of supraventricular tachycardia or pulmonary embolism and their absence after several hours have elapsed, imply that hemodynamics rather than hypertrophy are related to these changes.

Left Atrial Enlargement

Left atrial depolarization is responsible for the terminal portion of the T wave and therefore when left atrial enlargement occurs, this is manifest in the latter part of the P wave. The following criteria may be used.

1. INCREASED TERMINAL POSTERIOR FORCES. The most reliable indicator of left atrial enlargement is a late negative deflection in lead V_1. This deflection begins later than .04 sec after the onset of the P wave. In children and adults, if the terminal deflection in lead V_1 is greater than 1 mm deep and greater than .04 sec in duration, this indicates left atrial enlargement (Fig. 8-10A).[15] As the left atrial enlargement becomes more severe, the depth and duration of the terminal segment increase such that in the most severe left atrial enlargement in children, the mean depth of the P terminal segment in lead V_1 was 2.8 mm and the duration .08 sec.[16]

Increased terminal posterior forces are related more to left atrial volume than pressure. Similar to the changes in right atrial enlargement, the P waves may become abnormal with an abrupt increase in left atrial volume such as acute mitral insufficiency and then may return to normal shortly after the stress is removed, again implying that hypertrophy is not necessary for these changes. In general, the in-

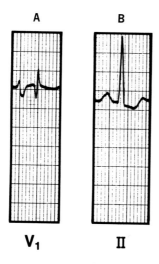

FIG. 8-10. Left atrial enlargement. A, Increased terminal negative deflection. The terminal portion of the P wave is 2.5 mm deep and .06 sec wide. B, Increased P wave duration.

crease in P terminal forces is a specific sign of left atrial enlargement, but there may be false negatives.[17] As with right atrial enlargement, if the pacemaker does not originate in the sinus node, left atrial enlargement should not be diagnosed on the electrocardiogram.

2. INCREASED P WAVE DURATION. This is a more nonspecific sign either of left atrial enlargement or of interatrial conduction delay which may be found in damage to the atrial myocardium due to myocarditis, fibrosis, or ischemia.[18] An abnormal P wave duration is defined as longer than .09 sec in children younger than age 3 and longer than .10 sec in children 3 years of age or older (Fig. 8-10B). This sign, similar to the increased terminal negative deflection, indicates abnormality when present, but it is not sensitive enough to diagnose most cases of left atrial enlargement in children detected echocardiographically.[17]

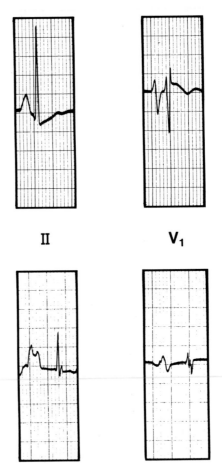

II   V$_1$

FIG. 8-11. Biatrial enlargement. *Top* tracings show P waves with increased positive amplitude in lead V$_1$, as well as a large terminal negative deflection in lead V$_1$. The P waves also have prolonged duration in addition to increased positive amplitude in lead II. *Bottom* tracings show P waves that are larger than the QRS complexes. The P wave is the first complex in each lead. The P wave in lead II begins with the sharp positive upstroke and is 6 mm tall. The P wave is .16 sec in duration. In lead V$_1$, there is also a large terminal negative deflection.

Biatrial Enlargement

Since the right and left atria depolarize sequentially causing different parts of the P wave, and since the signs of enlargement of one atrium do not distort the changes of enlargement in the other atrium, biatrial enlargement is diagnosed when the signs of right atrial enlargement coexist with the signs of left atrial enlargement.

1. ABNORMAL VOLTAGE AND DURATION. If the first .04 sec of the P wave are greater than 2.5 mm tall and the P wave is either prolonged for age or has a late terminal deflection in lead V_1 that is greater than 1 mm deep and .04 sec in duration, the diagnosis is biatrial enlargement (Fig. 8-11).

Self-Assessment Questions

Question 1: All of the following are criteria for right ventricular hypertrophy except:

A. QR pattern in the right chest leads
B. upright T wave in lead V_2 after one week of age
C. abnormally tall R wave in lead V_1
D. abnormally deep S wave in lead V_6
E. abnormal RS ratio in lead V_1

Question 2: Supportive evidence for left ventricular hypertrophy may be found in:

A. deep Q wave in lead V_6
B. absent Q wave in lead V_6
C. both
D. neither

Question 3: What is the electrocardiographic diagnosis in this 8-month-old (Fig. 8-12)?

A. right atrial enlargement
B. left atrial enlargement
C. both
D. neither

Question 4: What is the electrocardiographic diagnosis in this 3-month-old (Fig. 8-13)?

A. right ventricular hypertrophy
B. right ventricular hypertrophy with strain

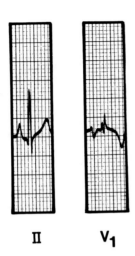

II V_1

FIG. 8-12. Question 3.

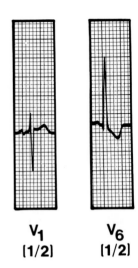

V_1 V_6
(1/2)   (1/2)

FIG. 8-13. Question 4.

C. normal
D. left ventricular hypertrophy
E. left ventricular hypertrophy with strain

Question 5: What is the electrocardiographic diagnosis in this 5-week-old (Fig. 8-14)?

A. right ventricular hypertrophy
B. right ventricular hypertrophy with strain
C. biventricular hypertrophy
D. left ventricular hypertrophy
E. left ventricular hypertrophy with strain

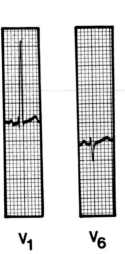

V_1 V_6

FIG. 8-14. Question 5.

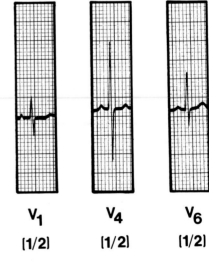

V_1 V_4 V_6
(1/2)   (1/2)   (1/2)

FIG. 8-15. Question 6.

Question 6: What is the electrocardiographic diagnosis in this 3-week-old (Fig. 8-15)?

A. right ventricular hypertrophy
B. right ventricular hypertrophy with strain
C. biventricular hypertrophy
D. left ventricular hypertrophy
E. left ventricular hypertrophy with strain

Question 7: What is the electrocardiographic diagnosis in this 10-year-old (Fig. 8-16)?

A. right atrial enlargement
B. left atrial enlargement
C. both
D. neither

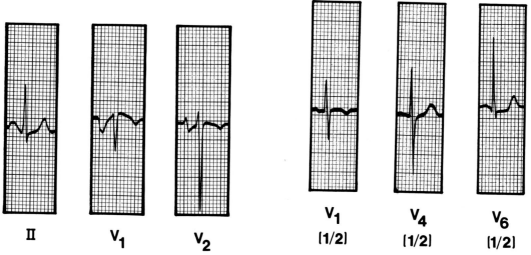

FIG. 8-16. Question 7.

FIG. 8-17. Question 8.

Question 8: What is the electrocardiographic diagnosis in this 11-year-old (Fig. 8-17)?

A. right ventricular hypertrophy
B. right ventricular hypertrophy with strain
C. biventricular hypertrophy
D. left ventricular hypertrophy
E. left ventricular hypertrophy with strain

Question 9: What is the electrocardiographic diagnosis in this 1-day-old (Fig. 8-18)?

A. right ventricular hypertrophy
B. right ventricular hypertrophy with strain

C. biventricular hypertrophy
D. left ventricular hypertrophy
E. left ventricular hypertrophy with strain.

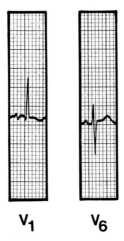

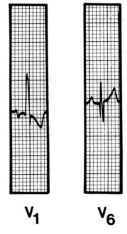

FIG. 8-18.   Question 9.   FIG. 8-19.   Question 10.

Question 10: What is the electrocardiographic diagnosis in this 4-month-old (Fig. 8-19)?

A. right ventricular hypertrophy
B. right ventricular hypertrophy with strain
C. biventricular hypertrophy
D. left ventricular hypertrophy
E. left ventricular hypertrophy with strain

Answers to Self-Assessment Questions

Answer 1: B
An upright T wave in lead V_1 (not V_2) after one week of age is indicative of right ventricular hypertrophy.

Answer 2: C
Deep Q waves are generally associated with left ventricular dilation and absent Q waves with concentric left ventricular hypertrophy. These are considered supportive evidence and weaker criteria than either the T wave changes of left ventricular "strain" or voltage criteria.

Answer 3: A
The P wave in lead II is taller than 2.5 mm. There is also an *early* negative component which is compatible with right atrial enlargement. There is no late negative component which would be indicative of left atrial enlargement.

Answer 4: E

This could be mistaken for right ventricular hypertrophy on the basis of the upright T wave in lead V_1. This is a reciprocal T wave change from the primary T wave change of left ventricular hypertrophy with strain. The voltage in lead V_6 exceeds the 98th percentile from Table A-9 (see Appendix) for this age (25 mm) thus R wave voltage criteria for diagnosis of left ventricular hypertrophy.

Answer 5: A

The upright T wave in lead V_1 is a primary change (note the T wave is positive in lead V_6) due to right ventricular hypertrophy. In addition, the R' wave voltage in lead V_1 exceeds 15 mm.

Answer 6: C

There is prominent midprecordial voltage with the total voltage (R + S) in lead V_4 exceeding the 98th percentile for age (51.2 mm) in Table A-14 (see Appendix). V_1 and V_6 are normal.

Answer 7: B

The P wave is .14 sec in duration. This is abnormally long for a 10-year-old (over .10 sec). There is also an abnormal terminal negative deflection. In V_2, the negative deflection begins later in the P wave, lasts at least .04 sec, and is more than 1 mm deep. All this indicates left atrial enlargement.

Answer 8: C

There is clear evidence for left ventricular hypertrophy in that the R wave in lead V_6 exceeds the 98th percentile for age (33 mm) (Table A-9, Appendix). In addition, the R wave in lead V_1 exceeds the *mean* for age (15.4 mm) (Table A-7, Appendix); in addition, there is right ventricular hypertrophy.

Answer 9: A

The height of the R wave in lead V_1 by itself is insufficient for the diagnosis of right ventricular hypertrophy but there is a small Q wave preceding the R wave indicating right ventricular hypertrophy in a newborn.

Answer 10: A

There is a QR pattern which indicates right ventricular hypertrophy. Although there is a deep Q wave in V_6, this *not* sufficient evidence for additional left ventricular hypertrophy.

References

1. Ellison R. C., Freedom R. M., Keane J. F., et al.: Indirect assessment of severity in pulmonary stenosis. Circulation *56*:15–20, 1977.
2. Wagner H. R., Weidman W. H., Ellison R. C., et al.: Indirect assessment of severity in aortic stenosis. Circulation *56*:20–23, 1977.

3. Liebman J., and Plonsey R.: Electrocardiography. *In* Heart Disease in Infants, Children and Adolescents. Edited by A. J. Moss, F. H. Adams, and C. G.. Emmanouilides. Baltimore, Williams & Wilkins, 1977, pp 18–61.

4. Cayler G. G., Ongley P., and Nadas A. S.: Relation of systolic pressure in the right ventricle to the electrocardiogram. N Engl J Med *258:*979–982, 1958.

5. Cooksey J. D., Dunn M., and Massie E.: Clinical Vectorcardiography and Electrocardiography. 2nd Ed. Chicago, Yearbook Medical Publishers, 1977, pp 9–112.

6. Burch G. E., and DePasquale N. P.: Electrocardiography in the Diagnosis of Congenital Heart Disease. Philadelphia, Lea & Febiger, 1967, pp 30–105.

7. Chou T.: Electrocardiography in Clinical Practice. New York, Grune & Stratton, 1979, pp 114–150.

8. Okuni M.: A proposal of new pediatric electrocardiographic criteria for ventricular hypertrophy. Jpn Heart J *23:*189–195, 1975.

9. Gerard R., Lasry F., Seichter J., et al.: Les critères éléctrocardiographiques de surcharge ventriculaire droite chez l'enfant. I. Les surcharges systoliques. Arch Mal Coeur *62:*1049–1071, 1969.

10. Morganroth J. Maron B. J., and Krovetz L. J.: Electrocardiographic evidence of left ventricular hypertrophy in otherwise normal children: clarification by echocardiography. Am J Cardiol *35:*278–281, 1975.

11. Cabrera C. E., and Monroy J. R.: Systolic and diastolic loading of the heart. II. Electrocardiographic data. Am Heart J *43:*669–680, 1952.

12. Katz L. N., and Wachtel H.: The diphasic QRS type of electrocardiogram in congenital heart disease. Am Heart J *13:*202–206, 1937.

13. Reynolds J. L.: The electrocardiographic recognition of right atrial abnormality in children. Am Heart J *81:*748–759, 1971.

14. Reeves W. C., Hallahan W., Schwiter E. J., et al.: Two dimensional echocardiographic assessment of electrocardiographic criteria for right atrial enlargement. Circulation *64:*387–391, 1981.

15. Morris J. J. Jr., Estes E. H. Jr., and Whalen R. E.: P wave analysis in valvular heart disease. Circulation *29:*242, 1964.

16. Sanyal S. K., Vijayalaxmi B., Sharma S., et al.: Evaluation of terminal P-V_1 index in assessment of left atrial enlargement in childhood. Indian J Med Res *61:*1868, 1973.

17. Biancaniello T. M., Bisset G. S., Gaum W. E., et al.: Left atrial size in childhood. J Electrocardiol *13:*11–16, 1980.

18. Sodi-Polares D., and Calder R. M.: New Bases of Electrocardiography. St. Louis, C. V. Mosby Co., 1956, pp 23–28.

9

Interventricular Conduction Disturbance

Conduction through the ventricles can be disturbed either by delay or by preexcitation, resulting in an abnormal sequence of ventricular activation.

Conduction Delay

RIGHT BUNDLE BRANCH BLOCK

Right bundle branch block results from delay in right ventricular activation. There is sequential activation of the right ventricle after the left ventricle, rather than simultaneous activation. The conduction delay can occur in the distal His bundle in fibers destined for the right bundle branch, or it can occur in the main portion of the right bundle branch (both are considered "central" lesions). Alternatively, the delay may be localized to the peripheral ramifications of the right bundle branch (a "distal" lesion). Regardless of the site of origin, the pattern is the same on the surface electrocardiogram: delayed, slurred activation oriented anteriorly and rightward.[1,2]

Complete Right Bundle Branch Block

The pattern of the QRS is most important for the diagnosis of complete right bundle branch block. There is an initial rapid deflection, followed by a slurred, slower terminal deflection. In lead V_1, the rapid component consists of an R wave and an S wave of varying magnitudes followed by a slurred tall R wave. There may be no S wave, resulting in an RR' complex (Fig. 9-1). In leads I and V_6, the late slurred terminal deflection causes a broad S wave. The rapid part of the complex results from normal left ventricular activation and is not changed by right ventricular surgery (Fig. 9-2).

The QRS complex in complete right bundle branch block can be divided into the following four separate time periods. (1) The .01 sec

119

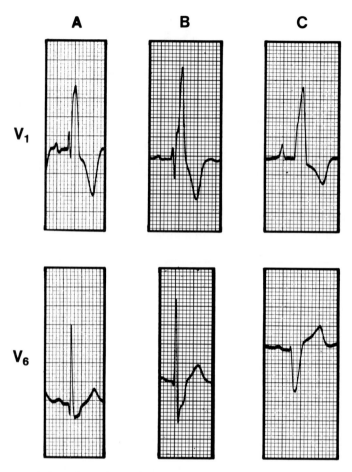

FIG. 9-1. Variations of complete right bundle branch block. A, Large R wave and small S wave. B, Small R wave and deeper S wave. C, R wave without an S wave. In lead V_1, the latter part of all three complexes has a slurred component which is the R' wave. All three tracings have broad terminal S waves in lead V_6.

septal vector (Fig. 9-3A). This is the same as the vector occurring with normal conduction and is oriented to the right, anteriorly, and superiorly. This results in an R wave in V_1 and possibly a small Q wave in leads I and V_6. When a Q wave appears in lead I preceding the RSR', it has the same significance as in the patient without complete right bundle branch block. (2) The .02 sec apicoanterior vector (Fig. 9-3B). This is directed to the left, anteriorly, and inferiorly causing an R wave in leads I and V_6, and this marks the termination of the small R wave in lead V_1. (3) The .03 and .04 sec left ventricular vector (Figs. 9-3C and D). This is the maximum leftward vector in complete right bundle branch block and is directed leftward, posteriorly, and inferiorly causing the completion of the R wave in leads I and V_6 and the end of the S wave in V_1. Thus far, the QRS complex could be similar to that found in the same patient without complete right bundle branch block. The dominant left ventricular forces and activation are identical in the patient with and without complete right bundle branch block, so the major

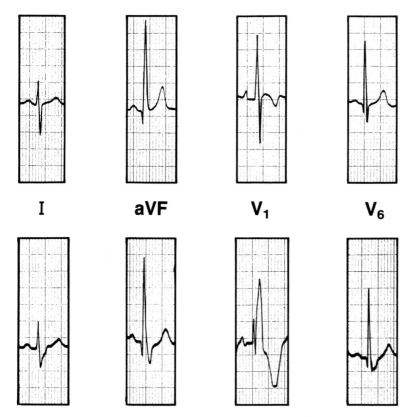

I   **aVF**   **V₁**   **V₆**

FIG. 9-2. Preoperative-postoperative comparison. **Top** tracings, The preoperative electrocardiogram of a patient with tetralogy of Fallot. There is right ventricular hypertrophy. **Bottom** tracings, Electrocardiogram from the same patient taken postoperatively;
there is complete right bundle branch block. The first .04 sec are the same in the preoperative and postoperative tracings in each lead.

forces of the QRS are similar. Because in normal conduction the anterior right ventricle is activated in the .02 or .04 sec vector, the *lack* of
right ventricular activation may contribute to minor changes in the
early part of the QRS in complete right bundle branch block, but these
are not usually observed. (4) The .05 to .12 sec terminal vector (Fig.
9-3E). The major difference from normal and complete right bundle
branch block is the late, relatively unopposed activation of the right
ventricle which spreads slowly across the septum and right ventricle
from the left ventricle resulting in a vector directed anteriorly, rightward, and horizontally. Thus the terminal vector results in a wide R′ in
V_1 and a broad terminal S wave in leads I and V_6.[3]

This pattern can be quantified so that the mean duration of the
"fast" component (RS of the RSR′) is 0.038 sec in adults and the time
from the end of the fast component to the peak of the R′ is 0.061 sec.
Essentially, in lead V_1 the R′ is twice the width of the RS, or in lead V_6
the S wave is twice the width of the R wave. This pattern of discrep-
ancy between the initial and terminal components is a more reliable
sign of complete right bundle branch block than the exact duration of
the total QRS complex, especially since 0.01 sec or even 0.02 sec may

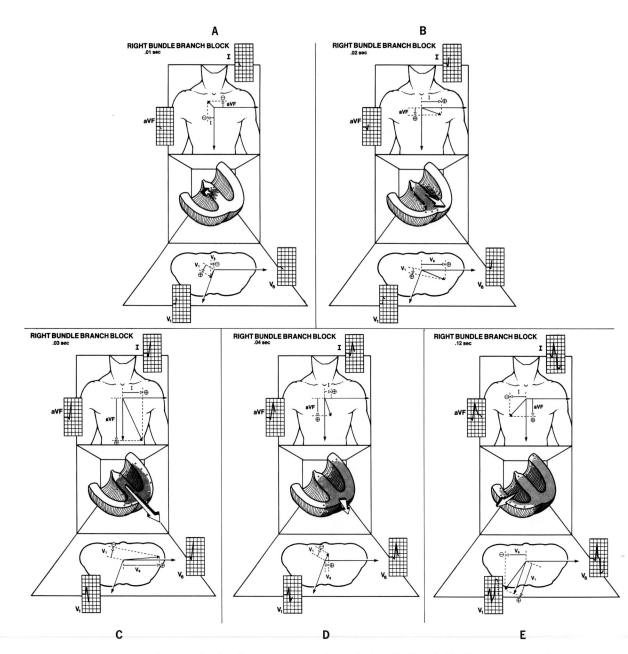

FIG. 9-3. Vectors of ventricular depolarization in complete right bundle branch block. **A**, .01 sec septal vector. **B**, .02 sec apicoanterior vector. **C**, .03 sec left ventricular lateral vector. **D**, .04 sec left ventricular posterior vector. **E**, .05 to .12 sec terminal vector. Further explanation of these figures is provided in Figures 4-1 and 4-4.

be difficult to measure accurately. The criteria for complete right bundle branch block are: (1) QRS duration prolonged for age: greater than .09 sec up to the age of 4 years and greater than .10 sec for 4 years to 16 years, (2) normal initial forces (first 0.04 sec), and (3) terminal conduction delay directed anteriorly and to the right.

The mean vector (or "axis") in complete right bundle branch block considers the frontal plane QRS axis calculated based upon the "fast" initial portion of the complex. Generally this is the first .04 msec; however, the initial rapid portion before the "break" to the terminal slow portion should be used, regardless of the specific timing (Fig. 9-4). If

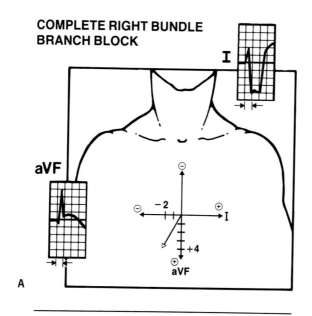

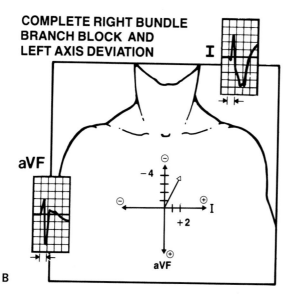

FIG. 9-4. Mean vector in right bundle branch block. The amplitude method has been applied to the first .04 sec (see Fig. 5-3). A, The frontal plane mean vector of the first .04 sec is +120°. Depending upon the age, this is designated either "complete right bundle branch block" or "complete right bundle branch block with right axis deviation." B, The mean frontal plane QRS vector of the first .04 sec is −60°. This is designated "complete right bundle branch block with left axis deviation."

the frontal plane axis of the initial "unblocked" portion is between -30 and $-90°$, this is considered to be left axis deviation in addition to complete right bundle branch block. This distinction is important in the diagnosis of bifascicular block and will be further discussed in that section of this chapter.

Attempts have been made to use the mean vector, as well as the absolute height and proportions of the R, S, and R' components, to diagnose hypertrophy in the presence of complete right bundle branch block. The correlation of these parameters with the ventricular pressure or free wall thickness is insufficient to permit the diagnosis of either right ventricular or left ventricular hypertrophy in the presence of complete right bundle branch block.[4,5]

The T wave changes in complete right bundle branch block are secondary to the abnormal sequence of depolarization. The T waves are opposite in direction to the QRS complexes. In right bundle branch block, ventricular repolarization proceeds in the same direction as depolarization. Opposite electrical processes occurring in the same direction result in discordant QRS and T waves. The major uncancelled voltage of the QRS consists of the terminal R', which is directed anteriorly and to the right. The T waves in complete right bundle branch block are therefore directed posteriorly and to the left. Since normal left ventricular repolarization is occurring at the same time as depolarization and repolarization of the right ventricle, there is an ST segment shift caused by the T wave of the left ventricle. Therefore, in complete right bundle branch block in lead V_1, there is a positive R' with a negative T wave and depressed ST segment. In lead V_6, there is a deep S wave with an elevated ST segment and a positive T wave.

ETIOLOGY OF COMPLETE RIGHT BUNDLE BRANCH BLOCK. The most common cause of complete right bundle branch block is surgery involving closure of a ventricular septal defect or right ventriculotomy.[2] In approximately half of the patients with right bundle branch block operated upon for repair of tetralogy of Fallot, the complete right bundle branch block is "central" due to injury occurring during closure of the ventricular septal defect and in the other half, it is "peripheral," occurring during ventriculotomy.[6] Congenital complete right bundle branch block is rare in children, but may occur with autosomal dominant inheritance. Isolated congenital complete right bundle branch block does not appear to progress to further conduction disturbances.[7,8] Complete right bundle branch block may also be a manifestation of inflammation from myocarditis or endocarditis and may progress to complete AV block.[1] In normal children, functional right bundle branch block or left bundle branch block may occur due to ventricular aberration of a supraventricular rhythm. However, rate-dependent bundle branch block is extremely rare in children and occurred in only 2% of children reported with supraventricular tachycardia.[9]

*"Incomplete Right Bundle
Branch Block" Pattern*

The RSR' pattern in lead V_1, in which the duration of the R' is approximately equal to the duration of the RS wave (i.e., no terminal conduction delay), has been referred to as the "incomplete right bundle branch block" pattern (Fig. 9-5). The duration of the QRS may be normal or slightly prolonged for age (up to .09 sec under the age of 4 years or .10 sec from 4 to 16 years). Approximately 7% of normal children over the age of 6 months have this pattern.[10] The only major pathologic cause of an incomplete right bundle branch block pattern in childhood is right ventricular diastolic volume overload, and this is found in 93% of children with a secundum atrial septal defect. In children with atrial septal defect, it has been demonstrated that the central right bundle conduction time is normal, which therefore implies that the pattern is due to more peripheral factors.[11] This pattern of terminal activation directed anteriorly and rightward is currently explained either by selective hypertrophy of the right ventricular outflow tract or by stretching of the peripheral specialized conduction fibers due to distention of the right ventricular outflow tract.[12] Numerous attempts have been made to distinguish normal children from those with atrial septal defect and among those with atrial septal defect to predict the size of the shunt or right ventricular pressure. These attempts have been unsuccessful with a few general exceptions. In children with an atrial septal defect, the R' tends to be slightly wider than in normal children; in those with an atrial septal defect with a small shunt, there is a deep S wave compared to those with larger shunts or high pulmonary pressure in whom both the R and R' waves

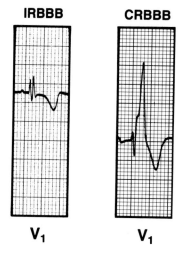

IRBBB　　**CRBBB**

V_1　　　V_1

FIG. 9-5. Distinction of "incomplete" from "complete" right bundle branch block. Left, Normal duration RSR' complex. There is no "break." The duration of the R wave and R' wave is almost the same. This is the "incomplete right bundle branch block pattern." Right, In the "complete right bundle branch block pattern," there is a definite break and the R' is three times the duration of the R wave.

become taller and the S wave disappears. Specifically, atrial septal defect was more common in those younger than 1 year of age if the R′ was greater than 15 mm and in those older than 1 year if the R′ was greater than 10 mm.[13,14] Despite these generalities, it may be impossible to distinguish normal from atrial septal defect by the electrocardiogram in an individual patient.[15]

LEFT BUNDLE
BRANCH BLOCK

Complete Left Bundle
Branch Block

Complete left bundle branch block results from delay in left ventricular activation. Since fibers of the left bundle branch initiate normal ventricular depolarization, if there is delay in left bundle branch conduction, the entire QRS is aberrant. This is different from the situation in right bundle branch block in which only the terminal portion is aberrant. In left bundle branch block, the right ventricle is activated first; therefore, the normal initial vector, due to left to right septal spread, is absent. The slow activation of the left ventricle occurs from the right ventricle and the resultant slurred QRS is directed to the left, posteriorly, and superiorly. The criteria for complete left bundle branch block are: (1) Abnormally wide QRS complex (greater than .09 sec in a child less than 4 years of age, or greater than .10 sec from 4 to 16 years), (2) absent normal initial forces (absent Q wave in leads I, aV_L, and V_6), and (3) notched, slurred QRS complexes directed leftward and posterior: in lead V_1 a QS or small R-deep S, and in lead V_6 a tall, notched R wave (Fig. 9-6).

The QRS complex in complete left bundle branch block can be divided into four time periods. (1) The .01 sec right ventricular vector (Fig. 9-7A). The first part of the heart activated is the right anterior papillary muscle by way of the right bundle branch. Activation proceeds anteriorly to the free wall and posteriorly to the septum. In less than half of patients with complete left bundle branch block, the anterior vector is expressed on the surface electrocardiogram as a small initial R wave in V_1. In the majority, the larger posterior spread into the septum predominates with a leftward and inferior vector cancelling out the anterior vector. In this case, a QS is inscribed in lead V_1 and a notched R wave in leads I and V_6. (2) The .02-.06 sec septal vector (Fig. 9-7B). Spread occurs through the septum from right to left and apex to base, giving a vector oriented leftward, inferiorly, and posteriorly. This causes the major downstroke of the QS in V_1 and the major initial upstroke in leads I and V_6. (3) The .07-.09 sec left ventricular vector (Fig. 9-7C). This is the maximum vector and is directed to the left, posteriorly, and either superiorly or inferiorly. It causes the second notch on the R wave in leads I and V_6 and the nadir of the S wave in lead V_1. (4) The .10-.12 sec terminal vector (Fig. 9-7D). The part of the left ventricle that is most distant from the septum and therefore activated last is

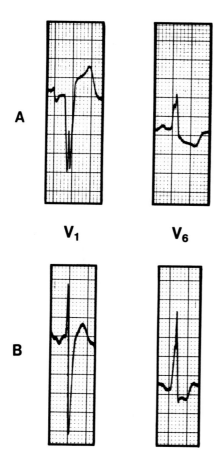

FIG. 9-6. Variations of complete left bundle branch block. A, QS pattern in lead V_1. B, RS pattern in lead V_1. In lead V_6, both tracings are similar and marked by the absence of a Q wave.

the anterolateral left ventricle. In leads I and V_6, this causes the downstroke of the R wave and in V_1, the terminal limb of the S wave. The T waves in complete left bundle branch block are approximately 180° discordant from the QRS for the same reasons as in complete right bundle branch block.

The frontal plane QRS mean vector in complete left bundle branch block is calculated based upon the major deflection of the QRS (Fig. 9-8). If the initial and terminal parts have different vectors, the terminal part of the QRS should be used. Adults with left bundle branch block and left axis deviation are more likely to develop complete AV block than those without left axis deviation.[16] These data are not available for children.

ETIOLOGY OF COMPLETE LEFT BUNDLE BRANCH BLOCK. Left bundle branch block is rare in children. The most common cause is surgery on the aortic valve or subvalve area. It may occur as a result of myocarditis, endocarditis, hypertrophic cardiomyopathy, or myocardial infarction.[1]

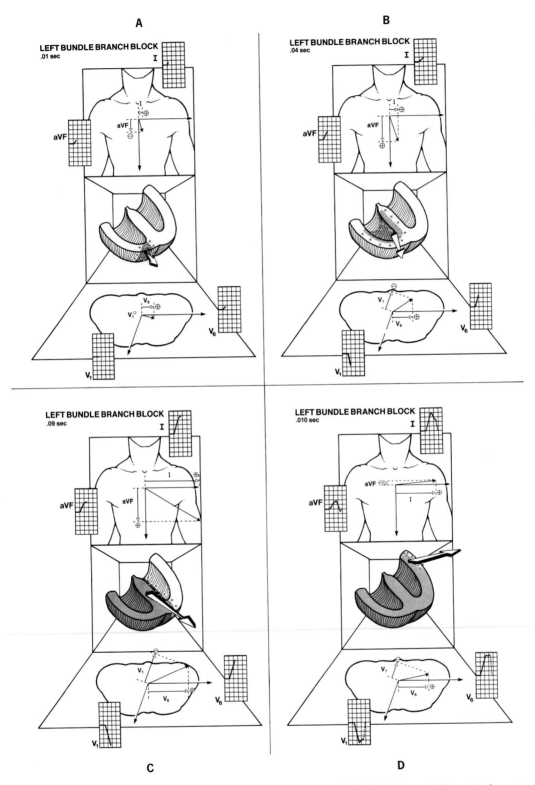

FIG. 9-7. Vectors of ventricular activation in complete left bundle branch block. A, .01 sec right ventricular vector. B, .02 to .06 sec septal vector. C, .07 to .09 sec left ventricular vector. D, .10 to .12 sec terminal vector.

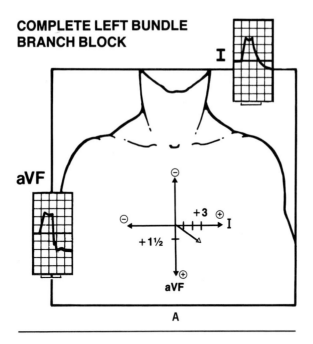

A

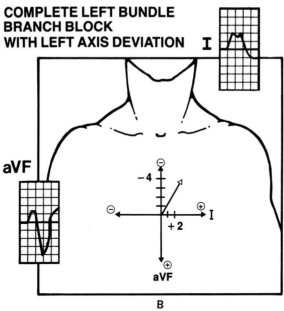

B

FIG. 9-8. Calculation of mean vector in left bundle branch block. The entire QRS complex is used for the calculation, and the amplitude method (Fig. 5-3) was used in this case. A, Frontal plane mean QRS vector +30°. This is designated "complete left bundle branch block." B, Frontal plane QRS mean vector −60°. This is designated "complete left bundle branch block with left axis deviation."

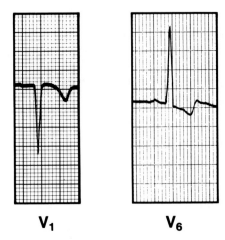

V_1 V_6

FIG. 9-9. "Incomplete left bundle branch block pattern" in an 11-year-old. There is an absent Q wave in lead V_6, a normal QRS duration, and no R wave in lead V_1.

*"Incomplete Left Bundle
Branch Block" Pattern*

Left ventricular hypertrophy may cause delayed left ventricular activation or stretching of the Purkinje fibers and produce a pattern of "incomplete left bundle branch block." The QRS duration may be normal or prolonged by 0.01 sec for age. There are absent Q waves and tall slurred R waves in leads I and V_6 (Fig. 9-9). On surface electrocardiogram, it is not possible to distinguish patients with incomplete left bundle branch block on the basis of left ventricular hypertrophy from those with mild conduction system disease.

FASCICULAR
BLOCK

Although the anatomic correlation is not exact, there are patterns on the surface electrocardiogram that correspond to lesions in the anterior and posterior fascicles of the left bundle branch and these patterns are called left anterior hemiblock and left posterior hemiblock, respectively.

*Left Anterior
Hemiblock*

The pattern of left anterior hemiblock results from asynchronous left ventricular activation in which the posterior-inferior wall is activated before the anterior-superior wall and there are two sequential vectors. The "earlier" activation of the posterior-inferior diaphragmatic surface of the left ventricle is directed inferiorly and slightly to the right at $+120°$ in the frontal plane. The "later" activation occurs in the opposite direction when the anterior-superior wall is activated at $-60°$ in the frontal plane (Fig. 9-10A). The QRS duration is prolonged by less than 0.02 sec in pure left anterior hemiblock because part of the left ventricle is activated normally and spread to the rest of the left ventricle occurs relatively rapidly through the endocardium. The criteria for left anterior hemiblock are the following. (1) Initial forces directed inferiorly and slightly to the right at $+120°$. (2) Major QRS forces directed superiorly and leftward. Left axis deviation resulting from a horizontal heart position may give a QRS axis of $-30°$; therefore, for the diagnosis of left anterior hemiblock, the frontal plane QRS axis must be to the left of $-30°$ (i.e., negative in lead II). In most children with left anterior hemiblock, the QRS axis is $-60°$. (3) Normal or minimally prolonged QRS duration (Fig. 9-11A).

The QRS complex in left anterior hemiblock can be divided into four major time periods. (1) The .01 sec septal vector. Septal activation probably occurs normally and is directed anteriorly and to the right, resulting in an initial Q wave in leads I and V_6. (2) The .02 sec posterior-inferior left ventricular vector. The abnormal unopposed activation of the posterior-inferior left ventricle by way of the left posterior fascicle causes forces that are directed to the right, posteriorly, and inferiorly and overshadow the normal septal and early right ventricular forces. These forces result in a Q wave in lead aV_L and may contribute to the Q wave in leads I and V_6. (3) The .04 sec left ventricular vector. This is directed leftward and superiorly and results from left ventricular endocardial to epicardial spread. (4) The .06 sec anterolateral left ventricular vector. The unopposed terminal activation of the anterolateral wall (served by the left anterior fascicle) causes the terminal superior leftward vector with tall R waves in aV_L and deep S waves in leads V_5 and V_6. The T waves in left anterior hemiblock are normal.

ETIOLOGY OF LEFT ANTERIOR HEMIBLOCK. In children, the most common cause of the left anterior hemiblock pattern is that found in association with congenital heart disease. This may be due either to elongation of the left anterior fibers, or to shortening of the left posterior fibers, or to a different orientation of the conduction system causing the posterior left ventricular wall to be activated before other parts of the heart.[17] These mechanisms may explain the left axis deviation found in endocardial cushion defects (including ostium primum atrial septal defect, AV canal, and single atrium), single ventricle, and double outlet right ventricle. Recent observations on tricuspid atresia suggest a different mechanism.[18] The activation times of the proximal left anterior and posterior fascicles were found to be normal and it has been postulated that in tricuspid atresia, selective hypertrophy of the basal anterolateral left ventricle is responsible for sufficient conduction delay to cause the pattern of left anterior hemiblock on the surface electrocardiogram.[19] In anomalous left coronary artery, the left axis deviation frequently observed may also be due to selective hypertrophy of noninfarcted superior portions of the left ventricle. This mechanism may also account for the occasional left axis deviation found in aortic stenosis, aortic insufficiency, or cardiomyopathy. Isolated injury

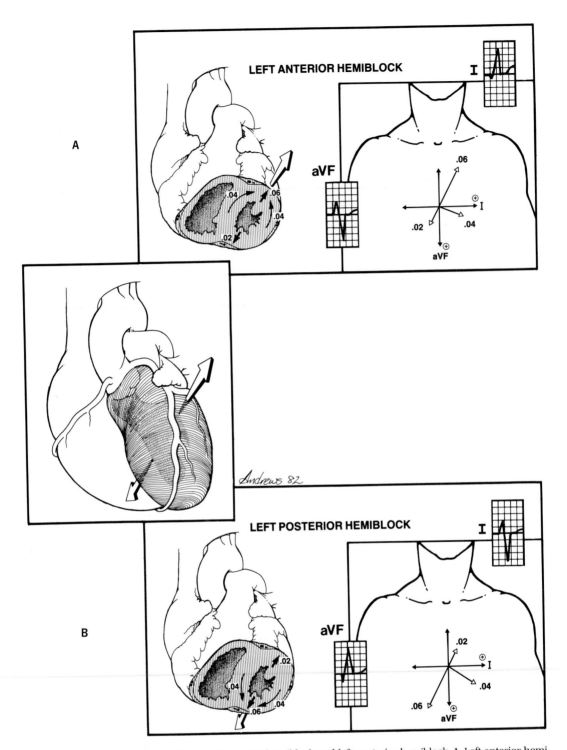

FIG. 9-10. Comparison of activation in left anterior hemiblock and left posterior hemiblock. A, Left anterior hemiblock. The initial .02 sec vector is directed at +120°, and the terminal .06 sec vector is directed at −60°. This causes an initial Q wave in lead I and a deep S wave in lead aV$_F$. A coronal section through the heart is shown with the posterior-inferior wall activated before the anterior-superior wall. The mean QRS vector is directed superiorly, as shown by the large arrow in the top diagram. B, Left posterior hemiblock. The initial .02 sec vector is directed at −60°, and the terminal .06 sec vector is directed at +120°. This causes a Q wave in lead aV$_F$ and a deep S wave in lead I. The anterior-superior wall is activated before the posterior-inferior wall. The mean QRS vector in the frontal plane is directed at +120°, as shown by the large arrow in the bottom diagram. The orientation of the posterior-inferior and anterior-superior walls is shown in the middle diagram.

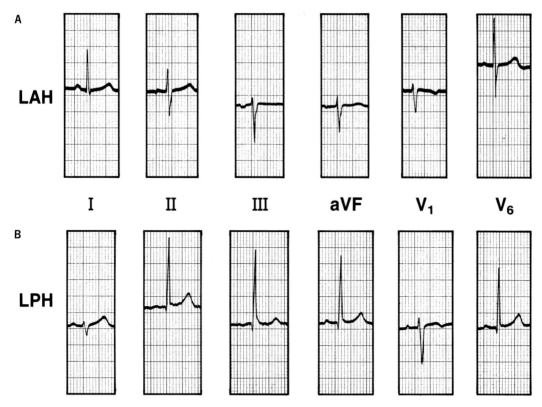

FIG. 9-11. Comparison of the electrocardiograms of left anterior hemiblock and left posterior hemiblock. **Top** tracings, Left anterior hemiblock. **Bottom** tracings, Left posterior hemiblock. Note the absence of right ventricular hypertrophy in this 15-year-old child with left posterior hemiblock.

to the left anterior fascicle resulting in left anterior hemiblock from myocarditis has been postulated as the cause of the left axis deviation observed in up to 50% of infants with the rubella syndrome. Left anterior hemiblock may also result from myocardial infarction, ventricular septal myectomy, aortic valve surgery, or subvalve aortic resection. Usually in closure of a ventricular septal defect, the left anterior hemiblock is accompanied by right bundle branch block (see the section on bifascicular block in this chapter). Left anterior hemiblock may rarely be familial and occur in otherwise normal children.[7]

Left Posterior
Hemiblock

The activation sequence in left posterior hemiblock is exactly the opposite to that found in left anterior hemiblock (Fig. 9-10B). The anterior-superior wall is activated first with a frontal plane QRS axis of $-60°$ and then the posterior-inferior wall is activated last with a frontal plane QRS axis of $+120°$. The criteria for left posterior hemiblock follow: (1) Initial forces directed superiorly (Q waves in leads II, III, aV$_F$), (2) major frontal plane QRS forces directed inferiorly and rightward with an axis of +90 to +180°, and (3) normal or minimally prolonged QRS duration (Fig. 9-11B). This constitutes a normal electrocardiogram in most children, so left posterior hemiblock is difficult to diagnose. Left posterior hemiblock can be diagnosed if the frontal plane QRS axis is between +120 and 180° in a child over the age of 1 year who does not have right ventricular hypertrophy or right atrial enlargement (i.e., another reason for right axis deviation). Left posterior hemiblock is quite rare in children and has been diagnosed mainly in cases due to surgical trauma, myocarditis, or endocarditis.[20]

BIFASCICULAR BLOCK

If the conduction system is considered as trifascicular and therefore comprised of the left anterior fascicle, left posterior fascicle, and right bundle branch, then bifascicular block is defined as block in any two of the three fascicles. In the strict sense of the term, complete left bundle branch block is a form of bifascicular block. The combination of right bundle branch and left posterior hemiblock is practically never diagnosed in children because the right bundle branch block is most often due to an operation on a lesion with preexistent right ventricular hypertrophy and right axis deviation. Therefore, in children, the term bifascicular block is almost synonymous with right bundle branch block plus left anterior hemiblock.

Right Bundle Branch Block-
Left Anterior Hemiblock Pattern

Left anterior hemiblock changes the first "fast" part of the QRS complex and right bundle branch block changes the terminal "slow" part. The criteria are the following. (1) Initial forces (first 0.02 sec) directed inferiorly and rightward at +120° in the frontal plane giving a Q wave in lead aV_L and possibly lead I. (2) Major axis of the "unblocked" initial part of the QRS to the left of −30° giving a dominant S wave in the initial part of lead II and possibly leads V_5 and V_6. (3) Slurred terminal portion of right bundle branch block directed to the right (Fig. 9-12).

ETIOLOGY OF RIGHT BUNDLE BRANCH BLOCK-LEFT ANTERIOR HEMIBLOCK PATTERN. The most common cause of right bundle branch block and left anterior hemiblock in children is surgery for tetralogy of Fallot and occurs in approximately 10% of such patients.[21] This pattern may also occur in any injury to the area of the distal His bundle or proximal right bundle branch since the right bundle branch and left anterior fascicle lie in such close proximity. This pattern may also be seen following other intracardiac operations involving surgery near the AV junction, or it may be found in myocarditis, cardiomyopathy, and endocarditis. Familial bifascicular block occurs and may progress to complete AV block.[22]

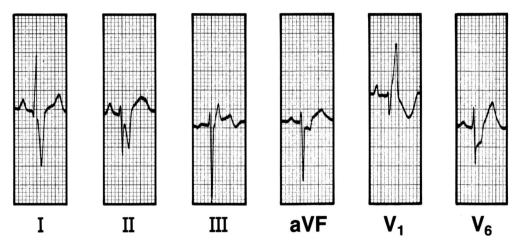

FIG. 9-12. Right bundle branch block with left axis deviation.

TRIFASCICULAR BLOCK

Trifascicular block is defined as delay in all three fascicles. It can only be diagnosed by intracardiac electrograms as a prolonged H-V interval and cannot be diagnosed on the surface electrocardiogram. The combination of right bundle branch block, left anterior hemiblock, and first-degree AV block has been erroneously termed trifascicular block. This combination has many different possible causes. Most children with this pattern have AV nodal delay and bifascicular block with a normal H-V interval.[23,24]

DIFFUSE INTERVENTRICULAR CONDUCTION DELAY

The QRS complex is prolonged for age but without a specific pattern of right bundle branch block or left bundle branch block. This may be found in children with quinidine or procainamide toxicity, myocarditis, hypoglycemia, myocardial ischemia, or hyperkalemia (Fig. 9-13).[25]

Preexcitation

Preexcitation is defined as an abnormally rapid transit of the wave of depolarization from atria to ventricles. In most cases of preexcitation, the ventricles are activated asymmetrically from a point other than the bundle of His, in addition to being activated via the normal conduction system. Since AV conduction can occur by two possible pathways, usually with different properties, one of the possible consequences of preexcitation is reciprocating supraventricular tachycardia.

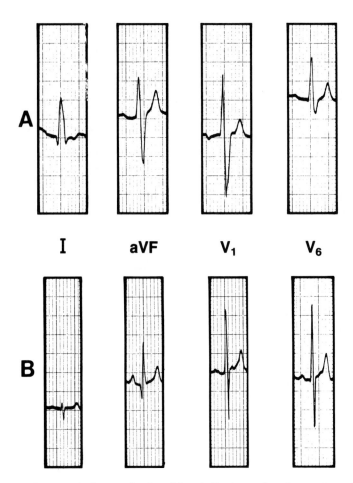

FIG. 9-13.   Interventricular conduction delay. A, Tracings taken from a 1-month-old child with renal failure who was hyperkalemic. B, Tracings taken from the same child after dialysis. The QRS complexes are similar in comparing the same leads, but they have a prolonged duration in the top tracings.

WOLFF-PARKINSON-WHITE

Wolff, Parkinson, and White first described the syndrome of short PR interval with a prolonged QRS duration in 1930.[26] It has since been demonstrated that the cause of this pattern is a direct muscular connection between the atria and the ventricles: "a Kent bundle" or "accessory atrioventricular connection." The accessory connection runs perpendicular to the AV ring and can be located anywhere around either valve orifice except the point of fibrous continuity between the mitral and aortic valves. Most Kent bundles conduct much faster than the AV node, so the atrial depolarization is transmitted to the ventricles prematurely resulting in a short PR interval. The ventricles then begin to depolarize from the point of insertion of the accessory connection. If there were no AV nodal conduction and the ventricles were completely excited by the accessory connection, the QRS complex would be similar to a premature ventricular contraction that originated at the site of insertion of the accessory connection (Fig. 9-14).

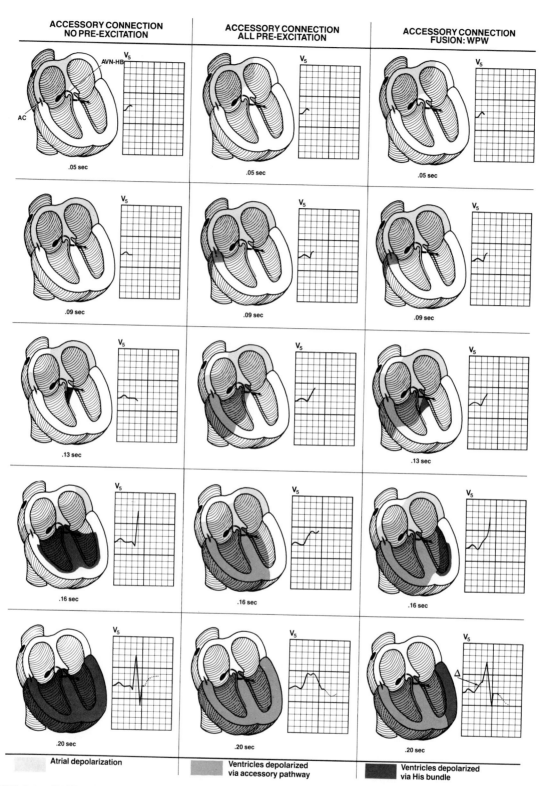

ACCESSORY CONNECTION NO PRE-EXCITATION

ACCESSORY CONNECTION ALL PRE-EXCITATION

ACCESSORY CONNECTION FUSION: WPW

FIG. 9-14. Wolff-Parkinson-White syndrome with varying degrees of conduction through the accessory connection and the AV node. The numbers refer to timing after the onset of the P wave. **Left column** of diagrams, The activation sequence in the patient with an accessory connection who is not conducting through the accessory connection but entirely through the AV node. Note the normal PR interval, the Q wave, and the lack of the delta wave. **Middle column,** The activation sequence of a patient who is conducting entirely through the accessory connection. Note the short PR interval and the wide QRS complex. There is no real "delta" wave because the entire QRS complex is wide. **Right column,** The usual situation of Wolff-Parkinson-White syndrome, in which a "fusion" complex results from conduction through both the accessory connection and the AV node. The parts of the ventricles activated through the AV node are shaded differently in the diagrams from those activated by the accessory connection. Note that there is a short PR interval and a delta wave (indicated by the "delta" at .16 sec in the right column of diagrams). The delta wave occurs because there is fusion of the completely wide QRS with the completely narrow QRS causing an abrupt change in slope. AC, accessory connection; AVN-HB, AV node-His bundle.

In most cases, the AV node *also* conducts the impulse from atria to ventricles and the depolarization wave resulting from the accessory connection and the AV node collide in the ventricles causing a "fusion" QRS complex (Fig. 9-14). The characteristics of this complex are that the beginning is more slurred (resulting from eccentric slow ventricular activation by the accessory connection) and the end of the complex is more normal (resulting from normal ventricular activation via the His bundle and bundle branches). In any individual child, the amount of the ventricles activated via the Kent bundle and the His bundle can vary from day to day, and this accounts for our observation that one third of children with Wolff-Parkinson-White had at least one electrocardiogram without any preexcitation (normal PR interval and normal QRS complex), which was later followed by the reappearance of Wolff-Parkinson-White.

The criteria for Wolff-Parkinson-White are: (1) Short PR interval for age (see Appendix, Table A-4), and (2) a QRS complex with initial slurring (the "delta wave"). All electrocardiographic leads may not show a short PR interval and delta wave if the vector of the delta wave is perpendicular to that lead (Fig. 6-6). Rosenbaum classified the Wolff-Parkinson-White pattern on surface electrocardiogram into types A and B in an attempt to predict localization of the Kent bundle.[27] In type A, the major QRS deflection is positive in lead V_1, predicting a left lateral accessory connection (Fig. 9-15A). This simulates right bundle branch block, but the two can be distinguished since the initial forces in Wolff-Parkinson-White are slow in comparison to the rapid initial forces in right bundle branch block. In type B, the major QRS deflection is negative in V_1, predicting a right-sided accessory connection (Fig. 9-15B). This simulates left bundle branch block except for the normal terminal forces indicating Wolff-Parkinson-White. Despite the general helpfulness of this classification scheme, we have not found that the exact site of the accessory connection can be predicted from the 15-lead surface electrocardiogram. Since Wolff-Parkinson-White is more common in children than left bundle branch block, the PR interval should be measured carefully in any child with a pattern similar to left bundle branch block.

LOWN-GANONG-LEVINE

Lown, Ganong, and Levine described the syndrome of short PR interval without a delta wave in sinus rhythm in 1952.[28] All their cases had associated supraventricular tachycardia. Although it does not cause interventricular conduction disturbance, we have included Lown-Ganong-Levine in this section because by our definition it results in ventricular preexcitation. The anatomic substrate for Lown-Ganong-Levine is thought to be a muscular connection between the atrium and the bundle of His, or atrio-His fiber.[29] This results in an AV nodal bypass and therefore a short PR interval is observed (Figs. 9-16 and 9-17). Since there are two possible pathways from atria to ventricles, supraventricular tachycardia may occur. The criteria for a short PR interval are age related (see Appendix, Table A-3). Lown-Ganong-

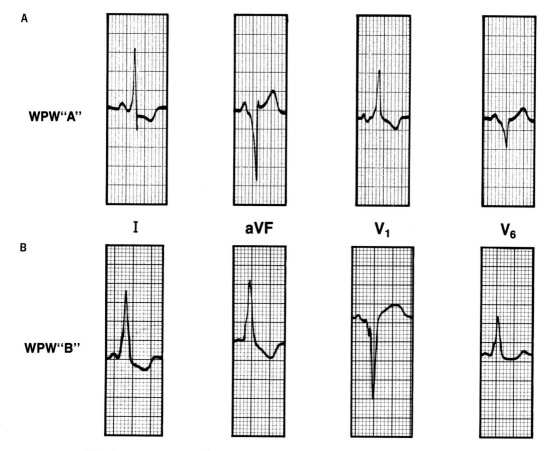

FIG. 9-15. Wolff-Parkinson-White syndrome. A, Rosenbaum "type A," and B, Rosenbaum "type B."

Levine should probably not be diagnosed in the absence of supraventricular tachycardia, since a short PR interval may be found in normal children without a predisposition to supraventricular tachycardia.[30] It is not currently possible to distinguish those with an anatomic bypass tract from those with rapid AV nodal conduction.

Short PR intervals are also observed in mannosidosis, Fabry's disease, and Pompe's disease (Fig. 9-18).[31–34] All these diseases may have in common an increase in cell size in the AV node; this may be related to rapid AV nodal conduction.[33] Since conduction is uniformly enhanced throughout the AV node and there is no bypass tract, patients with these diseases do not appear to be at risk for supraventricular tachycardia.

MAHAIM
CONDUCTION

Mahaim first described muscular connections between the His bundle and ventricular septum in 1938.[35] The definition of a Mahaim fiber has been broadened to include a fiber that originates in the AV

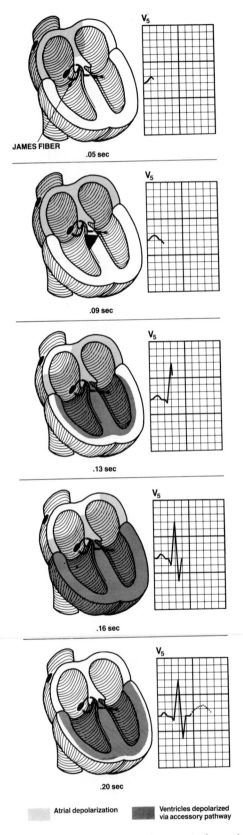

JAMES FIBER

FIG. 9-16. Lown-Ganong-Levine syndrome. The ventricular activation sequence is shown in a manner similar to Figure 9-14. The PR interval is short due to conduction through the James fiber, but the ventricular activation sequence is entirely normal.

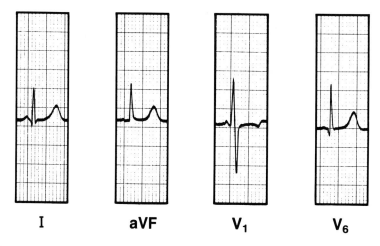

FIG. 9-17. Lown-Ganong-Levine syndrome. The PR interval is short and the QRS complex is normal in all leads.

node, His bundle, or proximal bundle branch and inserts in the ventricular muscle. This is a "bundle branch bypass" tract and results in preexcitation. Usually, the bundle inserts into the right ventricle, giving a left bundle branch block morphology to the QRS complex.[36] As conduction can also occur by way of the normal pathway (His bundle and bundle branches) and through the Mahaim fiber, there may be a fusion QRS similar to that seen in Wolff-Parkinson-White. However, with a Mahaim fiber, the PR interval is normal (Figs. 9-19 and 9-20). Since two pathways exist with different properties, reciprocating supraventricular tachycardia can occur.

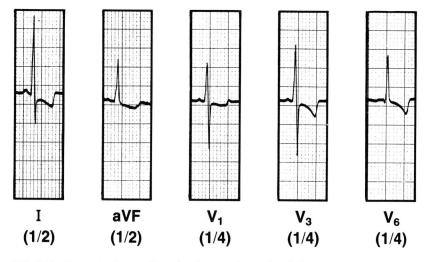

FIG. 9-18. Pompe's disease. Note the short PR interval and the extreme biventricular hypertrophy. 118 mm of deflection (at normal standardization) extend from the top of the R wave to the bottom of the S wave in lead V_3.

MAHAIM FIBER: FUSION

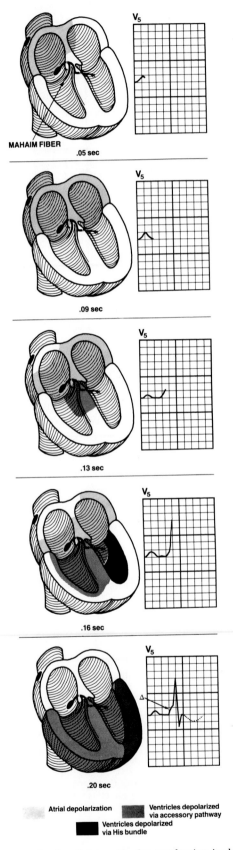

FIG. 9-19. Mahaim conduction. Interventricular conduction is shown for a Mahaim fiber. The PR interval is normal and a delta wave may result from fusion of the impulse passing through both the Mahaim fiber and the AV node.

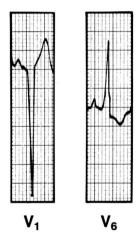

V₁   **V₆**

FIG. 9-20. Mahaim conduction. The PR interval is normal and there is a delta wave in lead V₆. The morphology of this complex is similar to left bundle branch block.

Self-Assessment
Questions

Question 1: The most important criterion for the diagnosis of complete right bundle branch block is:

A. initial rapid component followed by a delayed component directed toward the left
B. delayed initial and terminal components directed to the left
C. initial rapid component followed by a delayed component directed toward the right
D. delayed initial and terminal components directed toward the right
E. none of the above

Question 2: In left anterior hemiblock,

A. the initial forces are directed toward $+120°$ and the terminal forces toward $-60°$ causing a QR pattern in lead III
B. the initial forces are directed toward $-60°$ and the terminal forces toward $+120°$ causing a QR pattern in lead aV$_L$
C. the initial forces are directed toward $+120°$ and the terminal forces toward $-60°$ causing a QR pattern in lead aV$_L$
D. the initial forces are directed toward $-60°$ and the terminal forces toward $+120°$ causing a QR pattern in lead III

Question 3: Match the diagnosis with the electrocardiographic criteria:

_____ Wolff-Parkinson-White	A. short PR interval, normal QRS
_____ Lown-Ganong-Levine	B. short PR interval, delta wave
_____ Mahaim	C. normal PR interval, normal QRS
	D. normal PR interval, delta wave

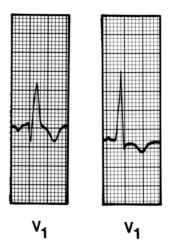

$$V_1 \qquad V_1$$

FIG. 9-21.   Question 4.

Question 4: The electrocardiographic diagnosis of the left tracing (11-year-old) is _____, and of the right tracing (12-year-old) is _____ (Fig. 9-21).

A. complete left bundle branch block, complete right bundle branch block
B. complete left bundle branch block, Wolff-Parkinson-White
C. Wolff-Parkinson-White, complete left bundle branch block
D. complete right bundle branch block, Wolff-Parkinson-White
E. Wolff-Parkinson-White, complete right bundle branch block

Question 5: What is the electrocardiographic diagnosis in this 16-year-old (Fig. 9-22)?

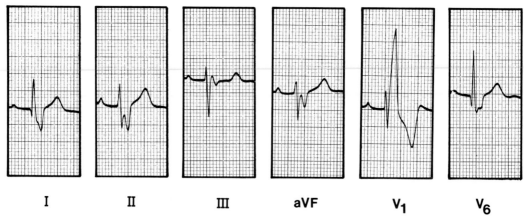

$$\text{I} \qquad \text{II} \qquad \text{III} \qquad \text{aVF} \qquad V_1 \qquad V_6$$

FIG. 9-22.   Question 5.

A. complete right bundle branch block, first-degree AV block
B. complete right bundle branch block, left axis deviation, first-degree AV block
C. trifascicular block
D. B or C

Question 6: The electrocardiographic diagnosis of the top tracings (12-year-old) is _____, and of the bottom tracings (4-year-old) is _____ (Fig. 9-23).

A. complete left bundle branch block, complete right bundle branch block
B. complete left bundle branch block, Wolff-Parkinson-White
C. Wolff-Parkinson-White, complete left bundle branch block
D. complete right bundle branch block, Wolff-Parkinson-White
E. Wolff-Parkinson-White, complete right bundle branch block

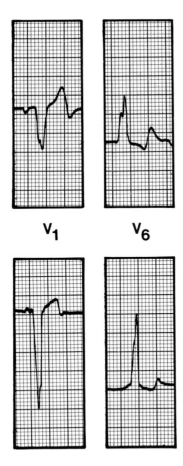

V₁   V₆

FIG. 9-23. Question 6.

Answers to Self-Assessment Questions

Answer 1: C
In complete right bundle branch block there is normal early activation of the left ventricle and then delayed activation of the right ventricle proceeding from left to right.

Answer 2: C
In left anterior hemiblock, the anterior left ventricular wall has delayed activation. Therefore initial forces are directed toward the posterior left ventricular wall at $+120°$ in the frontal plane causing a Q wave in lead aV_L; the delayed activation of the left anterior wall directed at $-60°$ causes the R wave in lead aV_L.

Answer 3:
In Wolff-Parkinson-White, there is a short PR interval because the accessory connection connects the atria and ventricles via a rapidly conducting pathway and bypasses the AV node. There is a delta wave because the ventricles are activated both via the accessory connection and the His bundle (answer B). In Lown-Ganong-Levine, there is a short PR interval because the AV node is bypassed but a normal QRS complex because the accelerated conduction pathway connects to the bundle of His and the ventricles are depolarized normally (answer A). In Mahaim conduction, there is a short PR interval because conduction is delayed normally in the AV node but a delta wave because the pathway connects the His bundle to the ventricular myocardium and bypasses the bundle branches. Some of the ventricles are also activated via the His bundle in the bundle branch system (answer D).

Answer 4: D
In Wolff-Parkinson-White, the initial part of the QRS complex is slow, whereas in complete right bundle branch block, the terminal part of the QRS complex is slow. In the tracing on the right, the PR interval is also short.

Answer 5: B
The frontal plane mean vector of the first 40 msec is $-45°$; therefore the patient has left axis deviation in addition to the complete right bundle branch block and first-degree AV block. Trifascicular block cannot be determined on the surface electrocardiogram.

Answer 6: B
In Wolff-Parkinson-White, usually the terminal part of the QRS complex is rapid, whereas in complete left bundle branch block the terminal portion is slow. The initial portion of the QRS complex in Wolff-Parkinson-White and complete left bundle branch block may be similar, but in Wolff-Parkinson-White, the PR interval is short. In children,

Wolff-Parkinson-White is so much more common that if the diagnosis of left bundle branch block is made, it is important to be sure that this is not actually Wolff-Parkinson-White.

References

1. Gumbiner C. H.: Bundle branch and fascicular block. *In* Pediatric Cardiac Dysrhythmias. Edited by P. C. Gillette and A. Garson. New York, Grune & Stratton, 1981, pp 405–419.
2. Gelband H., Waldo A. L., and Kaiser G. A.: Etiology of right bundle branch block in patients undergoing total correction of tetralogy of Fallot. Circulation 44:1022–1033, 1971.
3. Cooksey J. D., Dunn M., and Massie E.: Clinical vectorcardiography and electrocardiography. 2nd Ed. Chicago, Yearbook Medical Publishers, 1977, pp 9–112.
4. Brohet C. R., Styns M., Arraud P., et al.: Vectorcardiographic diagnosis of right ventricular hypertrophy in the presence of right bundle branch block in young subjects. Am J Cardiol 42:602–612, 1978.
5. Wasserburger R. H., Young W. P., Siebecker K., et al.: Further electrocardiographic observations on direct epicardial potentials in congenital heart lesions. Differential features of right ventricular preponderance and right bundle branch block. Circulation 26:561–573, 1962.
6. Garson A., Porter C. J., and Gillette P. C.: Ventricular tachycardia induction during electrophysiologic study after repair of tetralogy of Fallot. Circulation 64:860, 1981.
7. Husson G. S., Blackman M. S., and Rogers M. C.: Familial congenital bundle branch system disease. Am J Cardiol 32:365–369, 1973.
8. Esscher E., Hardell L., and Michaelson M.: Familial isolated complete right bundle branch block. Br Heart J 37:745–747, 1975.
9. Garson A.: Supraventricular tachycardia. *In* Pediatric Cardiac Dysrhythmias. Edited by P. C. Gillette and A. Garson. New York, Grune & Stratton, 1981, pp 177–254.
10. Burch G. E., and DePasquale N. P.: Electrocardiography in the Diagnosis of Congenital Heart Disease. Philadelphia, Lea & Febiger, 1967, pp 30–105.
11. Sung R. J., Tamer D. M., Agha A. S., et al.: Etiology of the electrocardiographic pattern of "incomplete right bundle branch block" in atrial septal defect: an electrophysiologic study. J Pediatr 87:1182–1186, 1975.
12. Boineau J. P., Spach M. S., and Ayers C. R.: Genesis of the electrocardiogram in atrial septal defect. Am Heart J 68:642, 1964.
13. Wasserburger R. H.: The Normal and Abnormal Unipolar Electrocardiogram in Infants and Children. Baltimore, Williams & Wilkins, 1963, pp 64–100.
14. Tapia F. A., and Proudfit W. L.: Secondary R waves in right precordial leads in normal persons and in patients with cardiac disease. Circulation 21:28–35, 1960.
15. Perloff J. K.: The Clinical Recognition of Congenital Heart Disease. Philadelphia, W. B. Saunders, 1970, p 237.
16. Scher A. M.: Excitation of the heart. *In* The Theoretical Basis of Electrocardiography. Edited by C. V. Nelson and D. B. Geselowitz. Oxford, Clarendon Press, 1976, pp 44–95.
17. Rosenbaum M. B., Elizari M. V., and Lazzari J. O.: The Hemiblocks. Oldsmar, Florida, Tampa Tracings, 1970, pp 30–60.
18. Boineau J. P., Moore E. N., and Patterson D. F.: Relationship between the electrocardiogram, ventricular activity and the conduction system in ostium primum atrial septal defect. Circulation 48:556–562, 1973.
19. Kulangara R. J., Boineau J. P., Moore H. V., et al.: Ventricular activation and genesis of QRS in tricuspid atresia. Circulation 64:225, 1981.
20. Schatz J., Krongrad E., and Malm J. R.: Left anterior and left posterior hemiblock in tricuspid atresia and transposition of the great arteries. Circulation 54:1010–1013, 1976.

21. Garson A., McNamara D. G., and Cooley D. A.: Postoperative tetralogy of Fallot. *In* Pediatric Cardiovascular Disease. Edited by M. A. Engle. Philadelphia, F. A. Davis, 1981, pp 407–430.

22. Schaal S. F., Seidensticker J., and Goodman R.: Familial right bundle branch block, left axis deviation, complete heart block, and early death. A heritable disorder of cardiac conduction. Ann Intern Med *79:*63–66, 1973.

23. Neches W. H., Park S. C., and Mathews R. A.: Management of surgical complete atrioventricular block in children. Am. J. Cardiol *43:*1175–1180, 1979.

24. Gillette P. C., Yeoman M. A., and Mullins C. E.: Sudden death after repair of tetralogy of Fallot: electrocardiographic and electrophysiologic abnormalities. Circulation *57:*566–577, 1977.

25. Garson A., Gillette P. C., and McNamara D. G.: A Guide to Cardiac Dysrhythmias in Children. New York, Grune & Stratton, 1980, p 10.

26. Wolff L., Parkinson J., and White P. D.: Bundle branch block with short PR interval in healthy young people prone to paroxysmal tachycardia. Am Heart J *5:*686–692, 1930.

27. Rosenbaum F. F., Hecht H. H., Wilson F. N., et al.: The potential variations of the thorax and esophagus in anomalous atrioventricular excitation (WPW syndrome). Am Heart J *29:*281–300, 1945.

28. Lown B., Ganong W. F., and Levine S. A.: The syndrome of short P-R interval, narrow QRS complex and paroxysmal rapid heart action. Circulation *5:*663–670, 1952.

29. Brechenmacher C.: Atrio-His bundle tracts. Br Heart J *37:*853–855, 1975.

30. Thapar M. K., and Gillette P. C.: Dual atrioventricular nodal pathways: a common electrophysiologic response in children. Circulation *60:*1369–1374, 1979.

31. Mehta J., and Desnick R. J.: Abbreviated PR interval in mannosidosis. J Pediatr *92:*599–600, 1978.

32. Roudebush C. P., Foerster J. M., and Bing O. H. L.: The abbreviated PR interval of Fabry's disease. N Engl J Med *289:*357, 1973.

33. Gillette P. C., Nihill M. R., and Singer D. B.: Electrophysiologic mechanism of the short PR interval in Pompe's disease. Am J Dis Child *128:*622–626, 1974.

34. Rodriguez-Torres R., Schureck L., and Klienberg W.: Electrocardiographic and biochemical abnormalities in Tay-Sachs disease. Bull NY Acad Med *47:*717, 1971.

35. Mahaim I., and Benatt A.: Nouvelles recherches sur les connexions supérieures de la branche gauche du faisceau de His-Tawara avec cloison intérventriculaire. Cardiologia *1:*61–71, 1938.

36. Gallagher J. J., Smith W. M., Kasell J. H., et al.: Role of Mahaim fibers in cardiac arrhythmias in man. Circulation *64:*176–189, 1981.

10

Ischemia, Injury, and Infarction

The major changes that occur with ischemia, injury, and early infarction involve the T waves and ST segments.

Primary and Secondary T Wave Changes

Primary T wave changes occur when repolarization is affected, independent of changes in depolarization. These may occur either (1) with uniform alteration in the shape or duration of all action potentials without a change in the sequence of depolarization (e.g., hyperkalemia), or (2) with nonuniform alteration in the shape or duration of the action potentials in different parts of the ventricle resulting in an altered sequence of repolarization (e.g., localized ischemia). The majority of the primary T wave changes occur with ischemia or other systemic alterations that have an effect on the heart.

Secondary T wave changes occur when altered repolarization is caused by an abnormal sequence of depolarization. In children, these are much more common than primary changes and occur in such conditions as bundle branch block, preexcitation, and hypertrophy. Frequently, a secondary T wave change is mistaken for a primary change because the minor QRS abnormality responsible for the secondary change is not recognized. Minor changes in the duration and shape of the QRS, especially in the terminal portion, may be responsible for significant secondary T wave changes. Therefore, before assigning a T wave change to the primary category, it is important to be sure the changes cannot be explained by an abnormal QRS complex.[1]

Functional T Wave Changes

The majority of these changes appear to have a link to the sympathetic nervous system. Fear and anxiety are known to cause inverted T waves without a change in coronary blood flow.[2] Sympathetic mechanisms are thought to be responsible for the T wave changes in hyperventilation. Ten percent of teenagers inverted the T wave in at least one chest lead after 10 to 15 seconds of hyperventilation and 70% inverted their T waves after 45 seconds.[3] The degree of alkalosis or hypocarbia could not be related to the T wave changes. Orthostatic T wave changes have been described in the inferior leads in 3% of normal adults who stand up after lying down for several minutes.[1] It is not known whether the postural change is due to catecholamines or a physical shift of the heart. Approximately 4% of normal adults develop flat or inverted T waves in several leads within 30 minutes of eating a high-carbohydrate meal or drinking a high-concentration glucose solution. If a child has flat or inverted T waves without known cause, the electrocardiogram might be repeated in the postabsorptive state.[4]

There are two other functional changes that are most common in adolescence. The "early repolarization syndrome" is recognized by J point elevation in several leads and may mimic true ST elevation. Usually, the T waves in early repolarization are very large. This pattern is due to the early appearance of the T wave while the ventricles are still depolarizing.[5] This eliminates the ST segment. Sympathetic stimulation either by exercise or by isoproterenol infusion generally normalizes the J point elevation (Fig. 10-1). Alternatively, in the asymptomatic patient, one can wait for several days and check another electrocardio-

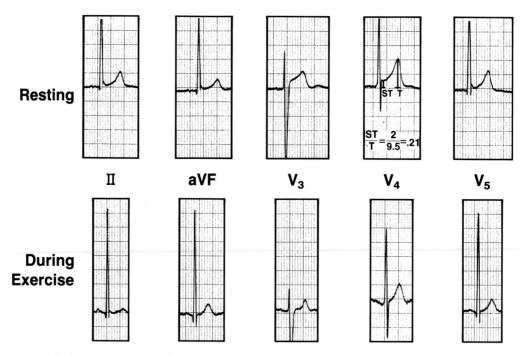

FIG. 10-1. Early repolarization syndrome. In the resting electrocardiogram shown in the top, there is J point elevation in the inferior and lateral leads. In this patient, leads I and aV$_L$ were normal. There was 1 mm of J point depression in aV$_R$. After 6 minutes of treadmill exercise, the bottom tracings were recorded. Note the normalization of all J point elevations. The exercise test was, therefore, helpful in supporting the diagnosis of early repolarization. Similarly, the ST/T ratios in leads I, V$_4$, and V$_5$ are .20, .21, and .15 respectively. Since these are less than .25, early repolarization is suggested.

gram. In early repolarization, the J point elevation is persistent, whereas in pericarditis, the other common cause of elevated ST segments in children, the changes evolve. One other sign that has been used in adults to distinguish between early repolarization and pericarditis is the ratio of the ST segment amplitude to the T wave amplitude (ST/T ratio) in either leads I, V_4, V_5, or V_6. The height of the ST segment and T wave were measured relative to the end of the PR segment at the beginning of the QRS complex. This measurement is based upon the observation that in early repolarization, the T waves are tall (therefore the ST/T ratio will be small) and in pericarditis, T waves are small (and the ST/T ratio will be large). Thus, in adults, if the ST/T ratio is .25 or greater, the patient is more likely to have pericarditis (compare Figs. 10-1 and 10-10).[6]

The second functional T wave change found in adolescence is the isolated inverted T wave in a midprecordial lead with an upright T wave in the leads on either side. This occurs in 1% of adolescents and has no pathologic correlate.[7] In general, benign T wave changes are labile.

Ischemia

Myocardial ischemia is manifest electrocardiographically by distortion of the T wave amplitude, configuration, and mean vector. In ischemic tissue, the action potential duration is prolonged by a long plateau. Therefore, ischemic tissue recovers more slowly than the surrounding normal tissue and the ischemic tissue is negatively charged relative to the surrounding tissue which has already recovered. Thus, the T wave vector points away from the ischemic tissue toward the positive potentials of the normal tissue. The first area to become ischemic in the heart is generally the subendocardium, and in cases of subendocardial ischemia, the T wave points toward the normal epicardial tissue overlying the ischemic area. In subendocardial ischemia, the T waves are symmetric and peaked with an increase in amplitude and duration in the leads overlying the ischemic area (Figs. 10-2 and 10-3). In subepicardial ischemia, the T waves are inverted, overlying the ischemic area. In transmural ischemia, the sequence of repolarization is abnormal and follows the depolarization sequence from endocardium to epicardium. This is the reverse direction from normal and therefore the T waves are inverted overlying an area of transmural ischemia (Fig. 10-4A).

Myocardial ischemia is rare in children. It can occur in the early stages of reduced coronary blood flow from neonatal stress, anomalous left coronary artery, or mucocutaneous lymph node syndrome (Kawasaki's disease) before infarction occurs. Subendocardial ischemia may occur in children with aortic stenosis or pulmonary stenosis. The flattened or inverted T waves that accompany rapid sinus tachycardia or supraventricular tachycardia may be due to ischemia but they may also be secondary T wave changes due to minor degrees of ventricular aberration obscured by the rapid rate. The persistence of

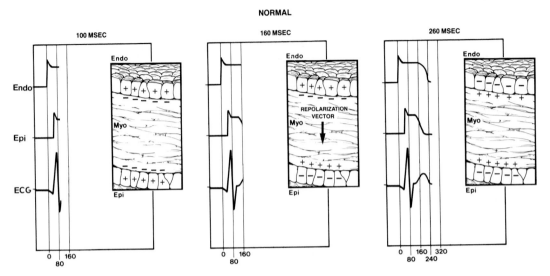

FIG. 10-2.   Genesis of the normal T wave. See Figure 4-7 for complete explanation.

these T wave changes up to days after the event may be related to potassium loss with slow replenishment of metabolic stores.[5] In 10% of children with mitral valve prolapse, there is T wave inversion in the inferior and lateral leads. These changes may be explained either by the presence of small ischemic areas due to traction interfering with the vascular supply or by uneven repolarization.[4] Other changes with mitral prolapse include a prolonged QT interval and prominent U waves.[8]

In pure left ventricular hypertrophy, the usual electrocardiographic pattern is an increase in the T wave amplitude; in advanced left ventricular hypertrophy, there is ST depression with inverted T waves: the "strain" pattern.[9] Thus, "strain" is different from subendocardial ischemia in which ST depression and upright or flat T waves are present. It has been suggested that "strain" is a primary T wave abnormality, is due to a difference in endocardial and epicardial conduction times, and has a different mechanism from ischemia.[10] Alternatively, the ST-T wave changes observed in hypertrophy and strain may be simply more severe changes in a spectrum from subendocardial to transmural ischemia.

Injury

Myocardial injury is evidenced electrocardiographically both by deviations from the baseline and by changes in the contour of the ST segment. In injured cells there is a release of potassium resulting in shortening of phase 2 of the action potential. This affects the ST segment. In subepicardial injury, the injured area is relatively positive compared to the underlying normal myocardium, and an electrode immediately over the area of subepicardial injury shows ST elevation

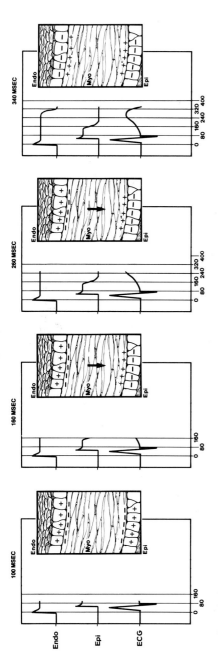

FIG. 10-3. Subendocardial ischemia. The action potential duration is prolonged so that at 260 msec after the onset of the QRS complex, the endocardium is still depolarized and a vector remains from the endocardium to the epicardium, causing a peaked T wave. The prolonged endocardial activation also results in a prolonged QT interval.

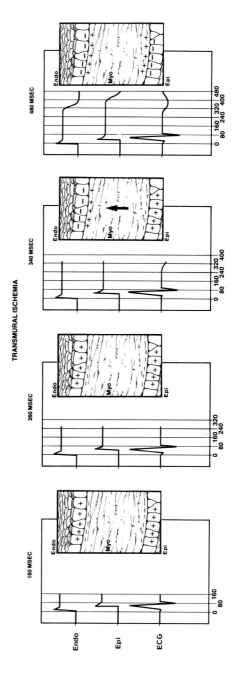

FIG. 10-4. Transmural ischemia. The epicardial action potentials are prolonged longer than the endocardial action potentials, resulting in a vector of repolarization directed in the direction opposite to normal. This causes T wave inversion in leads overlying transmural ischemia. There is also QT prolongation.

SUBEPICARDIAL INJURY

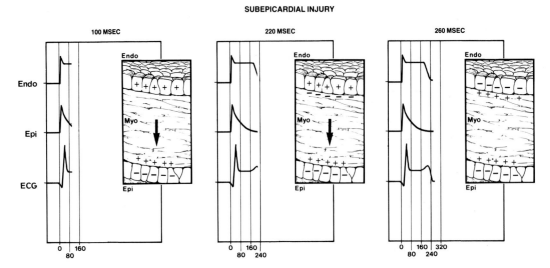

FIG. 10-5. Subepicardial injury. The epicardial action potential duration is shortened with a shortened plateau, resulting in early repolarization of the epicardium. This causes an ST segment shift toward the epicardial area of injury. The QT interval is normal because endocardial repolarization proceeds on schedule.

(Fig. 10-5). In subendocardial injury, the positive injured area has overlying normal myocardium which is relatively negative and the electrode immediately over this area shows ST depression (Fig. 10-6). Thus, with injury, the ST segment is displaced toward the injured surface. When the ST segment is elevated, the contour may be either upwardly convex or concave; with ST depression, the contour is usually concave or flat. In children, injury patterns that are not due to systemic alterations are found most frequently in pericarditis and ischemic episodes.

SUBENDOCARDIAL INJURY

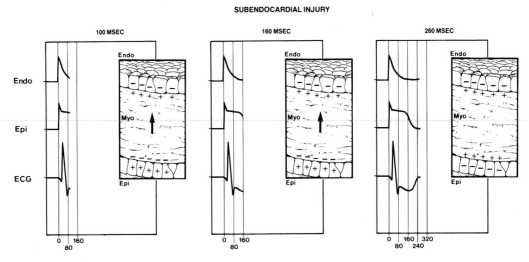

FIG. 10-6. Subendocardial injury. The endocardial action potentials are shortened with a shortened plateau. This results in early repolarization and an ST segment shift towards the endocardium, or ST depression in leads overlying subendocardial injury.

INJURY DUE TO
ISCHEMIA

It is rare to obtain an electrocardiogram from an infant or child who is undergoing an acute myocardial infarction, but this diagnosis should be included when considering ST elevation (Fig. 10-7). A more common kind of ST segment shift seen in children is the ST depression found in some infants with patent ductus arteriosus (Fig. 10-8). In 15 out of 19 severely ill infants who required patent ductus arteriosus ligation, ST depression of 2.5 to 10 mm was found in leads V_1 and V_2.

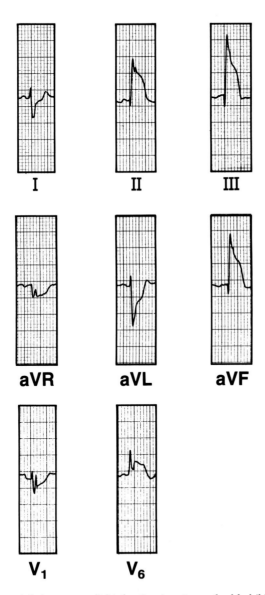

FIG. 10-7. Acute inferior myocardial infarction in a 3-month-old child with staphylococcal sepsis. At autopsy, extensive abscess was found in the left ventricle. There is considerable ST elevation in leads II, III, and aV_F and reciprocal ST depression in leads I, aV_L, aV_R, and V_1.

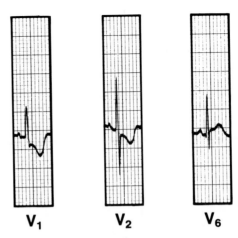

FIG. 10-8.   ST segment shift with patent ductus arteriosus. This tracing was taken from an 840-g infant with cardiomegaly due to a patent ductus arteriosus. Note the ST depression in leads V_1 and V_2 and ST elevation in lead V_6. The ST-T wave changes resolved after ductus ligation.

The ST change disappeared after ligation of the ductus. The explanation for these changes is a marked myocardial oxygen supply-demand imbalance primarily in the right ventricle: The supply is reduced due to the low aortic diastolic pressure with reduced coronary flow and the myocardial oxygen demand is increased due to the high pulmonary artery systolic pressure.[11]

INJURY DUE TO MYOCARDITIS

Cellular injury occurs with myocarditis. Approximately 70% of children with myocarditis have electrocardiographic changes.[12] An abnormal electrocardiogram implies myocardial damage; however, a normal electrocardiogram does not preclude severe injury. The electrocardiogram may normalize within two to three weeks of the onset of the disease, but it may remain abnormal for up to four months with later reversion to normal. A normal electrocardiogram after myocarditis also does not preclude severe residual damage.[5]

The most prominent electrocardiographic changes are flat or inverted T waves (primarily in the left chest leads) and "low voltage" QRS complexes (see Chapter 6, "Lower Limit of QRS Amplitude"). The T wave changes are probably due to altered repolarization of injured cells throughout the myocardium rather than to true ischemia. The QT interval may be prolonged. The low voltage QRS results from myocardial edema. Myocarditis also commonly results in ST depression due to extensive subendocardial injury. ST elevation is rare in myocarditis without pericarditis.[13] There have been several reports of the appearance of new Q waves in association with myocarditis. These have mostly been in children who have later died. The Q waves were accompanied by ST elevation in those patients. There was no characteristic electrocardiographic location for these changes. In different children, the Q waves were in the inferior, lateral, or anterior leads (Fig. 10-9). Pathologic studies have documented extensive areas of necrosis and scarring which correlate with the electrocardiographic location of the Q waves in these patients.[14,15]

AV block and interventricular conduction delay may occur in any type of myocarditis, but right bundle branch block is particularly common to the myocarditis due to Chagas disease. Premature ventricular contractions occasionally occur in myocarditis.[5]

INJURY DUE TO PERICARDITIS

Pericarditis is by far the most common pathologic cause of ST elevation in children. Other causes of primary ST changes include myo-

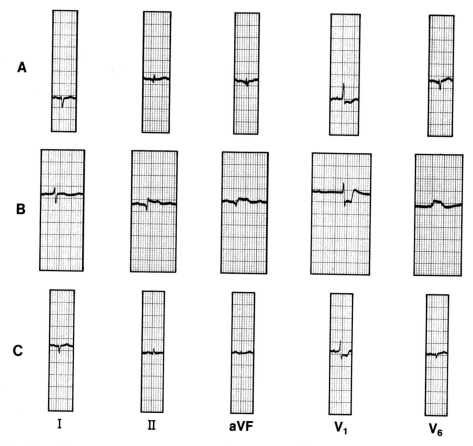

FIG. 10-9. Myocarditis in a 1-week-old infant. A, Low voltage QRS complexes are shown in both the limb leads and precordial leads. The T waves are concordant but decreased in amplitude. B, This electrocardiogram, taken 12 hours later, shows the development of complete AV block and deep, wide Q waves in leads II and aV$_F$ accompanied by ST elevation in leads II, aV$_F$, and V$_6$ with ST depression in lead V$_1$. This is compatible with an inferolateral myocardial infarction. C, The infant on the next day with even less voltage in the inferior and lateral leads. He died the following night and was found at autopsy to have diffuse areas of myocarditis and areas of necrosis throughout both ventricles.

cardial infarction, cor pulmonale, head injury, digitalis, hyperkalemia, emetine intoxication, pneumothorax, pneumopericardium, early ventricular repolarization, and normal atrial repolarization.

The electrocardiogram in pericarditis characteristically evolves through four stages (Fig. 10-10). Stage 1 is ST elevation. This is thought to be due to subepicardial myocarditis. The ST elevation occurs in leads facing the epicardium (leads II, aV$_F$, V$_3$ through V$_6$). Depending

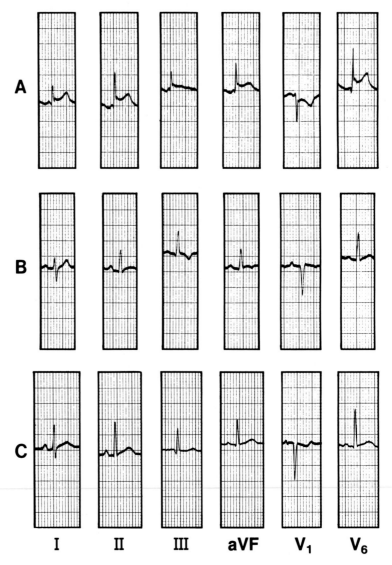

FIG. 10-10. Evolution of pericarditis in a 12-year-old. A, ST elevation with upright T waves in all leads except V$_1$. The ST/T ratios in leads I and V$_6$ are .42 and .33, respectively. Since these are greater than .25, pericarditis is suggested. B, The ST elevation is resolving and is replaced with T wave inversion in leads III and aV$_F$. This electrocardiogram was taken four days after the first electrocardiogram. C, Two weeks later, the ST-T wave changes are resolved but there is a Q wave in lead III which is wider than on previous tracings. This could indicate a small area of old inferior myocardial infarction.

upon the position of the heart, lead I or III may also be involved. The leads without epicardial representation, which are usually facing away from the left ventricle (leads aV_R and V_1), may show reciprocal ST depression. In neonates, the right ventricle constitutes more of the epicardial surface and the right chest leads may show ST elevation with the left chest leads showing ST depression.[5]

Pericarditis can usually be differentiated from acute myocardial infarction. In pericarditis, the ST elevation is found in numerous leads, whereas in myocardial infarction it is generally limited to a few leads; also, the ST elevation in pericarditis is associated usually with an upright T wave, whereas in myocardial infarction, beyond the hyperacute phase, the T wave is usually inverted. In pericarditis during the time of ST elevation, it may also be possible to detect PR segment elevation (greater than .8 mm) due to atrial subepicardial injury in leads overlying the right atrium, (aV_R and V_1) and reciprocal PR depression (greater than .5 mm) in those leads normally showing ST elevation.[4]

Stage 2 is characterized by normalization of ST segments with T wave flattening. This occurs as an intermediate stage to stages 1 and 3. In stage 3, there is T wave inversion in the same leads in which the ST elevation previously appeared. Stage 4 is resolution.

In a prospective study of adults, 92% had electrocardiographic changes in pericarditis. In only half of these, typical ST elevation occurred followed by T wave inversion. In those without preceding ST elevation, T wave inversion did not occur. PR segment elevation occurred in 64% of these adults, and in 10% this was the only change of pericarditis.[16] The QRS complex is generally not affected by pericarditis. Even in the presence of a large pericardial effusion, the QRS may have normal voltage in pericarditis.[4]

INJURY DUE TO
CARDIAC TUMORS

ST elevation and T wave inversion are the most common findings in metastatic tumors to the heart, because the pericardium is the most likely site for metastasis. If a primary cardiac tumor causes significant destruction of functioning myocardium, Q waves may appear; if the tumor is large enough, the QRS voltage may be decreased. Primary tumors of the heart can cause any type of arrhythmia, most notably ventricular tachycardia and AV block.[4]

Infarction

Infarcted muscle is electrically inert. The loss of electrical forces normally generated by the region of infarcted myocardium leaves unbalanced forces of unaltered magnitude in the opposite direction, resulting in Q waves overlying the area of infarction (Fig. 10-11). The earliest electrocardiographic manifestations of myocardial infarction

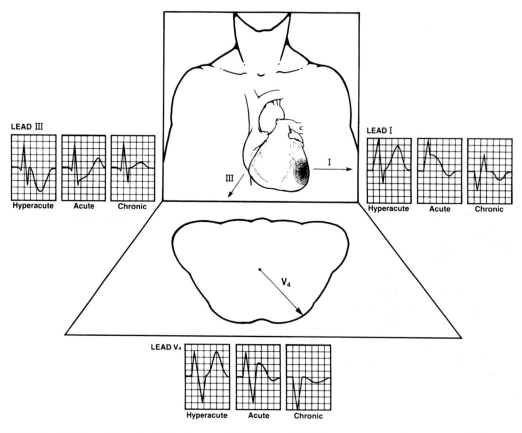

FIG. 10-11. Evolution of an anterolateral myocardial infarction. In the hyperacute stage there are peaked T waves in leads overlying the infarction (lead I), followed by ST elevation in the acute stage, and a Q wave in the chronic stage. Reciprocal ST depression is seen in lead III in the acute stage.

are "hyperacute," very tall, peaked T waves. These occur because in freshly infarcted tissue, the refractory periods have shortened considerably and the T wave points toward areas of shorter refractory period. Hyperacute T waves occur in the first minutes and are therefore infrequently observed. Soon thereafter, ST elevation is observed in leads overlying the infarction and a current of injury to that area is displayed. There may be reciprocal ST segment depression in leads opposite the infarction. Within several hours to days, the ST elevation is typically followed by the development of Q waves and inverted T waves in leads overlying the infarction. T wave inversion is due to eventual lengthening of the refractory periods of surviving cells in the region of the infarction. Q waves of myocardial infarction in children are wide (0.04 sec or more), similar to those found in adults (Fig. 10-12). In children, Q waves related to myocardial infarction may disappear. As growth occurs, the infarcted area may become relatively smaller compared to the greater total mass of the heart.

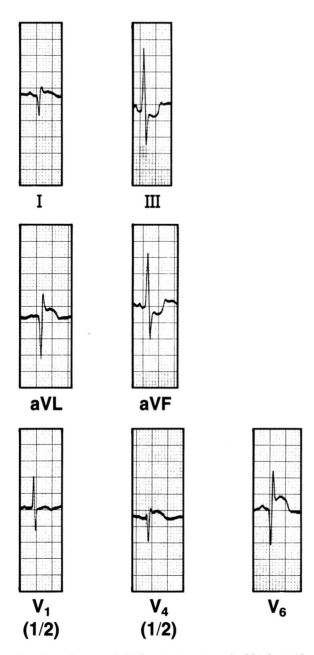

FIG. 10-12. Acute lateral myocardial infarction in a 4-month-old infant with anomalous left coronary artery originating from the pulmonary artery. The "acute" and "chronic" stages diagrammed in Figure 10-11 occurred simultaneously in this patient. Both ST elevation and the development of deep, wide Q waves occur in leads I, aV_L, and V_6.

ANOMALOUS LEFT CORONARY ARTERY ORIGINATING FROM THE PULMONARY ARTERY

Anomalous left coronary artery originating from the pulmonary artery is the most common congenital anomaly causing myocardial infarction in childhood. Most of the infants and children with anomalous left coronary artery have already infarcted some areas of the left ventricle by the time of their first electrocardiogram. The electrocardiograms may variously reflect healed myocardial infarction, ventricular growth around the infarction and varying degrees of acute and chronic ischemia.

In infancy, wide Q waves are more prominent than in later childhood.[17] Q waves are almost invariably present in lead I and are usually present in lead aV_L; they may extend from the mid to the lateral precordial leads (V_3 to V_6). There may be an abrupt loss of R wave in the midprecordium with a normal R wave in V_1, V_6, and V_7. In the frontal plane, the QRS mean vector is usually $+90°$.[18] The T waves are usually inverted in leads I and aV_L and in the lateral precordial leads. In older children, the Q waves become less prominent, resulting from compensatory hypertrophy of the posterobasal left ventricle. The major terminal QRS vector is superior, left, and posterior, frequently causing left axis deviation in the frontal plane. There may be loss of the normal right ventricular dominance and deep S wave in leads II, III, aV_F, and V_1 with tall R waves in leads aV_L, V_5, and V_6. The T waves are discordant in leads I, V_1, and V_5. Although this evolution is characteristic, an individual patient may present with any combination of these findings (Fig. 10-13).

PAPILLARY MUSCLE INFARCTION

Newborn infants with severe neonatal stress or infants with severe pressure or volume overload may develop papillary muscle infarction. Characteristic electrocardiographic findings have been found in infants with aortic stenosis or total anomalous pulmonary venous return who were proven at autopsy to have had anterior papillary muscle infarction of either the right ventricle or left ventricle. In these infants, Q waves were present in lead V_3R. There was also a progressive diminution of the R wave in lead V_3R on serial electrocardiographic tracings.[19] This is to be distinguished from the other major causes of Q waves in the right chest leads in infancy: severe right ventricular hypertrophy or reversed septal depolarization from ventricular inversion.

KAWASAKI'S DISEASE

Kawasaki's disease (or mucocutaneous lymph node syndrome) is the most common acquired cause of myocardial infarction in infants and children. Approximately 15% of such patients develop coronary artery aneurysms associated with a pancarditis in the first two weeks of the illness. In half of these, the aneurysms regress. Sudden death occurs in 2% of these patients, presumably due to myocardial infarction and resultant arrhythmia.[20] The Q waves that occur in Kawasaki's disease are abnormally deep and are usually abnormally wide.[21] Abnormally deep Q waves are defined in Chapter 6, which discusses the normal electrocardiogram. Q waves may develop in the first two weeks

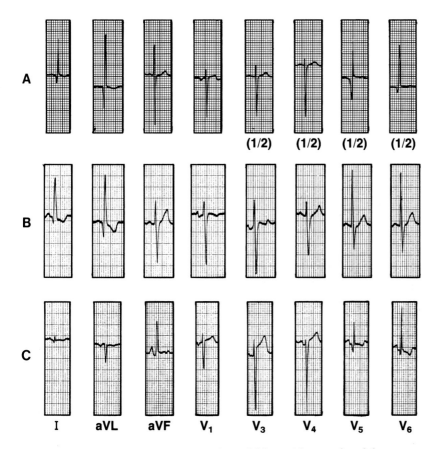

FIG. 10-13. Old myocardial infarction in three children with anomalous left coronary artery originating from the pulmonary artery. A, Tracings from a 7-month-old child demonstrating left axis deviation of the QRS mean vector in the frontal plane, a diminished R wave between lead V_3 and lead V_6, and deep, wide Q waves in leads I, aV_L, V_5, and V_6. B, Tracings from a 7-year-old girl. The findings are similar to those in the 7-month-old infant, except that there are no Q waves in leads V_5 and V_6, but deep S waves in those leads. These tracings, therefore, correspond more to the "adult" type of electrocardiogram in anomalous left coronary artery. C, Tracings taken from another 7-year-old, showing no left axis deviation, but deep Q waves in leads aV_L, V_5, and V_6. This is more consistent with the "infantile" pattern and demonstrates that the labels may not be helpful. All of these electrocardiograms show a loss of R wave in lead V_4, and both Q wave and T wave inversion in leads I and aV_L.

of the illness and may be due to severe myocarditis. These may subsequently resolve. If Q waves develop later than two weeks into the illness, this is usually associated with a coronary artery aneurysm and myocardial necrosis. In some patients, a serial deepening of the Q waves was the only sign of infarction (Fig. 10-14). The absence of Q waves does not imply an absence of aneurysms nor an absence of significant areas of myocardial necrosis at autopsy.[21]

PSEUDOINFARCTION

Other causes of abnormal Q waves, with or without ST-T wave changes, include the following. (1) Left ventricular hypertrophy with strain and a QS pattern in lead I along with ST elevation, with recipro-

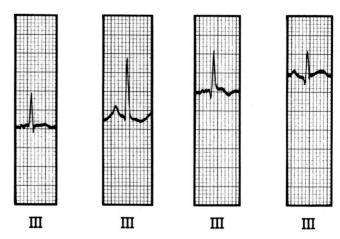

III   III   III   III

FIG. 10-14. Myocardial infarction in Kawasaki's disease. These tracings are from a 9-year-old boy who was hospitalized on the seventh day of the illness. The *first* tracing is from the day of admission. He was asymptomatic at the time. The *second* tracing was taken three days later. Note the development of small Q waves, which were not present previously, and the T wave inversion in lead III. Four days later, the Q waves have deepened and are now slightly wider. There is also ST elevation with the terminal portion of the T wave inverted. The day after the *third* tracing, the Q wave remains and the T waves have normalized. By radionuclide imaging, the entire inferior wall of the left ventricle was infarcted. This points out the subtle changes that may occur in an extensive myocardial infarction in a child. Although the depth of the Q wave in the *last* tracing is not distinctly abnormal, the new appearance of the Q wave is abnormal and the width of the Q wave is also abnormal.

cal ST depression in V_6. (2) Right ventricular hypertrophy with a QR pattern in lead V_1. (3) Ventricular inversion with normal anatomic left ventricular to right ventricular activation occurring in a right-to-left direction resulting in a narrow Q wave in lead V_1 and absent Q wave in V_6. (4) Clockwise rotation of the heart from lung disease or pneumothorax may move the transition leads leftward to leads V_5 or V_6, and therefore lead V_1 may have a QS pattern. (5) Hypertrophic cardiomyopathy with asymmetric septal hypertrophy. Deep and usually not wide Q waves are found in the lateral leads due to septal hypertrophy. (6) Replacement by nonfunctioning living tissue. Myocarditis, progressive muscular dystrophy, Friedreich's ataxia, scleroderma, and cardiac tumors. (7) Replacement with prosthetic material. When a large prosthetic patch is used on the right ventricular outflow tract, deep, wide Q waves may occur in the anterior chest leads (Fig. 10-15). (8) Left bundle branch block, causing a QS pattern in lead V_1. (9) Left anterior hemiblock, with Q waves in the lateral precordial leads. (10) Wolff-Parkinson-White with wide Q waves in the inferior leads. (11) Intracranial hemorrhage may produce a QS pattern in leads V_1 or V_2.

Aneurysm

The most common electrocardiographic feature of a ventricular aneurysm is persistent ST elevation in leads overlying the aneurysm.[22] This has been found in children with anomalous left coronary artery

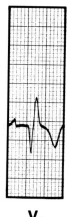

V$_1$

FIG. 10-15. Pseudoinfarction. This tracing was taken from a 20-year-old patient who had undergone intracardiac repair of tetralogy of Fallot. A deep, wide Q wave precedes the wide, slurred terminal activation of the right bundle branch block. This Q wave was most likely due to the 3-cm-by-8-cm patch that extended from the right ventricular anterior wall up to the pulmonary artery bifurcation. This is also compatible with an old anteroseptal myocardial infarction. There was no clinical evidence for myocardial infarction, however, nor was there electrocardiographic evolution of an infarction.

after myocardial infarction.[23] In a congenital aneurysm of the posterior left ventricular base, there was ST depression in the anterior chest leads (reciprocal from the posteriorly directed ST elevation), as well as diminished QRS voltage and T wave inversion in leads I, II, aV$_L$, V$_5$, and V$_6$.[24]

Self-Assessment Questions

Question 1: The most likely diagnosis in the 13-year-old patient with the following electrocardiogram is (Fig. 10-16):

A. acute myocardial infarction
B. early repolarization
C. pericarditis
D. cannot distinguish between A and C
E. cannot distinguish between B and C

Question 2: Match the electrocardiographic finding with the diagnosis:

_____ T wave inversion; long QT interval	A. subendocardial ischemia
_____ tall peaked T waves, long QT interval	B. subepicardial injury
_____ ST elevation	C. subendocardial injury
_____ ST depression	D. subepicardial ischemia
	E. B or C

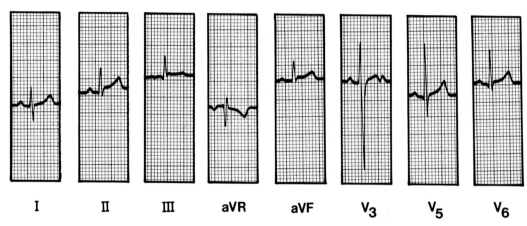

FIG. 10-16. Question 1.

Question 3: What is the most likely diagnosis in this 3-year-old patient (Fig. 10-17)?

A. left ventricular hypertrophy
B. myocardial infarction
C. Wolff-Parkinson-White
D. ventricular inversion
E. right ventricular hypertrophy

Question 4: What is the most likely diagnosis in this 11-month-old patient (Fig. 10-18)?

A. left ventricular hypertrophy
B. myocardial infarction
C. Wolff-Parkinson-White
D. ventricular inversion
E. right ventricular hypertrophy

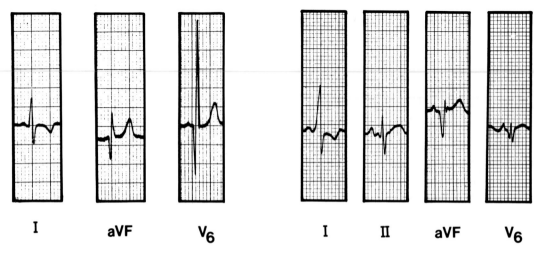

FIG. 10-17. Question 3.   **FIG. 10-18.** Question 4.

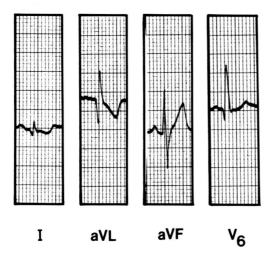

I   aVL   aVF   V₆

FIG. 10-19.   Question 5.

Question 5: What is the most likely diagnosis in this 9-month-old patient (Fig. 10-19)?

A. left ventricular hypertrophy
B. myocardial infarction
C. Wolff-Parkinson-White
D. ventricular inversion
E. right ventricular hypertrophy

Answers to Self-Assessment Questions

Answer 1: E
This could represent either early repolarization (J point elevation) or pericarditis (ST elevation). The ST/T ratios in V_5 and V_6 are .24, which are borderline. The elevation occurs in so many leads that acute myocardial infarction is unlikely.

Answer 2: D, A, B, C
T wave inversion occurs over the area of transmural or subepicardial ischemia (answer D), while tall T waves indicate subendocardial ischemia (answer A). With injury, the ST segment is displaced toward the injured surface, therefore ST elevation results from subepicardial injury (answer B) and ST depression from subendocardial injury (answer C).

Answer 3: A
This patient had a ventricular septal defect and subaortic stenosis. The Q wave, although deep, is only 30 msec long.

Answer 4: C

The short PR interval and delta wave are most apparent in lead I. The delta wave is the peak following the P wave in lead II. The negative delta wave in leads aV_F and V_5 causes the Q waves. With preexcitation interpretation of the electrocardiogram for hypertrophy or infarction should not be attempted since the ventricles are activated asymmetrically.

Answer 5: B

The Q wave in lead I is 40 msec long and the Q wave in lead aV_L is 35 msec long. In a child, a Q wave of this duration is strongly suggestive of old myocardial infarction.

References

1. Cooksey J. D., Dunn M., and Massie E.: Clinical Vectorcardiography and Electrocardiography. 2nd Ed. Chicago, Yearbook Medical Publishers, 1977, pp 9–112.
2. Awa S., Linde L. M., Oshima M., et al.: The significance of late-phased dart T wave in the electrocardiogram of children. Am Heart J *80*:619–628, 1970.
3. Thomsen J. H., and Wasserburger R. H.: Effect of hyperventilation on precordial T waves of children and adolescents. Circulation *36*:700–707, 1967.
4. Chou T.: Electrocardiography in Clinical Practice. New York, Grune & Stratton, 1979, pp 114–150.
5. Hoffman, J. I. E.: Primary T wave changes in children. Praxis *64*:803–811, 1975.
6. Ginzton L. E., and Laks M. M.: The differential diagnosis of acute pericarditis from the normal variant: new electrocardiographic criteria. Circulation *65*:1004–1009, 1982.
7. Awa S., Linde L. M., Oshima M., et al.: Isolated T wave inversion in the electrocardiogram of children. Am Heart J *81*:158–165, 1971.
8. Bissett G. S., Schwartz D. C., and Meyer R. A.: Clinical spectrum and long-term follow-up of isolated mitral valve prolapse in 119 children. Circulation *62*:423–428, 1980.
9. Mashima, S., Fu L., and Fukushima K.: The ventricular gradient and the vectorcardiographic T loop in left ventricular hypertrophy. J Electrocardiol *2*:55–62, 1969.
10. Grant R. P., Estes E. H., and Doyle J. T.: Spatial vector electrocardiography. The clinical characteristics of ST and T vectors. Circulation *3*:182–197, 1951.
11. Way G. L., Pierce J. R., Wolfe R. R., et al.: ST depression suggesting subendocardial injury in neonates with respiratory distress syndrome and patent ductus arteriosus. J Pediatr *95*:609–611, 1979.
12. Sachder J. C., and Puri D.: Electrocardiographic alterations in diphtheria. Indian J Pediatr *34*:429–431, 1967.
13. Rodriguez-Torres R., Lin J., and Berkovitch S.: A sensitive ECG sign in myocarditis associated with viral infection. Pediatrics *43*:846–851, 1969.
14. Gross, H., Rubin I. L., and Dardick I.: Abnormal Q waves in a child with myocarditis. N.Y. State J Med *67*:283–287, 1967.
15. Dominguez P., Lendrum B. L., and Pick A.: False "coronary patterns" in the infant electrocardiogram. Circulation *19*:400–419, 1959.
16. Bruce M. A., and Spodick D. H.: Atypical electrocardiogram in acute pericarditis: characteristics and prevalence. J Electrocardiography *13*:61–66, 1980.
17. Puri P. S., Rowe R. D., and Neill C. A.: Varying vectorcardiographic patterns in anomalous left coronary artery arising from the pulmonary artery. Am Heart J *71*:616–626, 1966.
18. Perloff, J. K.: The Clinical Recognition of Congenital Heart Disease. Philadelphia, W. B. Saunders, 1970, p 237.

19. Kangos J. J., Ferrer I., Franciosi R. A., et al.: Electrocardiographic changes associated with papillary muscle infarction in congenital heart disease. Am Heart J *23*:801–809, 1969.

20. Fukushige J., Nihill M. R., and McNamara D. G.: The spectrum of cardiovascular lesions in the mucocutaneous lymph node syndrome. Am J Cardiol *45*:98–107, 1980.

21. Fujiwara, H., Chen C., Fujiwara T., et al.: Clinicopathology of abnormal Q waves in Kawasaki disease. Am J Cardiol *45*:797–805, 1980.

22. Dubnow M. H., Burchell H. B., and Titus J. L.: Postinfarction ventricular aneurysm. Am Heart J *70*:753–760, 1965.

23. Keith J. D.: Anomalous left coronary artery from the pulmonary artery. Br Heart J *21*:149–156, 1959.

24. Franco-Vasquez S., Sutherland R. D., Fowler M., et al.: Congenital aneurysm of the left ventricular base. Chest *57*:411–415, 1970.

11

Effect of Systemic Alterations on the Electrocardiogram

Action Potential Changes Reflected in the Electrocardiogram

The majority of systemic alterations exert their effect on the electrocardiogram by changing all the action potentials in a similar manner. It is therefore important to understand how changes in action potentials cause changes in the electrocardiogram. The most important alterations, diagrammed in Figure 11-1, are as follows: (1) A decrease in the upstroke velocity of the action potential (Vmax of phase 0) causes a decrease in ventricular conduction velocity and uniform QRS widening (e.g., hyperkalemia). (2) Because the end of the ventricular action potentials corresponds to the end of the T wave, prolonged action potential duration causes a long QT interval (e.g., quinidine); short action potential duration causes a short QT interval (e.g., epinephrine). (3) A long plateau (phase 2) causes a long ST segment (e.g., hypocalcemia); a short plateau causes a short ST segment (e.g., hypercalcemia). (4) Increased velocity of the initial phase of repolarization abolishing the plateau causes disappearance of the isoelectric portion of the ST segment and therefore deviation of the ST segment from the baseline (e.g., digitalis). (5) An abrupt transition from phase 2 to phase 3 combined with an increase in the slope of phase 3 results in an abrupt onset of the T wave with an increased amplitude and decreased duration, causing the T wave to appear peaked (e.g., hyperkalemia). (6) Loss of plateau caused by uniform repolarization approaching a straight line causes a decrease in T wave amplitude (e.g., barbiturates). (7) Prolonged terminal repolarization of the ventricles causes U waves (e.g., hypokalemia). The effects of systemic alterations on the electrocardiogram are summarized in Table 11-1.

170

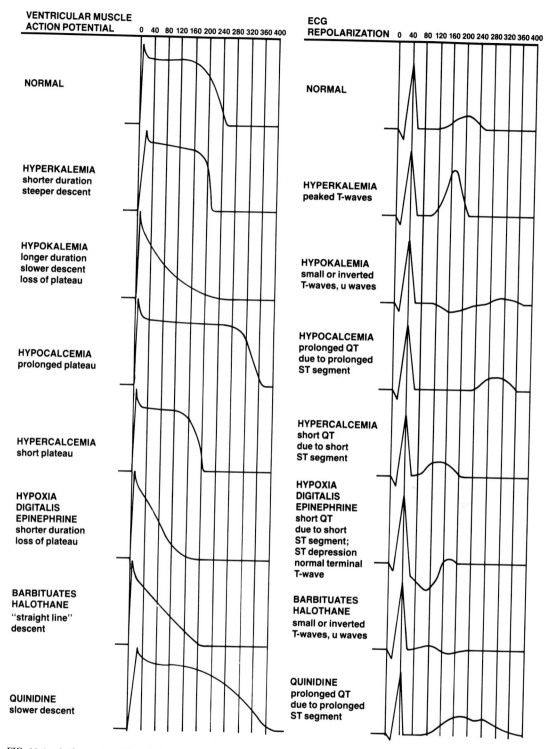

FIG. 11-1. Action potential and electrocardiographic changes in systemic alterations. In the *left* column are drawn sample ventricular muscle action potentials associated with each condition. The effect on repolarization of the electrocardiogram is shown in the *right* column. Effects on the QRS are not shown. The times are milliseconds after the onset of the ventricular muscle action potential and the corresponding QRS complex. (Adapted from Surawicz B: Primary and secondary T wave changes. Heart Bull *15*:31–35, 1966.)

TABLE 11-1. *Systemic Effects on the Electrocardiogram**

	SHORT QT	LONG QT-U	PROLONGED QRS	ST-T CHANGES	SINUS TACHY	SINUS BRADY	AV BLOCK	ATRIAL FLUTTER	V. TACHY	MISC
Chemistry										
Hyperkalemia			X	X			X		X	low voltage P waves
Hypokalemia		X	X	X						
Hypercalcemia	X					X	X		X	
Hypocalcemia		X			X		X			
Hypermagnesemia							X			
Hypomagnesemia		X								
Hypoglycemia			X	X			X		X	
Hypoxia, acidosis			X	X			X		X	
Drugs										
Digitalis	X			X		T	X		T	
Quinidine		X	X			T	T		T	
Phenytoin	X									
Propranolol	X					X	X			
Verapamil						X	X			
Halothane	X					X			T	
Cyclopropane									T	
Phenothiazines		T							T	
Tricyclics		T	T	T	T		T			
Imipramine							T	T	T	
Organophosphates		T			T	T	T		T	
CNS										
Jervell-Lange-Nielsen		X				X				
Romano-Ward		X				X				
CNS injury		X		X	X	X	X			
Neuromuscular										
Friedreich's ataxia				X	X			X		deep Q V6 tall RV1
Duchenne's				X	X			X		deep Q V6 tall RV1
Myotonic dystrophy			X	X	X		X			low voltage P waves
Misc										
Collagen disease				X			X		X	
Hypothyroid						X				low voltage + "Mosque"
Hyperthyroid			X	X	X		X			
Adrenal insufficiency		X		X						
Pheochromocytoma		X		X	X					
Peritoneal irritation				X	X					
Sarcoid			X				X	X	X	

*Note: X = present; T = present only with drug toxicity; Brady, bradycardia; CNS, central nervous system; Misc, miscellaneous; V. Tachy, ventricular tachycardia.

Body
Chemistry

HYPERKALEMIA

Hyperkalemia is most commonly due to renal failure, salt losing adrenogenital syndrome, or iatrogenic overdose.[2] The serum potassium level can be predicted from the electrocardiogram because of the different effects on the action potential. At a level of 5.5 to 6.5 meq/L, the velocity of phase 3 of the action potential increases and the T waves on the electrocardiogram become tall and peaked. This is a poor sign because many normal children have "peaked" T waves and many children with hyperkalemia do not have peaked T waves. At a serum potassium level over 6.6 meq/L, the cellular resting membrane potential is decreased (more toward zero) and therefore the conduction velocity (and Vmax) is decreased. This causes interventricular conduction delay. This may be manifested as diffuse QRS widening or it may have a specific bundle branch block or fascicular block pattern. These are generally very bizarre QRS complexes and may be combined with ST elevation, leading to the mistaken diagnosis of ventricular tachycardia if preceding P waves are missed (Fig. 11-2). If P waves are seen, these complexes may also be mistaken for acute myocardial infarction or pericarditis. At a level over 7.0 meq/L, intra-atrial conduction delay becomes manifest with prolongation of the P wave. At a level over 8.5 meq/L, the P wave may disappear. Direct conduction from the sinus node through atrial Purkinje fibers to the AV node and the ventricles has been hypothesized. The sinus node and atrial Purkinje fibers are most resistant to hyperkalemia. Since the ordinary atrial muscle fibers are depressed by the hyperkalemia, they neither conduct nor contract. Therefore, there may be no P wave despite conduction through the atrium. This has been termed "sinoventricular conduction." At approximately 9.0 meq/L, arrhythmias begin: AV block, ventricular tachycardia, and ventricular fibrillation.

HYPOKALEMIA

Hypokalemia is most often found in vomiting, diarrhea, endocrine disease (Cushing's disease, hyperaldosteronism, cortisone treatment), acquired renal disease, iatrogenic lack of intake, and most importantly to cardiologists, diuretic treatment. Hypokalemia causes a lengthening of phase 3 of the action potential with a loss of the plateau and a slower descent. At a level of 2.7 to 3.0 meq/L, the electrocardiograms in 35% of adults have demonstrated abnormalities of hypokalemia and at a level below 2.7 meq/L, 78% are abnormal.[3] The most prominent changes are the decrease in the T wave amplitude (occasionally with ST depression) and an increase in the U wave amplitude. Therefore, hypokalemia causes a broadened T wave and U wave with a normal onset to the T wave (Fig. 11-3). Other causes of prominent U waves are: bradycardia, ischemia, left ventricular hypertrophy, quinidine, pro-

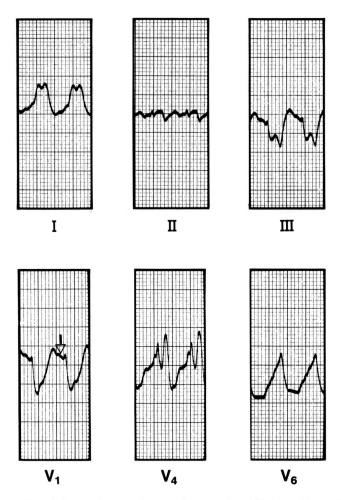

FIG. 11-2. Hyperkalemia. These tracings are from a 2-day-old infant with renal failure and hyperkalemia. The QRS complex is similar to left bundle branch block. The small P waves are marked with an arrow in lead V_1, indicating that this is sinus rhythm.

cainamide, phenothiazines, and cerebrovascular accidents. Hypokalemia may cause a minimally prolonged QRS duration. Arrhythmias are rare with hypokalemia unless the patient is receiving digitalis. In this case, hypokalemia enhances the arrhythmogenic effects of digitalis.

HYPERCALCEMIA

Hypercalcemia may be due to hyperparathyroidism, hypophosphatasia, hypervitaminosis D, idiopathic hypercalcemia, or iatrogenic overdose with rapid infusion of calcium. Hypercalcemia shortens phase 2 of the action potential and therefore shortens the QT interval by shortening the ST segment. It may be difficult to diagnose hypercalcemia on the electrocardiogram in sinus rhythm, because the QT interval may be normal and only the ST segment is shortened (Fig. 11-4). The most common effect of hypercalcemia is on the sinus node, with

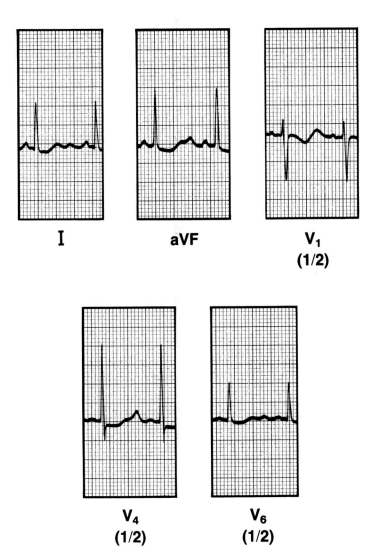

FIG. 11-3. Hypokalemia. These tracings are from a 4-year-old with the nephrotic syndrome. Note the prominent U waves in all leads with ST depression and T wave inversion in leads I, aV$_F$, V$_4$, and V$_6$.

slowing of the sinus rate, sinoatrial block, or sinus arrest. AV block and ventricular arrhythmias are uncommon unless the patient is taking digitalis. In this case, hypercalcemia potentiates digitalis effect and digitalis-induced arrhythmias.

HYPOCALCEMIA

Hypocalcemia can be due to malabsorption, hypoparathyroidism, vitamin D deficiency, stress in the newborn period, or iatrogenic lack of intake. This causes a prolongation of phase 2 of the action potential and prolongation of the ST segment on the electrocardiogram. Hypocalcemia, therefore, has a different effect from hypokalemia, which

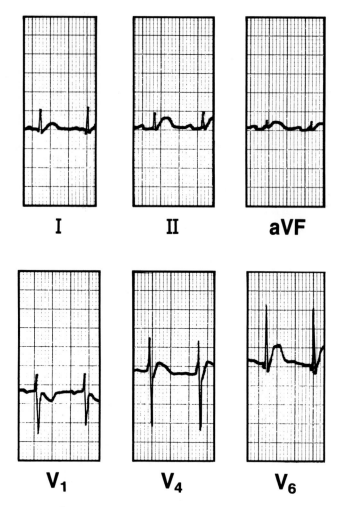

FIG. 11-4. Hypercalcemia in a 1-year-old who had an iatrogenic overdose of calcium. The QT interval is short due to the absence of the ST segment.

prolongs phase 3. In hypokalemia, the onset of the T wave occurs at the normal time, the T wave duration (including the U wave) is prolonged, and the QT (or QU) interval is prolonged. In hypocalcemia, the T wave duration is normal and the QT interval is prolonged because there is a prolonged ST segment and a prolonged *onset* of the T wave (Fig. 11-5). The interval from the onset of the QRS to the onset of the T wave (Q-OT interval) correlates well with serum calcium in newborn babies (see Fig. 6-17). In prematures, the normal corrected Q-OT (Q-OT/square root of the RR) is 0.20 or less, and in full term infants it is 0.19 or less.[4] On the basis of these parameters, if the Q-OT$_C$ interval is normal, the serum calcium concentration is normal in 98% of babies; if the Q-OT$_C$ is prolonged, 70% are hypocalcemic with a total serum calcium concentration less than 7.5 mg/dl. The remainder of the infants with a prolonged Q-OT$_C$ interval have undergone severe neonatal stress.[5] Although patients with hypocalcemia have a prolonged QT interval, arrhythmias are rare, perhaps because repolarization is

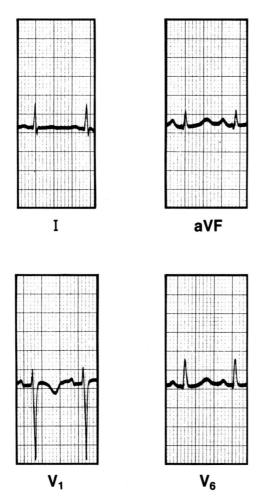

FIG. 11-5. Hypocalcemia in a 13-year-old with the nephrotic syndrome. The ST segment is long. The Q-OT$_C$ interval is prolonged at .24, and the QT$_C$ interval is prolonged at .46.

uniformly prolonged throughout the ventricles. AV block may occasionally occur.

HYPERMAGNESEMIA

Hypermagnesemia decreases the upstroke velocity of the action potential and shortens the duration of phase 2, simulating hypercalcemia. Isolated hypermagnesemia produces few changes on the electrocardiogram, although individual cases of prolonged PR interval and interventricular conduction delay have been reported.[6]

HYPOMAGNESEMIA

The effects of hypomagnesemia on the action potential and the electrocardiogram are similar to those of hypokalemia. In newborns, hypomagnesemia may coexist with hypocalcemia. In these infants, the electrocardiographic pattern is similar to combined hypocalcemia and hypokalemia: prolonged plateau and slower descent. These produce a summation of effects to delay repolarization and therefore large U waves are observed with flattened T waves.

HYPERNATREMIA AND HYPONATREMIA

In the tissue bath, the effects of sodium on the action potential are considerable with an increased sodium concentration causing an increase in the slope of phase 0 (increased $\dot{V}$max) and prolonged phase 3. A decrease in sodium concentration causes the opposite effect. However, in the range of serum sodium concentrations that are physiologically possible in the body, these effects are not usually seen on the electrocardiogram. The effects of sodium may be demonstrated in the patient with a prolonged QRS duration due to quinidine or hyperkalemia, in whom sodium infusion improves interventricular conduction and shortens the QRS duration.

HYPOGLYCEMIA

The electrocardiographic changes of hypoglycemia are thought to be caused by the associated hyperkalemia that is frequently present. In hypoglycemia, insulin secretion is inhibited and hyperkalemia may result.

HYPOXIA AND ACIDOSIS

The effects on the action potential of hypoxia and acidosis are similar to those of increased extracellular potassium and the changes may be due, in part, to leakage of potassium out of the cell.[7] The QRS duration prolongs, as does the QT interval. All types of atrial and ventricular arrhythmias may occur in addition to AV block.

Antiarrhythmic Drugs

DIGITALIS

Digitalis shortens phase 2 of the action potential and also shortens the action potential duration. The ST-T wave changes can be explained by the effect of digitalis to hasten repolarization. Digitalis tends to cause all layers of the ventricle to repolarize simultaneously, resulting in greater cancellation of the repolarization vector and flat

T waves. With moderate amounts of digitalis effect, primarily the onset of repolarization is affected, as represented in the ST segment. The ST segment is depressed most in the leads facing the left ventricle; taller R waves are generally associated with more ST depression.[7] The late part of repolarization is still unaffected. Therefore, the terminal parts of the T waves are normal and concordant with the QRS complex, although the overall QT_C interval may be shortened (Fig. 11-6A). With increasing amounts of digitalis effect, the entire process of repolarization is reversed (from endocardium to epicardium) and the same leads with ST depression also show T wave inversion. The T waves are coved and the descending limb of the ST segment and T wave has an angle of 90° with the ascending limb (Fig. 11-6B).[3]

The effect of digitalis on impulse formation and conduction results from a combination of direct and vagotonic effects. The cellular basis of these effects has been reviewed by Reder and Rosen.[8] The overall effect of digitalis is to slow the sinus rate, speed intra-atrial conduction, decrease atrial automaticity, and prolong AV conduction. This may be manifest on the electrocardiogram as sinus bradycardia and a prolonged PR interval.

Digitalis toxicity results in further slowing of the sinus rate, sino-atrial block or sinus arrest, and second-degree AV block (usually type 1—Wenckebach) or third-degree AV block. These manifestations are more common in children than those that result in increased atrial, junctional, or ventricular automaticity, namely, premature atrial contractions, supraventricular tachycardia, nonparoxysmal junctional tachycardia, premature ventricular contractions, or ventricular tachycardia.[9,10] If AV block and premature ventricular contractions occur on the same electrocardiogram, digitalis toxicity should be suspected (Fig. 11-7). Digitalis toxicity (especially associated with hypokalemia) has been associated with "bidirectional tachycardia." This has the morphology of constant complete right bundle branch block with alternating right axis deviation and left axis deviation (Fig. 11-8). Bidirec-

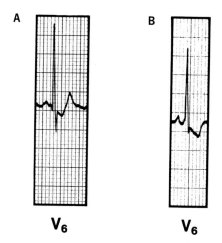

FIG. 11-6. Digitalis effect. A, ST depression with normal terminal portion of the T wave. B, Coved initial portion, with complete inversion of the T wave.

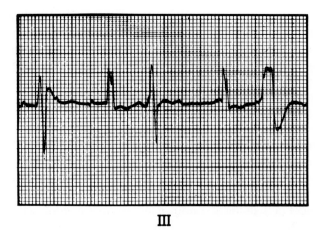

III

FIG. 11-7. Digitalis intoxication. Complete AV block with idioventricular escape rhythm (second and fourth QRS complexes) and multiform premature ventricular contractions (first, third, and fifth QRS complexes).

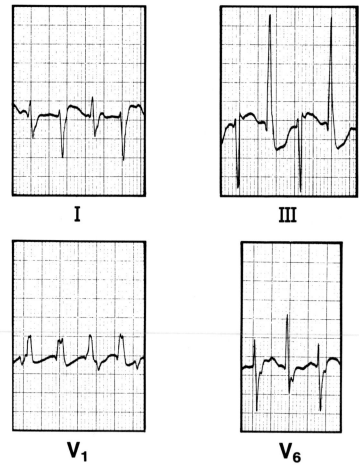

I   III

V₁   V₆

FIG. 11-8. Bidirectional tachycardia in a 5-year-old child. This was due to digitalis intoxication and hypokalemia. There is constant right bundle branch block in lead V_1 with alternating right axis and left axis deviation shown in the limb leads.

tional tachycardia is probably ventricular tachycardia with alternating exit pathways, rather than junctional tachycardia with alternating bundle branch block.[11]

QUINIDINE, PROCAINAMIDE, AND DISOPYRAMIDE

These drugs are class I antiarrhythmic agents and have similar actions. Quinidine's effects will be used as examples of the other type I agents. Quinidine decreases the upstroke velocity (reduced $\dot{V}$max) of all action potentials, prolongs phase 3 (resulting in a prolonged action potential duration), and reduces automaticity. The decreased upstroke velocity results in interventricular conduction delay and a prolonged QRS duration. This may result in a diffusely widened QRS, or a specific right or left bundle branch block pattern. The effects on the T waves are both "secondary" (to the interventricular conduction delay) and "primary" (due to prolongation of the action potential). Since the terminal part of repolarization is most affected, the early part of the T wave may have decreased amplitude and the terminal part may be increased. This is difficult to distinguish from a U wave. The QT (or QU) interval is prolonged. Because of its vagolytic properties, quinidine may shorten the PR interval slightly.

Quinidine toxicity is manifest on the electrocardiogram as the following: (1) A decreased atrial rate usually due to sinoatrial exit block; (2) prolongation of the P wave duration due to intra-atrial conduction delay; (3) prolongation of the PR interval due to prolongation of His-Purkinje conduction; (4) prolongation of the QRS complex to 125% or more of the original QRS duration (Fig. 11-9); (5) further prolongation of

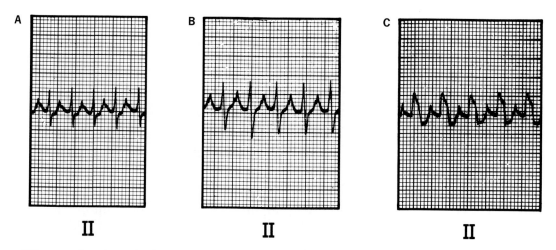

FIG. 11-9. Procainamide effect and toxicity. A, Before medication, this 5-month-old girl had supraventricular tachycardia due to an atrial ectopic focus at a rate of 270/min. The QRS duration was .05 sec. B, After 70 mg of procainamide, the rate slowed to 225/min and the QRS duration increased to .08 sec. C, After 80 mg of procainamide, the rate did not change, but the QRS duration increased to .10 sec with a pattern of left bundle branch block.

the QT interval due to an increase in refractory period dispersion throughout the ventricles;[12] and (6) premature ventricular contractions and ventricular tachycardia.[13] The ventricular tachycardia in quinidine toxicity may have a similar morphology to that sometimes found in other patients with prolonged QT intervals and is called "Torsade de Pointes" (Fig. 11-10).[14]

LIDOCAINE AND PHENYTOIN

These drugs increase the slope of phase 0 (increase V̇max) in diseased tissue (improving conduction) and shorten action potential duration but have very little effect on the surface electrocardiogram. Rarely with high doses of phenytoin the PR and QT intervals may shorten due to accelerated AV conduction and shortened ventricular refractoriness. If phenytoin is given to a patient with a prolonged QT interval for prevention of ventricular tachycardia, effective antiarrhythmic treatment may occur without shortening the QT interval.[15]

PROPRANOLOL

Propranolol decreases the upstroke velocity of phase 0 (reduces V̇max), shortens the action potential duration, and decreases automaticity. In the patient, propranolol's effects are mainly antiadrenergic. The sinus rate is slowed, the PR interval is prolonged, and the QT interval may be shortened. Similar to phenytoin, propranolol may not shorten the QT interval in a patient with a prolonged QT interval, but it may be effective in preventing ventricular tachycardia and sudden death.[15]

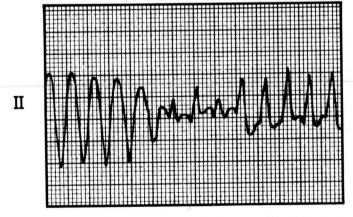

FIG. 11-10. Torsade de Pointes due to quinidine toxicity. The tachycardia has two different polarities, separated by a narrower transition QRS.

VERAPAMIL

Verapamil is a calcium antagonist with primary effects on the sinus node and AV node. It decreases the slope of phase 0 (reduced V̇max), prolongs the action potential duration, and reduces automaticity. The electrocardiographic findings are a slowed sinus rate and prolonged PR interval.

Anesthetic Agents

Halothane decreases the action potential duration slightly by increasing the slope of phase 2 and phase 3. These effects are rarely seen on the electrocardiogram but occasionally the QT interval is shortened and there may be a decrease in T wave amplitude. Halothane sensitizes the heart both to vagal and sympathetic stimulation. Therefore, bradycardia and ventricular arrhythmias may occur. Methoxyflurane, teflurane, and enflurane have effects on the electrocardiogram similar to those of halothane.

Chloroform, ethyl chloride (given by inhalation), trichloroethylene, and cyclopropane all may cause ventricular arrhythmias. Diethyl ether and other ethers have no effect on the electrocardiogram.[16]

Psychotropic Drugs

Phenothiazines cause shift of potassium inside the cell, thus decreasing the extracellular potassium and therefore prolonging phase 3 of the action potential.[17] These changes are similar to those found with quinidine: The T waves have reduced amplitude with prominent terminal depolarizations. It is difficult to distinguish a U wave from broad notched T waves with an increased terminal component. The QT (or QU) interval is prolonged.[18] In therapeutic doses, arrhythmias are rarely observed with phenothiazines, but in overdosage ventricular arrhythmias may occur.

The electrocardiographic changes with tricyclic antidepressants occur in 20% of adult patients taking the drugs. The most common manifestations are sinus tachycardia, prolonged PR interval, and flat T waves. Less commonly observed are QRS prolongation, QT prolongation, and ST-T wave changes. Overdosage with tricyclic antidepressants may cause any atrial or ventricular arrhythmias or AV block.[19]

Imipramine (Tofranil) causes an imbalance of intracellular and extracellular potassium with an increase in serum potassium. In one reported case of an overdosage in a child, atrial flutter, AV block, interventricular conduction delay, and ventricular tachycardia were observed in the same patient.[20]

Organophosphorous Insecticides

Poisoning with organophosphorous insecticides causes inhibition of acetylcholinesterase and pseudocholinesterase, resulting in a buildup of acetylcholine. Clinically, poisoning has been traditionally thought to have two electrophysiologic effects—an early intense sympathetic discharge, resulting in sinus tachycardia followed by a parasympathetic discharge which may last several days and results in sinus bradycardia and AV block. Recently, a third phase has been described which can occur as late as five days after the poisoning. It is marked by prolongation of the QT interval and Torsade de Pointes ventricular tachycardia.[21]

Central Nervous System Effects

CONGENITAL PROLONGATION OF THE QT INTERVAL

Jervell and Lange-Nielsen[22] and Romano[23] and Ward[24] described syndromes that have in common congenital prolongation of the QT interval, syncope or sudden death, and hereditary transmission. In the Jervell-Lange-Nielsen syndrome, the hearing is abnormal and the heredity is autosomal recessive; in the Romano-Ward syndrome, the hearing is normal and the heredity is autosomal dominant. The electrocardiograms are similar. The T waves may be inverted or biphasic and may vary in both shape and amplitude from minute to minute. The T waves frequently have bizarre shapes with greater amplitude at the terminal portion of the T wave (Fig. 11-11).

Although the exact mechanism of the prolonged QT interval is uncertain, central and peripheral nervous system sympathetic imbalance is involved. Normally, innervation to the heart is asymmetric: Fibers project from the right hypothalamus to the right stellate ganglion and supply the anterior surface of the cardiac ventricles; fibers from the left hypothalamus project to the left stellate ganglion and supply the left lateral and posterior wall of the cardiac ventricles. Experimental stimulation of the left stellate ganglion prolongs the QT interval and causes ST depression.[7] In patients with a congenitally prolonged QT interval, left stellate ganglionectomy may shorten the QT interval and eliminate episodes of syncope, adding strength to the concept of neural imbalance as a cause of this syndrome.

CENTRAL NERVOUS SYSTEM INJURY

In children with moderate to severe head trauma or those who have undergone neurosurgical procedures, the electrocardiogram has

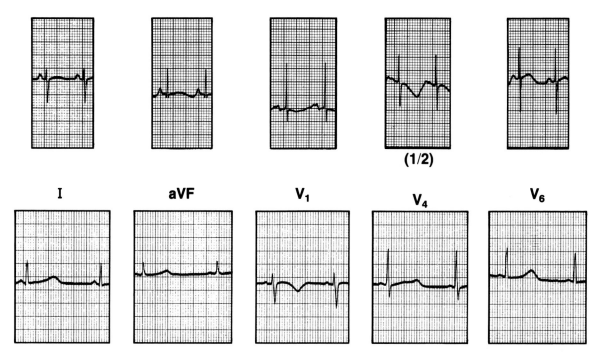

FIG. 11-11. Congenital prolongation of the QT interval. **Top** tracings, From a 9-day-old infant with a history of ventricular tachycardia and ventricular fibrillation at the age of 4 days. All the T waves are abnormal; the T waves in lead V_4 (at half standard) are especially bizarre, however. **Bottom** tracings, From a 12-year-old child who had his first episode of syncope at age 10. He was being treated for a "familial seizure disorder," although the actual cause of the "seizures" was probably ventricular tachycardia. Note that the terminal portion of the T wave in lead V_4 is greater in amplitude than the initial portion.

been reported to be abnormal in 75%.[25] The most common abnormalities are a prolonged QT interval with either notched, bizarre-shaped T waves or prominent U waves. Occasionally, the T waves are diffusely flattened in the lateral leads or even inverted with ST depression.[26] ST elevation is rare in central nervous system lesions but has been reported.[27] "J" or "Osborne" waves are occasionally found (see "Hypothermia" in this chapter). These repolarization changes are thought not to be due to increased intracranial pressure but rather to differential stimulation or suppression of the cortical representations of the sympathetic fibers. In some patients with central nervous system lesions, there is evidence at autopsy for cardiac abnormalities, primarily subendocardial ischemia. Identical lesions can be produced by catecholamine infusion.[28]

Any arrhythmia can occur with central nervous system injury. Vagal tone is enhanced and there may be alternating sympathetic stimulation. The bradyarrhythmias (sinus bradycardia, wandering atrial pacemaker, junctional rhythm, and type 1 second-degree AV block) generally respond to atropine, supporting the theory of their central vagal origin. Sinus tachycardia may occur in addition to any of the pathologic tachyarrhythmias.

Hypothermia

A J wave (or Osborne wave) occurs on the electrocardiogram of patients with a body temperature below 25° C. This is a slowly inscribed extra deflection between the QRS and the early ST segment (Fig. 11-12).[29] The PR and QT intervals prolong and there may be ST depression or ST elevation. Initially, the sinus node slows but at approximately 29°, 50 to 60% of adult patients with hypothermia have atrial fibrillation.

Neuromuscular Disorders

The electrocardiogram in Duchenne's progressive muscular dystrophy is abnormal in about 75% of patients. The abnormalities are most specific to Duchenne's and occur less frequently in the other forms of muscular dystrophy.[30] The usual findings are tall R waves in the right precordial leads (with or without interventricular conduction delay) and deep narrow Q waves in the left precordial leads (Fig. 8-4). These changes are thought to be due to selective scarring of the posterobasal left ventricle, rather than right ventricular hypertrophy, pulmonary hypertension, or septal hypertrophy.[31] The scarring could be due to continued stress on the left AV ring due to poor support of the mitral valve from abnormal cardiac muscle. These electrocardiographic changes do not correlate with the degree of involvement in the skeletal muscles or the degree of cardiomyopathy. Late in the disease, when cardiomyopathy is present, any type of active arrhythmias may occur—sinus tachycardia, premature atrial contractions, atrial flutter, premature ventricular contractions, or ventricular tachycardia.

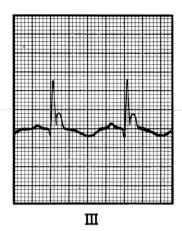

III

FIG. 11-12. Hypothermia. This tracing was taken from a 3-month-old with hypothermia and severe brain damage. The J wave is the rounded, second portion of the QRS complex. The heart rate is slow for an infant of this age. The PR interval, QRS duration, and QT interval are also prolonged.

In Friedreich's ataxia, the electrocardiogram is abnormal in 90% of the patients, most commonly manifesting QRS-T discordance; 20% have asymmetric septal hypertrophy as the cause of deep Q waves in the lateral precordial leads.[19] Either left ventricular hypertrophy or right ventricular hypertrophy may also occur. The arrhythmias are similar to those in muscular dystrophy.

The electrocardiogram in myotonic dystrophy is abnormal in about half of the patients, with low voltage P waves, prolonged PR interval, left axis deviation, left bundle branch block, and ST-T wave changes. Atrial fibrillation is common.

Connective Tissue Disease

In patients with scleroderma or systemic lupus erythematosus, pulmonary hypertension may cause right ventricular hypertrophy and systemic hypertension may cause left ventricular hypertrophy. In addition, ST elevation and T wave changes may occur from pericarditis. Chronic pericarditis with fibrin insulation or diffuse myocardial fibrosis may lead to low voltage QRS complexes. Supraventricular tachycardia, ventricular tachycardia, AV block, and bundle branch block are common in later stages of these diseases.

Metabolic Diseases

HYPOTHYROIDISM

The classic sign of hypothyroidism is the "mosque" sign (appropriately originally described in Turkey by Ertugrul in 1966)[32]: a dome-shaped symmetric T wave with an absent ST segment (Fig. 11-13). This was present in 37% of children with hypothyroidism. Therefore, if present, the mosque sign is helpful in the diagnosis; if it is absent, the patient still may have hypothyroidism. Low voltage of the P waves, QRS complexes, and T waves is also common and most likely due to myocardial edema, rather than myxomatous pericarditis which is exceedingly rare.[33] Sinus bradycardia occurs in children with hypothyroidism, usually after 3 years of age.

HYPERTHYROIDISM

The majority of children with hyperthyroidism have sinus tachycardia, and approximately 50% have left ventricular hypertrophy.[34] Less commonly observed are prolonged PR interval, nonspecific ST-T wave changes, and right bundle branch block. These changes may take up to a year to reverse after the patient becomes euthyroid.

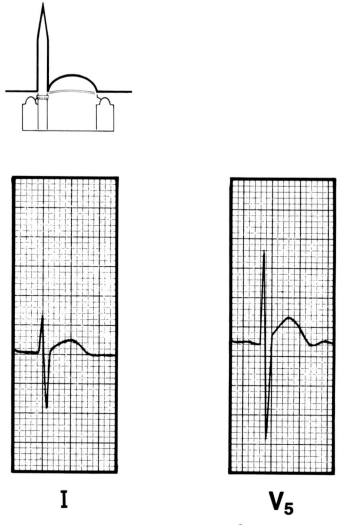

I   **V₅**

FIG. 11-13. Hypothyroidism. The "mosque" sign is demonstrated by an absence of the ST segment and a symmetrically rounded T wave.

ADRENAL INSUFFICIENCY

Patients with adrenal insufficiency may have QT prolongation with inverted T waves. These changes can be reproduced in adrenalectomized animals, but when the hearts are removed from the body, the cardiac action potentials are normal.[3] These changes are therefore thought to be due to autonomic imbalance.

PHEOCHROMOCYTOMA

Excess catecholamines are responsible for the prolonged QT interval and T wave inversion occasionally encountered in patients with pheochromocytoma.

Miscellaneous Diseases

PERITONEAL INFLAMMATION

Peritonitis, appendicitis, and ileus may be associated with nonspecific ST-T wave changes. These are thought to be due to vagally mediated reflexes.[3]

SARCOID

The granulomas of sarcoidosis have a predilection for the conduction system. The most common lesions are complete AV block and right bundle branch block. Premature atrial contractions and premature ventricular contractions also occur.[19]

Self-Assessment Questions

Question 1: A prolonged QT (or QU) interval can be produced by which *ones* of the following:

A. hypercalcemia
B. hypokalemia
C. hypermagnesemia
D. quinidine
E. phenothiazines
F. Jervell-Lange-Nielsen
G. CNS injury
H. hypothyroidism
I. pheochromocytoma

Question 2: AV block (first-, second-, or third-degree) can be produced by which *ones* of the following:

A. hypokalemia
B. hypomagnesemia
C. digitalis
D. propranolol
E. halothane
F. CNS injury
G. neuromuscular disease
H. hypothyroidism

Question 3: Bundle branch block can be produced by which *ones* of the following:

A. hypermagnesemia
B. hyponatremia

C. hyperkalemia
D. hypokalemia
E. hypoglycemia
F. phenytoin
G. quinidine
H. myotonic dystrophy
I. hypothyroidism

Question 4: A short QT interval can be produced by which *ones* of the following:

A. hyperkalemia
B. hypercalcemia
C. digitalis
D. quinidine
E. CNS injury
F. pheochromocytoma

Question 5: ST-T wave changes can be produced by which *ones* of the following:

A. hypokalemia
B. hypomagnesemia
C. digitalis
D. halothane
E. tricyclic antidepressants
F. CNS injury
G. neuromuscular disease
H. hypothyroidism
I. peritoneal irritation

Question 6: A 2-day-old infant had the electrocardiogram recorded in the top tracings. In the bottom tracings, the same infant is shown after resolving the problem. Which systemic effect most likely resulted in the top tracings (Fig. 11-14)?

A. digitalis intoxication
B. hypercalcemia
C. Romano-Ward
D. hyperkalemia
E. phenothiazines

Question 7: Which systemic effect most likely resulted in this electrocardiogram (Fig. 11-15)?

A. hypermagnesemia
B. sarcoid
C. digitalis
D. imipramine
E. verapamil

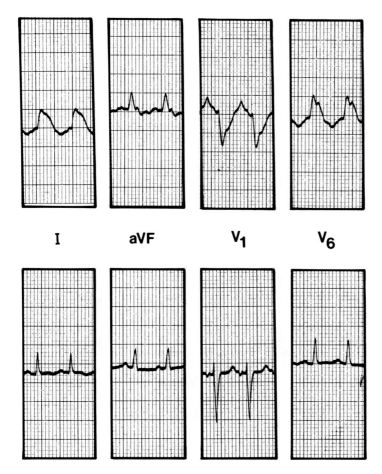

I   aVF   V$_1$ V$_6$

FIG. 11-14.   Question 6.

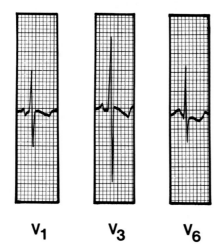

V$_1$ V$_3$ V$_6$

FIG. 11-15.   Question 7.

Question 8: Which systemic effect most likely resulted in this electro-cardiogram (Fig. 11-16)?

A. hyperkalemia
B. Jervell-Lange-Nielsen
C. digitalis
D. halothane
E. phenytoin

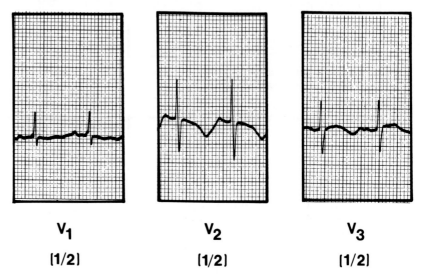

V_1

[1/2]

V_2

[1/2]

V_3

[1/2]

FIG. 11-16.   Question 8.

Answers to Self-Assessment Questions

Answer 1: B, D, E, F, G, I
Systemic effects causing a prolonged QT, or QU, interval are: hypoka-lemia, hypocalcemia, hypomagnesemia, quinidine, phenothiazines, tricyclic antidepressants, Jervell-Lange-Nielsen syndrome, Romano-Ward syndrome, CNS injury, adrenal insufficiency, and pheochromo-cytoma.

Answer 2: C, D, F, G
Systemic effects causing AV block are: hyperkalemia, hypercalcemia, hypocalcemia, hypermagnesemia, hypoglycemia, hypoxia, digitalis, quinidine, propranolol, verapamil, tricyclic antidepressants, imipra-mine, CNS injury, neuromuscular disease, hyperthyroidism, and sarcoid.

Answer 3: C, D, E, G, H
Systemic effects causing bundle branch block are: hyperkalemia, hy-pokalemia, hypoxia, hypoglycemia, tricyclic antidepressants, myo-tonic dystrophy, hyperthyroidism, and sarcoid.

Answer 4: B, C
Systemic effects that may cause a short QT interval are: hypercalcemia, digitalis, phenytoin, propranolol, halothane, and methoxyflurane.

Answer 5: A, C, E, F, G, I
Systemic effects causing ST-T wave changes are hyperkalemia, hypokalemia, hypoglycemia, hypoxia, digitalis, tricyclic antidepressants, CNS injury, neuromuscular disease, systemic lupus erythematosis, hyperthyroidism, adrenal insufficiency, pheochromocytoma, and peritoneal irritation.

Answer 6: D
This electrocardiogram simulates ventricular tachycardia but is actually sinus tachycardia with bundle branch block due to hyperkalemia. All of the other answers are conditions that are prone to ventricular tachycardia but not to bundle branch block.

Answer 7: C
This electrocardiogram demonstrates digitalis effect with a short QT interval and the early part of the T wave inverted. The other answers are conditions that do not affect the T waves.

Answer 8: B
The QT interval is prolonged. All the other answers are conditions that may shorten the QT interval.

References

1. Surawicz B.: Primary and secondary T wave changes. Heart Bull *15*:31–35, 1966.
2. Miller B. L., Dumas P. A., and Victorica B. E.: Office electrocardiography in general pediatrics VII: electrolyte effects. Clin Pediatr *9*:72–78, 1970.
3. Surawicz B.: Relationship between the electrocardiogram and electrolytes. Am Heart J *73*:814–825, 1967.
4. Colletti R. B., Pan M. W., Smith E. W. P., et al.: Detection of hypocalcemia in susceptible neonates: the Q-OT$_C$ interval. N Engl J Med *290*:931–935, 1974.
5. Giacoia C. P., and Wagner H. R.: Q-OT$_C$ interval and blood calcium levels in newborn infants. Pediatrics *61*:877–882, 1978.
6. Cooksey J. D., Dunn M., and Massie E.: Clinical Vectorcardiography and Electrocardiography. 2nd Ed. Chicago, Yearbook Medical Publishers, 1977, pp 9–112.
7. Hoffman J. I. E.: Primary T wave changes in children. Praxis *64*:803–811, 1975.
8. Reder R. F., and Rosen M. R.: Basic electrophysiologic principles: application to treatment of dysrhythmias. In Pediatric Cardiac Dysrhythmias. Edited by P. C. Gillette and A. Garson. New York, Grune & Stratton, 1981, pp 121–143.
9. Larese R. J., and Mirkin B. L.: Kinetics of digoxin absorption and relation of serum levels to cardiac arrhythmias in children. Clin Pharmacol Ther *15*:387–396, 1974.
10. Hayes C. J., Butler V. P., and Gersony W. M.: Serum digoxin studies in infants and children. Pediatrics *52*:561–568, 1973.
11. Morris S. N., and Zipes D. P.: His bundle electrocardiography during bidirectional ventricular tachycardia. Circulation *48*:32–38, 1973.
12. Di Segni E., Klein H. O., David D., et al.: Overdrive pacing in quinidine syncope and other long QT interval syndromes. Arch Intern Med *140*:1036–1040, 1980.
13. Castellanos A., and Salhanick P.: Electrocardiographic patterns of procainamide toxicity. Am J Med Sci *253*:52–60, 1967.

14. Horowitz L. N., Greenspan A. M., Spielman S. R., et al.: Torsades de Pointes: electrophysiologic studies in patients without transient pharmacologic or metabolic abnormalities. Circulation 63:1120–1128, 1981.
15. Schwartz P. J., Periti M., and Malliani A.: The long Q-T syndrome. Am Heart J 89:378–390, 1975.
16. Rollason W. N.: Electrocardiography for the Anesthetist. 3rd Ed. London, Blackwell Scientific Publications, 1976, pp 63–80.
17. Wolpert A., and Farr D.: Psychotropics and their effect on the electrocardiogram in children. Dis Nerv Syst 36:435–436, 1975.
18. Burda C. D.: Electrocardiographic abnormalities induced by Thioridazine (Mellaril). Am Heart J 76:153–156, 1968.
19. Chou T.: Electrocardiography in Clinical Practice. New York, Grune & Stratton, 1979, pp 114–150.
20. Fouron J., and Chicoine R.: ECG changes in fatal imipramine (Tofranil) intoxication. Pediatrics 48:777–781, 1971.
21. Ludomirsky A., Klein H., and Kaplinsky E.: QT prolongation and polymorphous ventricular arrhythmias associated with organophosphorous insecticide poisoning. Am J Cardiol 49:1654–1658, 1982.
22. Jervell A., and Lange-Nielsen F.: Congenital deafmutism, functional heart disease with prolongation of the Q-T interval and sudden death. Am Heart J 54:59–68, 1957.
23. Romano C., Gemme G., and Pongiglione R.: Aritmie cardiache rare dell'eta' pediatric a. II. Accessi sincopali per fibrillazoine ventricolare parossistica. Clin Pediatr 45:656–683, 1963.
24. Ward O. C.: A new familial cardiac syndrome in children. J Irish Med Assoc 54:103–106, 1964.
25. Rogers M.C., Zakha K.G., Nugent S.K., et al.: Electrocardiographic abnormalities in infants and children with neurological injury. Crit Care Med 8:213–214, 1980.
26. Millar K., and Abildskov J. A.: Notched T waves in young persons with central nervous system lesions. Circulation 37:597–603, 1968.
27. Anderson G. J., Woodburn R., and Fisch C.: Cerebrovascular accident with unusual electrocardiographic changes. Am Heart J 86:395–398, 1973.
28. Bordiuk J. M., Gelband H., Steeg C. N., et al.: Electrocardiographic changes in children undergoing pneumoencephalography. Neurology 19:1217–1222, 1969.
29. Emslie-Smith D., Sladden G. E., and Stirling G. R.: The significance of changes in the electrocardiogram in hypothermia. Br Heart J 21:343–355, 1959.
30. Durnin R. E., Ziska J. H., and Zellweger T.: Observations on the electrocardiogram in Duchenne's muscular dystrophy. Helv Paediatr Acta 26:331–339, 1971.
31. Perloff J. K., Roberts W. C., DeLeon A. C., et al.: The distinctive electrocardiogram of Duchenne's progressive muscular dystrophy. Am J Med 42:179–188, 1967.
32. Ertugrul A.: A new electrocardiographic observation in infants and children with hyperthyroidism. Pediatrics 37:669–672, 1966.
33. Malecka-Dymnicka S., and Bittel-Dobrzynska N.: Electrocardiographic changes in children with hyperthyroidism. Pol Med J 5:540–545, 1966.
34. Pilapil V. R., and Watson D. G.: The electrocardiogram in hyperthyroid children. Am J Dis Child 119:245–248, 1970.

12

Arrhythmias

This chapter is divided into two parts, each with a different approach to the diagnosis of an arrhythmia. In the first part, "The Electrophysiologic Approach," the major arrhythmias are discussed according to their site of origin and mechanism. After this overview, which will be helpful in understanding the arrhythmias, a systematic method is presented in the second part, "The Morphologic Approach," which will be helpful in reading the actual electrocardiograms.

Ladder Diagrams

Each tracing is accompanied by a "ladder diagram." These ladder diagrams are presented to simplify the various arrhythmias. Each P wave and QRS complex in the electrocardiogram is included on a ladder diagram. These are drawn on electrocardiographic paper to facilitate comparison.

Each ladder diagram is divided into three vertical sections corresponding to activity in the atrium, AV junction (AV node and His bundle), and ventricle. The vertical distance is arbitrary: 1 cm for each section. The horizontal distance corresponds exactly to the time, or estimated time, the impulse takes to enter and leave either the atrium, AV junction, or ventricle.

Sinus rhythm is diagrammed in Figure 12-1A. Each impulse begins high in the atrium. The PR interval in the middle complex is .10 sec. We have assumed a .04 sec intra-atrial conduction time, leaving .06 sec for conduction time through the AV node and bundle of His. The sum of these two times describes the PR interval. In this example, the intraventricular conduction time (QRS duration) is .08 sec. A prolonged QRS duration (for example, that found in complete left bundle branch block) of .12 sec is diagrammed as a prolonged intraventricular conduction time (Fig. 12-8D). The QRS complex of Wolff-Parkinson-White syndrome is a fusion QRS complex resulting from abnormally rapid atrioventricular conduction through a bundle of Kent and normal AV nodal conduction. This is diagrammed in Figure 12-15.

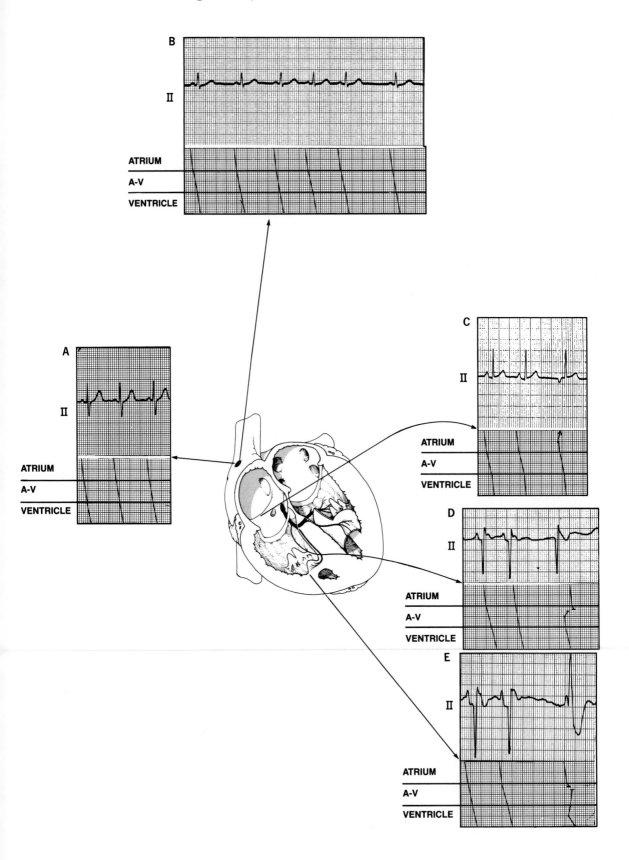

In rhythms that originate from a point in the heart different from the sinus node, a black circle indicates the point of origin; for example, low right atrial (Fig. 12-1C), junctional (Fig. 12-1D), or ventricular (Fig. 12-1E). The cellular mechanism of arrhythmias is not implied in these diagrams. Therefore, although the black circle indicates the site of origin of a rhythm, it does not imply reentry or abnormal automaticity.

If such an abnormal rhythm causes atrial depolarization, an arrow toward the top of the atrium is diagrammed (Fig. 12-1C). Atrial flutter is shown as a prolonged activation of the atria (Fig. 12-37) and atrial fibrillation as a continuous activation of the atria (Fig. 12-39).

Finally, atrioventricular block is diagrammed as a horizontal bar in the region of the AV junction. Block of antegrade impulses that originated in the atria and are not conducted to the ventricles is shown in Figure 12-52. Block of retrograde impulses that originate in the AV junction or ventricle and are not conducted to the atria is shown in Figure 12-3C. The actual site of atrioventricular block (whether within the AV node or His-Purkinje system) is not implied in these diagrams.

All times that are written on ladder diagrams are in seconds. (For example, in Figure 12-8, the RR intervals are .90 and .53 sec. This corresponds to 900 and 530 msec.)

The Electrophysiologic Approach

Arrhythmias in children can be grouped into four major electrophysiologic classes: escape rhythms, premature beats, tachyarrhythmias, and finally, arrhythmias that result from AV block. These are discussed after an introduction to normal sinus rhythm.

FIG. 12-1. Escape rhythms. Each rhythm in this figure is diagrammed with its approximate site of origin. The tracings are taken from children under the age of 3 years. A, Sinus rhythm. A P wave precedes each QRS complex, and the P waves are identical. The RR intervals are regular. The rate is approximately 95/min. The RR intervals vary by less than .04 sec. B, Sinus arrhythmia. Each QRS is preceded by a P wave with the same mean vector. The RR intervals are irregular. The shortest RR interval corresponds to a rate of approximately 95/min, and the longest RR interval corresponds to a rate of approximately 72/min. C, Atrial escape beat. The first two beats are sinus beats at a rate of 100, and then there is a pause. The pause is ended by a beat with an inverted P wave in lead II and a normal QRS. This is an atrial escape beat. It occurs .78 sec after the preceding P wave. This corresponds to a rate of 80/min. D, Junctional escape beat. After two sinus beats at a rate of 120/min, a pause follows, which is ended by a QRS complex that has a morphology similar to the preceding QRS complexes. No P wave precedes the escape beat. This is therefore a junctional escape beat. This occurs at a cycle length of .9 sec following the preceding QRS complex. This corresponds to a rate of 67/min. Note in the ladder diagram that the time of origin of the junctional escape beat occurs before the visible QRS on the surface electrocardiogram. The time of activation of the ventricles in the ladder diagram corresponds to the onset of the QRS complex. This diagram implies that the origin of the escape beat is in the AV junction and that approximately 20 to 40 msec are required for the impulse to conduct from the His bundle to the ventricles, thus beginning the QRS complex. E, After two sinus beats at a rate of 85/min, there is a pause, which is ended by a QRS complex that is different from the sinus QRS complexes. This is a ventricular escape beat. It occurs 1.15 sec after the preceding QRS complex. This corresponds to a rate of 54/min. The ventricular escape beat is preceded by a sinus P wave. One can see from the sinus beats preceding the escape beat that the normal PR interval is .16 sec. Therefore, for a P wave to conduct to the ventricles in this patient requires approximately .16 sec. The P wave preceding the ventricular escape beat occurs .07 sec before the QRS complex. Thus, although the sinus P wave occurs before the ventricular escape beat, the P wave does not cause the QRS complex, since it requires approximately another .09 sec for the P wave to reach the ventricles and they have already been depolarized by the ventricular escape beat at this time.

SINUS
RHYTHM

The sinus node is normally the most rapid pacemaker in the heart. Since it is located high in the right atrium, impulses originating from the sinus node produce P waves that are positive in leads I and aV_F. In normal sinus rhythm a P wave precedes each QRS complex. The P wave morphology may vary slightly but the mean vector of sinus P waves must be between 0 and $+90°$. The rate is normal for the age of the patient (see Appendix, Table A-2). The rhythm is regular with a variation in rate of .08 sec or less between RR intervals.

ESCAPE BEATS
AND ESCAPE RHYTHMS

An escape beat is one that originates from normal pacemaking tissue at a rate that is normal for that tissue. Normal inherent automaticity is present not only in the sinus node, but also in areas in the atria, AV junction (probably the His bundle), and ventricular Purkinje system (see Chapter 2). Normally, the sinus node suppresses the "subsidiary pacemakers" in the atria, AV junction, and ventricle. However, if the sinus node is suppressed (most commonly by output from the vagus nerve), an escape beat will result from the next highest pacemaking tissue in the hierarchy (i.e., the atrium is faster than the AV junction, which is faster than the ventricle) (Fig. 12-1). If two or more beats in a row occur from a subsidiary pacemaker, this is called an "escape rhythm."

The rate of escape rhythms depends not only on the site of origin but also on the age of the child. It is known that newborns with congenital complete AV block have a junctional escape rhythm.[1] This rhythm does not develop because of sinus suppression but rather because of a lack of conduction of atrial impulses to the ventricles. The junction is therefore the highest pacemaker available to pace the ventricles. The rate of this junctional rhythm usually varies between 50 and 80/min.[2,3] In older children, the junctional escape rate varies between 40 and 60/min.[4,5] The data for normal atrial and ventricular escape rates are not available in children; therefore, the figures in Table 12-1 are approximate. The rates of escape rhythms vary with sympathetic influence, just as the sinus node does, increasing with exercise and decreasing with sleep.

Sinus
Arrhythmia

In the strict sense of the word, sinus arrhythmia may be seen as an escape rhythm. Within the sinus node, there may be pacemaking cells with several different rates. With sinus arrhythmia, it is possible that the most rapid cells are cyclically depressed, with respiration allowing

TABLE 12-1. *Rates of Normal Escape Rhythms*

	AGE	
	Newborn–3 yr	Over 3 yr
Atrial	80–100/min	50–60/min
Junctional	50–80/min	40–60/min
Ventricular	40–50/min	30–40/min

Abbreviations: min—minute; yr—years

the slightly slower cells to become the pacemakers. Still, since all these cells are within the sinus node, the P wave morphology does not change. Therefore, in sinus arrhythmia there is a similar mean vector of the P waves that precede each QRS complex, but the P wave rate is irregular with more than .08 sec variation in PP interval (Fig. 12-1).

Atrial
Escape

If the entire sinus node is suppressed, the next most rapid normal pacemakers are in the atria. If the suppression occurs for one beat, the result is an atrial escape beat; if the suppression continues, an atrial escape rhythm may develop. Since these pacemaking cells are necessarily slower than the sinus node, in an atrial escape rhythm, the rate is slower than the sinus rate. A P wave still precedes each QRS complex, but the P wave morphology and mean vector are different from sinus rhythm (Figs. 12-1 and 12-2).

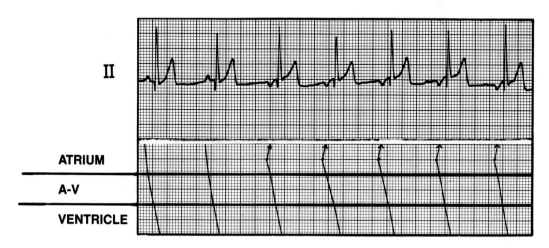

FIG. 12-2. Atrial escape rhythm. This tracing is taken from a 2-year-old child. There is mild sinus bradycardia in the first two beats with a rate of 72/min. An atrial escape rhythm then begins with an inverted P wave in lead II, indicating the site of origin low in the atria. The rate of the escape rhythm is between 75 and 80/min. Note the black dot in the ladder diagram, indicating a site of origin in the atria other than the sinus node. The arrow indicates that the atria are depolarized by this rhythm.

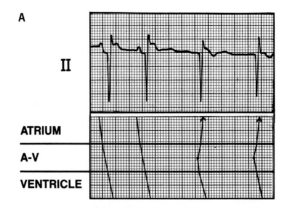

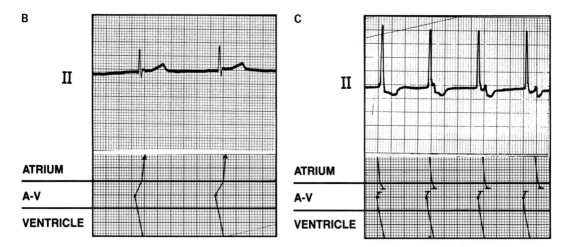

FIG. 12-3.   Junctional escape rhythms. A, Junctional rhythm without visible P waves. The tracing is taken from a 2-year-old child. Following two sinus beats, two successive QRS complexes are seen without preceding P waves. This is a junctional escape rhythm. It occurs at a rate of approximately 72/min. In the ladder diagram, it is assumed that there are no visible P waves because they are "buried" in the QRS complex. That is, they occur at exactly the same time as the QRS complexes. It is also possible that the sinus P waves block in the antegrade direction and cannot depolarize the ventricles since they have already been depolarized by the junctional escape rhythm. It is possible, from this tracing, that the atria were depolarized retrogradely by the junctional rhythm (see B, below) but that the retrograde conduction time was so short that no visible P wave appeared on surface electrocardiogram. The diagram could have been drawn to show retrograde block of the junctional impulse not conducting to the atrium (see C). A final possibility is that there was a profound sinus bradycardia and no atrial activity occurred after the last sinus P wave. This would be much rarer than the preceding two possibilities. B, Junctional rhythm with retrograde P waves. The tracings are from a 6-year-old. An inverted P wave follows each QRS complex. The rate is 50/min. C, Junctional rhythm with sinus bradycardia and AV dissociation. The tracings are taken from a 2-year-old. The junctional rate is absolutely regular at 84/min. The atrial rate is 75/min and unrelated to the junctional rate. The P waves appear to "walk through" the QRS complexes. These P waves are positive in lead II, indicating a sinus origin. It is not immediately apparent that a P wave forms the upstroke of the first QRS complex, but inspection of the three other QRS complexes reveals that the beginning of the complex is different when the P wave is not immediately preceding it.

Junctional
Escape

If both the sinus node and atria are suppressed, a junctional escape beat (Fig. 12-1) or junctional escape rhythm may develop at a rate slower than the atrial rhythm. Each QRS complex is not preceded by a

P wave. Junctional rhythm originates in the bundle of His and conducts to the ventricles with a normal QRS complex; if this rhythm also conducts retrogradely through the AV node, it will excite the atria beginning from the region of the AV node. If the retrograde conduction time through the AV node is rapid, the P waves may be "buried" within the QRS complexes and no P waves are visible (Fig. 12-3A) or a "retrograde" P wave may be visible following each QRS complex (Fig. 12-3B). If there is no retrograde conduction through the AV node, then the junctional rhythm will conduct only to the ventricles and not disturb the atria. In a junctional escape rhythm due to sinus bradycardia, if there is no retrograde conduction, sinus P waves can be seen at their own rate completely dissociated from the QRS complexes (Fig. 12-3C). A slow junctional or ventricular escape rhythm is only one cause of "AV dissociation," which literally means that the P waves and QRS complexes are unrelated. The other two causes of AV dissociation are junctional tachycardia and AV block.[6] Since there are three causes for AV dissociation and any of the three, or all of the three, may occur simultaneously in the same patient, it is not sufficient to write "AV dissociation" as the interpretation on an electrocardiogram. The abnormality causing the AV dissociation must also be specified.

Ventricular
Escape

If the sinus node, atria, and AV junction are suppressed, then the last subsidiary pacemaker to take over is in the ventricles. Depending on whether this is a single beat or multiple beats, this is called either a ventricular escape beat or an idioventricular rhythm. Unlike the preceding rhythms, in this rhythm, the QRS complex is different from the sinus QRS, indicating the origin from the ventricles (Figs. 12-1 and 12-4). Similar to junctional rhythm, in an idioventricular rhythm, there may be either no visible P waves, or retrograde P waves may follow each QRS complex, or sinus P waves may be completely dissociated from the QRS complexes.

Escape with
Aberrancy

Any of the supraventricular escape rhythms may conduct to the ventricles with aberrancy (Fig. 12-5). Since it is impossible on the surface electrocardiogram to distinguish junctional rhythm with aberrancy from an idioventricular rhythm, if the QRS complex is wide and not preceded by a P wave, it is designated as having a ventricular origin (see "The Morphologic Approach" in this chapter).[7] This is an arbitrary decision but it eliminates interpretations such as "junctional rhythm with aberrancy or idioventricular rhythm." If the aberrant QRS has the same morphology as the QRS on conducted beats, then this can be diagnosed as junctional with aberrancy.

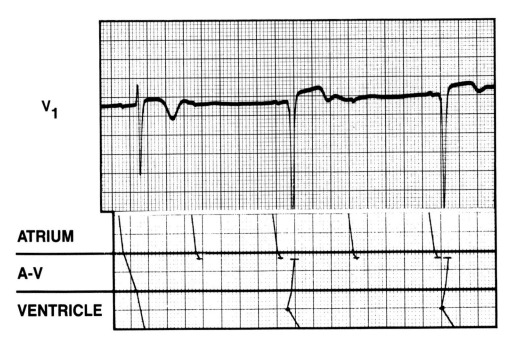

FIG. 12-4. Ventricular escape rhythm. The tracing is taken from an 11-year-old. The atrial rate is 72/min. The first QRS complex is conducted from the atria. This QRS has a normal duration and morphology. The remaining atrial beats are not conducted, indicating high grade AV block. Two successive QRS complexes with a morphology different from the sinus QRS occur at a rate of 36/min. A sinus P wave precedes each of the escape QRS complexes, but these P waves are not conducted to the ventricles. If the P waves had conducted and caused these QRS complexes, the QRS complexes should have the same morphology as the conducted QRS in the first beat. Also, the PR interval on conducted beats is usually similar or may get progressively longer. The PR interval on the conducted beat is .20 sec. The PR interval preceding the first ventricular escape beat is .17 sec and preceding the second ventricular escape beat is .14 sec. If we know that the first beat was conducted and required .20 sec to reach the ventricles, it is doubtful that the second and third QRS complexes were conducted in a shorter time. This shortening in PR interval also suggests AV dissociation and that the P waves do not cause the following QRS complexes.

Wandering Pacemaker

In normal children, whether awake or asleep, the pacemaker frequently shifts from sinus to atrial to junctional. This is called "wandering pacemaker" (Fig. 12-5). The pacemaker normally does not shift into the ventricles. Therefore, ventricular escape beats and idioventricular rhythm are abnormal and indicate decreased automaticity in the AV junction, since the AV junction should always depolarize before the ventricles.

Sinus Bradycardia

Sinus bradycardia can be defined as an abnormally low sinus rate on either routine electrocardiogram (see Appendix, Table A-2) or on 24-hour electrocardiogram while asleep. On 24-hour electrocardiogram, an abnormally slow sinus rate (counted over 6 sec) is 60/min for a baby, 50/min for a child, and 40/min for a teenager (see Fig. 12-6).[8]

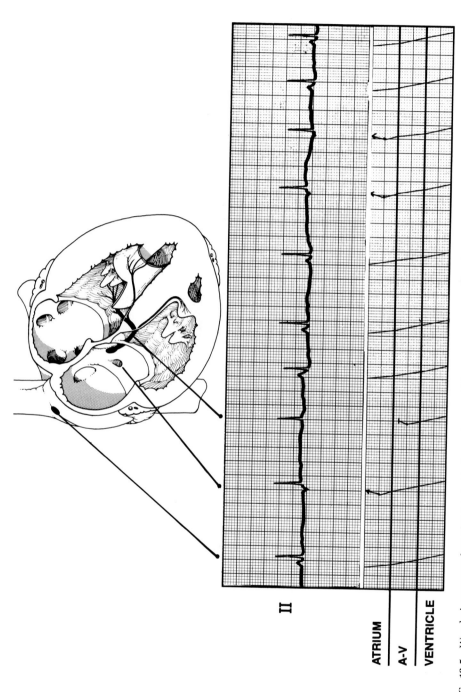

II

ATRIUM

A-V

VENTRICLE

FIG. 12-5. Wandering pacemaker. This tracing is from a 7-year-old boy. The approximate site of origin of each of the beats is diagrammed. All of these beats have a supraventricular origin since the QRS complexes are narrow and have a similar morphology. The first three beats are a sinus beat, followed by an atrial escape beat, followed by a junctional escape beat. The remaining beats are sinus and atrial beats. The RR intervals correspond to rates varying from 58 to 88/min.

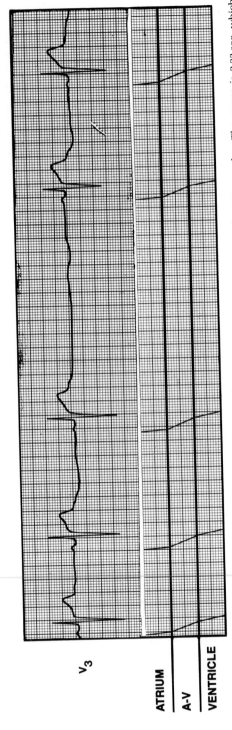

FIG. 12-6.   Sinus bradycardia. This tracing is taken from a 16-year-old boy. A P wave precedes each QRS complex. The pause is 3.32 sec, which corresponds to a sinus rate of 18/min.

Sinus bradycardia not only indicates disease of the sinus node, but it may also indicate loss of subsidiary pacemakers. For example, an infant with sinus bradycardia at a rate of 45/min also may have decreased atrial and AV junctional automaticity since the AV junction should be firing at least at 50/min. If an escape rhythm occurs at a rate below the lower limit for age and site of origin, this should be designated as bradycardia. For example, a newborn with a junctional rate of 40/min should be designated as having "junctional bradycardia."

CAUSES OF ESCAPE RHYTHMS. It is important to emphasize that most children with escape rhythms are normal. Junctional rhythm occurred for at least 3 consecutive beats in 19% of normal newborns and 45% of healthy teenagers on 24-hour electrocardiogram.[3–5] In the majority, this occurred at night and was explained by a normal increase in vagal tone. Junctional rhythm rarely occurs in normal children when awake.[3–5] The more extreme bradyarrhythmias are usually caused either by abnormally heightened vagal tone such as that found in increased intracranial pressure or by right atrial disease such as that found following Mustard's operation for transposition of the great arteries where the sinus node, atrial muscle, and AV junction (all right atrial structures) are diseased and the manifestation of the disease is reduced automaticity. The causes of escape bradyarrhythmias are listed in Table 12-2.

PREMATURE
BEATS

A premature beat is defined as a depolarization of the atrium, AV junction, or ventricle that occurs "earlier" than would normally be expected from its site of origin. Thus, the difference between an escape beat and a premature beat is that the escape beat occurs at a normal cycle length for a particular age and site of origin, whereas the premature beat occurs with a shorter cycle length than the escape beat (Figs. 12-7 and 12-8). The criteria for prematurity are inexact because the degree of sympathetic tone may vary. This definition of a premature beat is independent of the underlying rhythm. In a regular

TABLE 12-2. *Causes of Escape Rhythms*

ACUTE

Abnormally increased vagal tone (increased intracranial pressure, increased blood pressure, pharyngeal stimulation, ocular pressure, abdominal distention, idiopathic), hypoxia, hypothermia hypercalcemia, hypoglycemia

CHRONIC

Normal variant
Trained athletes
Surgery: following any open heart procedure, especially atrial operations
Drugs: digitalis or propranolol effect

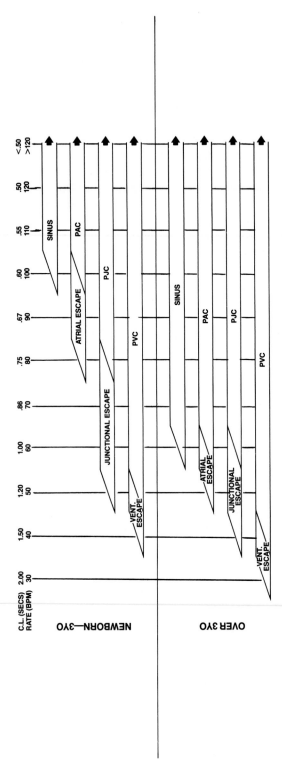

FIG. 12-7. Approximate rates for distinguishing between a normal escape beat and an abnormal premature beat. The rates are only approximate. Note that the transition points are inexact since they depend on sympathetic tone. See Figure 12-8 for an example in the use of this chart. BPM, beats per minute; C.L., cycle length; PAC, premature atrial contraction; PJC, premature junctional contraction; PVC, premature ventricular contraction; SECS, seconds; YO, years old.

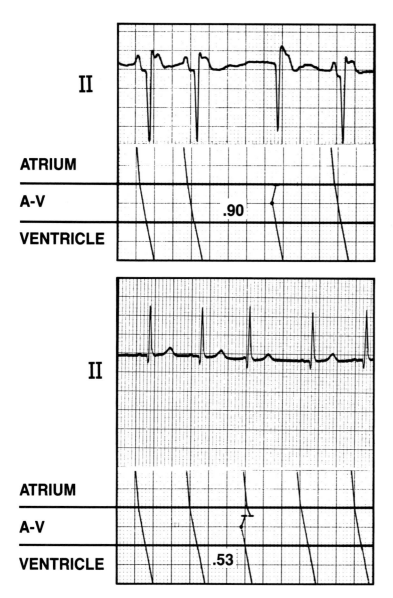

FIG. 12-8. Escape beat versus premature beat. **Top,** Junctional escape beat in a 2-year-old child. After two sinus beats at a rate of 120/min, a junctional escape beat occurs .90 sec after the preceding QRS complex. This corresponds to a rate of 67/min. **Bottom,** Premature junctional contraction in a 2-year-old child. Following two sinus beats at a rate of 110/min, a QRS occurs .53 sec after the preceding QRS. This corresponds to a rate of 113/min. The QRS complex has the same morphology as the sinus QRS but is not preceded by a premature P wave. This is therefore a premature junctional contraction. There is a sinus P wave, which is almost buried in the QRS complex. Since the sinus P wave has already depolarized the atria, the premature junctional contraction cannot conduct retrogradely to the atria.

sinus rhythm at a normal rate, there is usually no difficulty in distinguishing a premature beat; the premature beat occurs at least .09 sec before the next expected sinus beat.[7] However, in the case of an irregular rhythm, it is not possible to tell when the next expected beat should occur and a premature beat must be diagnosed by whether it is "too early" for a normal escape beat. What is "too early" depends upon the site of origin and the age of the patient (Fig. 12-7).

Premature beats may originate from either the atrium, AV junction, or ventricle. While the manifestations of these beats on the electrocardiogram only indicate an electrical "depolarization" and not necessarily "contraction" of the heart, the terminology of "premature contraction" is so ingrained that it is used here.

Premature Atrial Contractions

A premature atrial contraction is manifest on the surface electrocardiogram as a premature P wave. Premature atrial contractions usually have a different morphology and mean vector from sinus P waves.

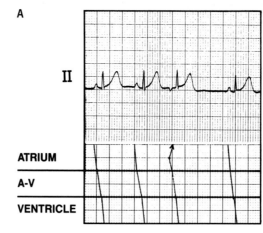

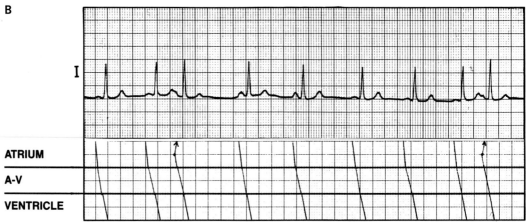

FIG. 12-9. A, Tracing taken from a 6-year-old. Following two sinus P waves, a premature P wave occurs .56 sec after the preceding P wave. This has a different mean vector and morphology from the sinus P waves and is a premature atrial contraction. This conducts to the ventricle, causing a normal supraventricular QRS complex. B, Tracing taken from an 8-year-old showing premature atrial contractions with sinus arrhythmia. The underlying rhythm is slightly irregular with RR intervals varying from .82 sec to .94 sec. In the underlying rhythm, a P wave with a similar mean vector precedes each of the QRS complexes, indicating that the underlying rhythm is sinus arrhythmia. Intermittently, the PP interval and RR interval shorten abruptly to .47 sec. These are premature atrial contractions, since they occur "too early" for normal atrial rhythm in an 8-year-old (see Fig. 12-7).

C

II

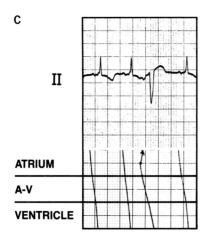

D

III

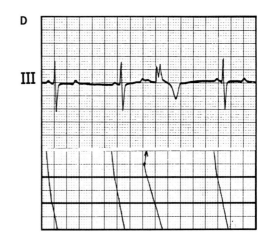

ATRIUM

A-V

VENTRICLE

FIG. 12-9. Cont'd C, Tracing taken from a 6-month-old showing premature atrial contraction with aberration. Following two sinus P waves, a premature P wave occurs, which is buried in the preceding T wave. At first glance, this appears to be a premature ventricular contraction; however, the preceding premature P wave indicates that this is a premature atrial contraction. D, Tracing taken from a 13-year-old showing premature atrial contraction with aberration. The buried P wave is even more subtle in this tracing.

In regular sinus rhythm at a normal rate, a P wave that occurs more than .08 sec before the next expected P wave is a premature atrial contraction (Fig. 12-9A). However, in a patient with sinus arrhythmia, a premature atrial contraction can be distinguished from an atrial escape beat by its timing (Fig. 12-9B). Normal atrial escape rates should be less than 100/min (cycle length longer than .6 sec) in a newborn. This means that if a nonsinus P wave (P wave mean vector +91 to −1°) occurs less than .6 sec after the preceding P wave, this is a premature atrial contraction (Figs. 12-7 and 12-9). If a nonsinus P wave occurs more than .6 sec after the preceding P wave, it is an atrial escape beat. In a child older than 3 years, the atrial escape rate should be less than 60/min (cycle length over 1.0 sec). Therefore, if a nonsinus P wave occurs less than 1.0 sec after the preceding P wave, it is a premature atrial contraction. If a nonsinus P wave occurs more than 1.0 sec after the preceding P wave, this an atrial escape beat (Figs. 12-7 and 12-9).

A premature atrial contraction may be conducted to the ventricles normally (premature P wave followed by a premature normal QRS complex), or it may be conducted with ventricular aberration if the impulse is able to conduct through the AV node but finds one of the bundle branches refractory (premature P wave followed by a wide QRS complex) (Fig. 12-9). In children, since the refractory periods of the bundle branches are so similar, premature atrial contractions may be conducted with either right bundle branch block or left bundle branch block aberration.[9] If the T waves preceding aberrant QRS complexes are not searched for buried P waves, these beats will be diagnosed incorrectly as premature ventricular contractions. Finally, a premature atrial contraction may be blocked (usually in the AV node) and not conduct to the ventricles at all (premature P wave not followed by a QRS). This is called a "nonconducted" or "blocked" premature atrial contraction (Fig. 12-10). If a blocked premature atrial contraction occurs after every sinus beat, this is called "blocked atrial bigeminy."

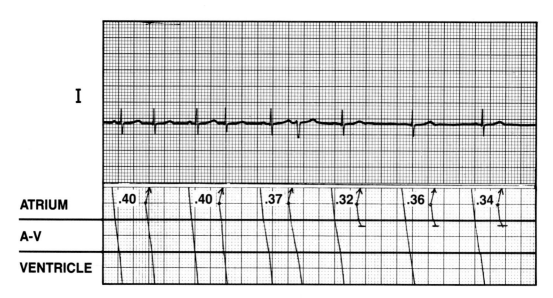

I

ATRIUM

A-V

VENTRICLE

FIG. 12-10. Blocked premature atrial contractions. The tracing is taken from a 1-day-old infant. The first beat is of sinus origin. This is followed by a premature atrial contraction. The baseline is completely flat immediately following the sinus T wave, after which there is a slight undulation in the baseline, indicating the premature P wave of the premature atrial contraction. This conducts to the ventricle normally. The premature atrial contraction occurs .40 sec after the preceding P wave. This sequence is repeated in the next two beats. Following the third sinus beat, the T wave is more peaked, indicating the premature P wave. This occurs .37 sec after the preceding P wave and conducts to the ventricles with aberration. This would be called a premature ventricular contraction if the T wave were not carefully searched for the P wave. It is possible that many cases of supposed premature ventricular contractions in newborns could actually represent premature atrial contractions with aberrancy, since the P waves may be difficult to find. Following the aberrant QRS, another sinus beat occurs. The sinus T wave has a different shape than the other sinus T waves, which indicates that a P wave is buried in the T wave. The premature P wave occurs .32 sec after the preceding sinus P wave. This is too early for conduction to the ventricles to occur, so the premature P wave is not followed by a QRS complex. This is called a "blocked premature atrial contraction." Blocked premature atrial contractions occur following the next two sinus beats. This simulates sinus bradycardia.

Frequently, the blocked P wave occurs within the T wave and the only clue to the diagnosis is that every other T wave has a different shape (Fig. 12-11). This is frequently misdiagnosed as sinus bradycardia.

CAUSES OF PREMATURE ATRIAL CONTRACTIONS. Most often, premature atrial contractions are idiopathic. They occur in 14% of normal infants (all having less than 12 premature beats per hour) and 13% of normal children on 24-hour electrocardiograms.[3-5] Other causes of premature atrial contractions are listed in Table 12-3.

Premature Junctional
Contractions

A premature junctional contraction is manifest on the surface electrocardiogram as a premature normal QRS complex (similar to the sinus QRS complex) that is not preceded by a premature P wave (Fig. 12-8A). A sinus P wave may occur before a premature junctional contraction but in this case the P wave is not premature. Premature junctional contractions may originate in the AV node or bundle of His so they are collectively referred to as "junctional."[10] A premature junc-

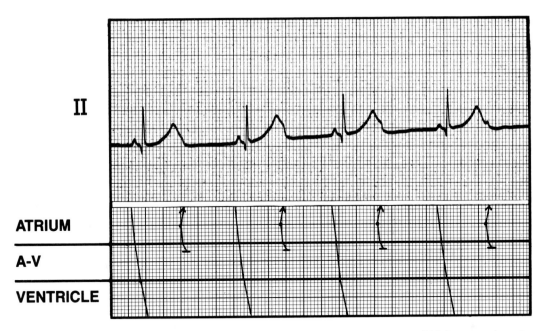

II

ATRIUM

A-V

VENTRICLE

FIG. 12-11. Blocked atrial bigeminy. After each sinus beat, there is a premature P wave which is not conducted to the ventricles. Although this is not immediately apparent in the first beat, with each successive beat the premature P wave becomes more obvious. In retrospect, the first T wave has an abrupt change in slope, which is not characteristic of normal T waves. This simulates sinus bradycardia.

tional contraction can be distinguished from a junctional escape beat by its timing (Fig. 12-8). In a newborn, the junctional escape rate should be less than 80/min (cycle length over .75 sec). Therefore, if a normal QRS without a preceding premature P wave occurs less than .75 sec after the preceding QRS complex, it is a premature junctional contraction (Fig. 12-7). If it occurs more than .75 sec after the preceding QRS complex, it is a junctional escape beat. In a child older than 3 years, the junctional escape rate should be less than 60/min (cycle length over 1.0 sec). If a QRS without a preceding premature P wave occurs less than 1.0 sec after the preceding QRS, it is a premature junctional contraction. If it occurs later than 1.0 sec after the preceding QRS, it is a junctional escape beat (Fig. 12-7).

TABLE 12-3. *Causes of Premature Atrial Contractions and Premature Junctional Contractions*

ACUTE

Mechanical (central venous pressure monitor), hypokalemia, hypercalcemia, hypoxia, hypoglycemia

Drugs: digitalis, sympathomimetic amines, imipramine

CHRONIC

Otherwise normal heart, atrial enlargement

Surgery: following atrial surgery

If a premature junctional contraction conducts to the ventricles with aberration, this appears on the surface electrocardiogram as a premature wide QRS complex without a preceding premature P wave. Because it is impossible to distinguish between a premature junctional contraction with aberration and a premature ventricular contraction, we have arbitrarily classified all such beats as premature ventricular contractions.

CAUSES OF PREMATURE JUNCTIONAL CONTRACTIONS. Premature junctional contractions are much less common than premature atrial contractions. The causes for both types of beats are similar (see Table 12-3). This would be expected since the AV node and proximal bundle of His are atrial structures (see Chapter 1).

Premature Ventricular Contractions

A premature ventricular contraction is manifest on the surface electrocardiogram as a premature abnormal QRS (not similar to the sinus QRS complex) that is not preceded by a premature P wave. A sinus P wave may occur before a premature ventricular contraction but in this case the P wave is not premature. Premature ventricular contractions may originate from either ventricle. In general, premature ventricular contractions that originate from the right ventricular free wall have left bundle branch morphology and those that originate from the septum or left ventricle have right bundle branch morphology. However, the relationship between morphology and site of origin is not exact enough to predict one from the other in an individual case.[11,12] This is because, for example, in a premature depolarization that begins in the right ventricle, activation of the left ventricle is delayed, and the pattern is similar to the left bundle branch block. While most premature ventricular contractions have a prolonged duration for the age of the patient, some premature ventricular contractions are not absolutely prolonged but do have a different morphology from the sinus QRS (Fig. 12-12). Premature ventricular contractions may show "fusion," thus confirming their ventricular origin.[13] A fusion complex is one in which the QRS morphology is intermediate between two QRS morphologies. In any case of fusion, it is important to identify the two "pure" QRS morphologies showing that the fusion complex has characteristics of both (Fig. 12-13). In order for fusion of QRS complexes to occur, the ventricles must be activated simultaneously from two different directions. In sinus rhythm, if fusion occurs between a normal QRS and a different QRS, the complexes with the different morphology must have originated in the ventricles in order to collide with the normal QRS which originated in the His bundle. Therefore, if premature beats show fusion, they are premature ventricular contractions. By the same logic, fusion could occur between two types of premature ventricular contraction. In contrast, fusion would not be seen if a sinus beat occurred at about the same time as a premature junctional contraction because each would produce the same QRS with activation via the His bundle.

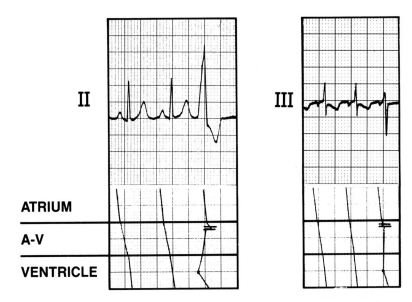

FIG. 12-12. Premature ventricular contractions. Left, Tracing taken from a 2-year-old. Following two sinus beats, a premature QRS complex occurs which has a different morphology from the sinus QRS complexes. The QRS duration of the premature QRS is .14 sec. It is not preceded by a premature P wave. We can assume that the normal sinus QRS occurred on time and did not conduct to the ventricles because a premature QRS complex depolarized the ventricles and part of the AV conduction system. Right, "Narrow premature ventricular contraction." This tracing is taken from a 3-day-old infant. Following two sinus beats, there is a premature QRS complex. The duration of the premature QRS complex is .06 sec, which is longer than the .04 sec of the sinus QRSs; however, it is still normal duration for the age of the patient. The important distinguishing point is that the QRS complex has a different morphology from the sinus QRS complexes. The premature QRS is preceded by a P wave. This is not a premature P wave but the normal sinus P wave.

A premature ventricular contraction can be distinguished from a ventricular escape beat by its timing. In a newborn, the ventricular escape rate should be less than 50/min (cycle length over 1.2 sec) (Fig. 12-7). Therefore, if an abnormal QRS without a preceding premature P wave occurs less than 1.2 sec after the preceding QRS complex, it is a premature ventricular contraction. If it occurs more than 1.2 sec after the preceding QRS complex, it is a ventricular escape beat. In a child older than 3 years, the ventricular escape rate should be less than 40/min (cycle length over 1.5 sec). Therefore, if an abnormal QRS complex without a preceding premature P wave occurs less than 1.5 sec after the preceding QRS complex, it is a premature ventricular contraction. If it occurs more than 1.5 sec after the preceding QRS complex, it is a ventricular escape beat (Fig. 12-7).

CAUSES OF PREMATURE VENTRICULAR CONTRACTIONS. Southall et al. found premature ventricular contractions to be approximately equal in frequency to premature atrial contractions in the newborn period.[3-5] They occur in 1 to 2% of normal newborns or older children on routine electrocardiogram. In older children with an otherwise normal heart, approximately 26% had premature ventricular contractions on 24-hour electrocardiograms.[3-5] The other common causes of premature ventricular contractions are shown in Table 12-4.

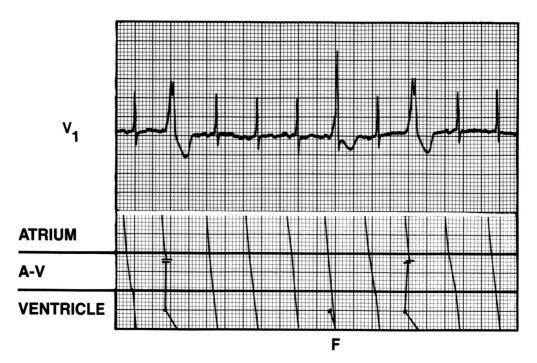

FIG. 12-13. Premature ventricular contractions: fusion. The second and eighth beats are premature ventricular contractions. The sixth beat is a fusion complex (labelled "F"). Note that the beginning of the fusion complex is similar in morphology to the beginning of the premature ventricular contraction. On the ladder diagram, the ventricle begins depolarization with the premature ventricular contraction. The end of the fusion QRS complex is similar to the normal sinus QRS. Also on the ladder diagram, the ventricular depolarization of the fusion is shown ending with the sinus QRS. Therefore, the fusion complex occurs from depolarization via two sites, one from the premature ventricular contraction and the other from conduction of the normal sinus P wave.

Differential Diagnosis
of Premature Beats

If a QRS complex is premature and has the same morphology as the sinus beats, it is either a premature atrial contraction or a premature junctional contraction. If there is a preceding premature P wave (look carefully in the T wave), the diagnosis is premature atrial contraction; it not, the diagnosis is premature junctional contraction.

TABLE 12-4. *Causes of Premature Ventricular Contractions*

ACUTE

Mechanical (catheters or pacing wires), hypoxia, hypoglycemia, hyperkalemia, hypokalemia, hypercalcemia

Drugs: toxic manifestations of digitalis, quinidine, sympathomimetic amines, halothane, phenothiazines, tricyclic antidepressants, imipramine

CHRONIC

Otherwise normal heart, structural congenital heart disease (especially postoperative), cardiomyopathy, myocarditis, congenitally prolonged QT interval, ventricular tumor

If a QRS complex is premature and has a different morphology from the sinus QRS, there are four possibilities. The only one of these in which the QRS is preceded by a premature P wave is a premature atrial contraction with aberration. One method that has been used to distinguish a premature atrial contraction with aberrancy from a premature ventricular contraction is the effect on the prevailing rhythm. Premature ventricular contractions were thought to produce a fully compensatory pause in the rhythm (i.e., the sum of the RR interval before the premature beat plus the RR interval after the premature beat is equal to twice the RR interval of the prevailing rhythm) (Fig. 12-14). Premature atrial contractions were thought to produce less than a compensatory pause.[6] Although this is generally true, exceptions are frequent enough to render it invalid (Fig. 12-14).[15]

If there is not a preceding premature P wave, the diagnosis could be either a premature junctional contraction with aberrancy (which cannot be proven on surface electrocardiogram), a premature ventricular contraction, or intermittent antegrade conduction through a Kent bundle (intermittent Wolff-Parkinson-White). If there is no preceding P wave, the diagnosis is premature ventricular contraction. However, if there is a preceding sinus P wave, it could be either a late diastolic premature ventricular contraction or intermittent conduction over a Kent bundle with a short PR interval and abnormal QRS complex. The transition to Kent bundle conduction may occur gradually over several beats showing several intermediate fusion QRS morphologies between the normal and the preexcited QRS. The maximally preexcited QRS complex should occur at the end of the sequence (Fig. 12-15). The change to Kent bundle conduction usually accompanies a change in rate of the prevailing rhythm, either with an increase or a decrease in the rate. Inspection of prior electrocardiograms in sinus rhythm with obvious Wolff-Parkinson-White may reveal a similar morphology. The diagnosis of premature ventricular contractions is more certain if there is no rate change or if there are single premature beats all with a similar morphology. If any of these beats occur without a preceding P wave, then all are likely to be premature ventricular contractions.

A special situation in the differential diagnosis exists when the supraventricular rhythm is not sinus, but atrial flutter or atrial fibrillation. In this case, since it is not possible to identify the preceding premature P wave, this criterion cannot be used to differentiate between the premature wide QRS complex due to aberrancy of the supraventricular rhythm and the premature wide QRS complex due to a premature ventricular contraction. Schamroth has listed four different points that are applicable to children.[16] Favoring aberrant conduction of the supraventricular rhythm are the following: (1) A relatively fast mean ventricular rate. Premature ventricular contractions tend to occur more often with slower ventricular rates. (2) QRS variability. The rapid atrial impulses occur during all stages of the cardiac cycle and therefore encounter different phases of recovery in the conduction system. This results in varying degrees of aberrancy. Premature ventricular contractions, on the other hand, usually have one or two fixed patterns. (3) Variation of coupling interval. Premature ventricular contractions usually have fixed coupling. (4) No attempt at a compensa-

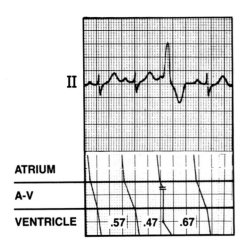

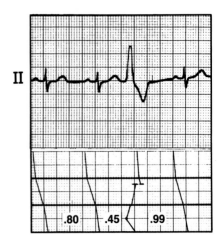

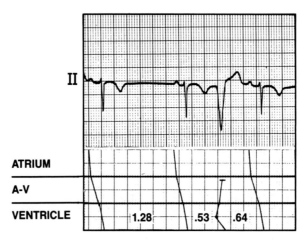

FIG. 12-14. Premature ventricular contractions. **Top left,** Premature ventricular contraction with fully compensatory pause. Following two sinus beats with an RR interval of .57 sec, a premature ventricular contraction occurs .47 sec after the preceding QRS complex. There is a pause following the premature ventricular contraction of .67 sec until the next sinus QRS complex. The interval from the last sinus QRS to the premature beat of .47 sec plus the interval from the premature beat to the next sinus QRS of .67 sec is 1.14 sec. This is exactly twice the basic sinus interval of .57 sec. The reason for this fully compensatory pause can be seen in the ladder diagram. The sinus P wave occurs at the normal time. This slightly precedes the premature QRS. Since the atrium and AV node are already depolarized by the sinus P wave, the premature QRS does not conduct retrogradely to the atrium. Therefore, the atrial activity is not disturbed and the normal sinus P wave occurs on time, thus resulting in a fully compensatory pause. **Top right,** Premature ventricular contraction with less than a compensatory pause. Two sinus beats occur with an RR interval of .80 sec. The premature ventricular contraction occurs .45 sec later, and the pause following the premature ventricular contraction results in an RR interval of .99 sec. The interval from the last sinus QRS to the premature beat of .45 sec plus the interval from the premature beat to the next sinus QRS of .99 sec is 1.44 sec. This is less than twice the sinus RR interval of .80 sec. The reason for the less than fully compensatory pause is sinus arrhythmia. This is diagrammed on the ladder diagram as a variation in the PP interval. **Bottom,** Interpolated premature ventricular contraction. The premature ventricular contraction occurs .53 sec after the last sinus QRS. The next sinus QRS occurs .64 sec after the premature ventricular contraction. These intervals add up to less than a single normal RR interval. In this case, there is much less than a compensatory pause. In fact, the sinus rhythm is not disturbed at all. In order for this to occur, the premature ventricular contraction does not conduct back to the atrium, and it also occurs early enough that the next sinus P wave can be conducted to the ventricles. The prematurity interval (.53) plus the interval to the next sinus QRS (.64) is even less than the basic sinus interval (1.28). This is because of sinus arrhythmia.

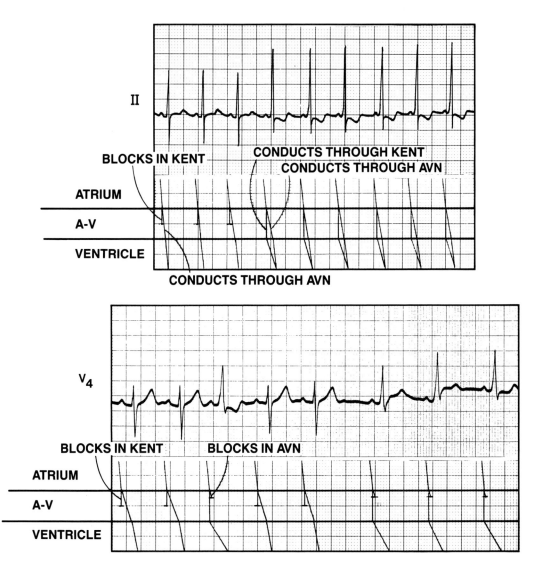

FIG. 12-15. Intermittent Wolff-Parkinson-White simulating premature ventricular contractions. **Top,** The first three beats are sinus rhythm and are normally conducted. The PR interval is .12 sec. As can be seen in the ladder diagram, these three beats do not conduct through the Kent bundle but conduct normally through the AV node. Beginning with the fourth beat, the PR interval shortens to .08 sec. The QRS complex has a slightly different morphology and the T wave is completely different. As shown in the ladder diagram, there is no delay of the atrial impulse through the Kent bundle, and this conducts directly to the ventricular myocardium initiating the QRS complex. The end of the QRS is somewhat similar to the sinus QRS, and this is therefore drawn as a fusion beat. The ventricles are activated both via the Kent bundle and the AV node-His bundle. **Bottom,** The first two beats are normal with a PR interval of .17 sec. These block in the Kent bundle and are conducted through the AV node. The third beat has a PR interval of .14 sec. In the ladder diagram, this has been drawn as if it conducts only through the Kent bundle and blocks completely in the AV node. It is possible that there was some AV nodal conduction, but the QRS complex is so different from the sinus QRS that at least most of the QRS was formed by conduction via the Kent bundle. Then there are two beats that conduct through the AV node, followed by three that conduct through the Kent bundle. The PR interval in the beats that conduct through the Kent bundle is not abnormally short for a 4-year-old child (.14 sec). However, it is shorter than the PR interval in normally conducted beats. It is possible that these are premature ventricular contractions. However, since the PR interval in the three successive aberrant beats at the end of the tracing is constant despite a variation in the PP interval, this indicates that the atria and ventricles are related and that each P wave is probably causing the following QRS complex. The most likely explanation for this is conduction through a Kent bundle.

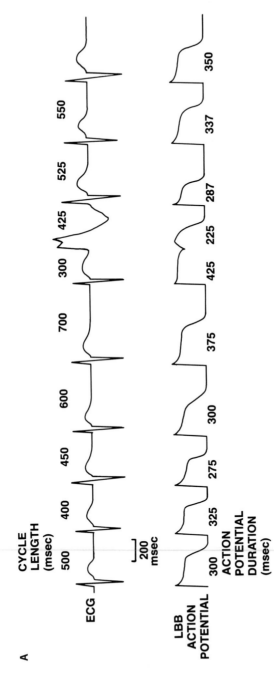

FIG. 12-16. Atrial fibrillation with premature ventricular contractions. A. Explanation of "Ashman" phenomenon. A hypothetical lead I electrocardiogram is shown during atrial fibrillation. The RR intervals in milliseconds (msec) are shown. Below is a corresponding drawing of a left bundle branch (LBB) intracellular action potential. Note that the action potential duration depends upon the preceding cycle length (e.g., the action potential duration of the second beat is 325 msec). This depends on the RR interval of 500 msec. The action potential of the third beat is shorter—275 msec—because the preceding RR interval of 400 msec is shorter. The cycle length preceding the sixth beat is the longest. This should give rise to an action potential duration of 425 msec. However, an impulse passes through the AV node and arrives at the left bundle branch 300 msec after the last impulse. This finds the left bundle branch partially refractory since it occurs on the downslope of the action potential. The resultant action potential of the early beat is slowly conducted and results in a left bundle branch block pattern on the surface electrocardiogram. Thus, the short cycle following a long cycle caused the aberrancy.

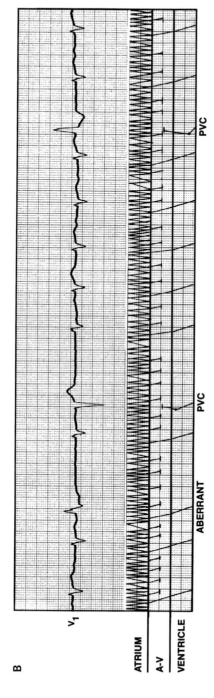

FIG. 12-16. Cont'd B, The RR interval is irregularly irregular and no two RR intervals are the same. This fact, combined with the absence of discrete atrial activity, makes for the diagnosis of atrial fibrillation. There are three beats that occur with short preceding cycle lengths and have QRS complexes that differ from the normal QRS. These could be either conducted beats with aberration or premature ventricular contractions. Each of these three beats has features that are compatible with either diagnosis. Each beat is followed by a pause that could be taken as a "compensatory pause." This would favor the diagnosis of a premature ventricular contraction. However, each beat follows a relatively long pause and could therefore be a supraventricular beat conducted with aberration due to the "Ashman" phenomenon. The fact that all three beats have a different morphology favors at least some of them being aberrant conduction. An intracardiac electrophysiologic study was performed on this patient and the morphology of these beats was identified. The first in the series is an aberrantly conducted supraventricular impulse. The last two are premature ventricular contractions. These are multiform premature ventricular contractions. In the ladder diagram, these are diagrammed as originating from different sites in the ventricles. However, it is known that these could actually originate from the same site but have different conduction, causing them to appear multiform.

tory pause. Premature ventricular contractions are usually followed by a compensatory pause. Finally, aberrant beats tend to occur if a short cycle follows a particularly long cycle. This is known as the "Ashman phenomenon" (Fig. 12-16A).[6] The refractory period of cardiac structures (e.g., the bundle branches) is dependent upon the action potential duration of the preceding beat. The action potential duration is dependent upon the duration of the interval that precedes the beat: the longer the preceding interval, the longer the action potential is. Therefore, if there is a long interval, the beat that terminates the long interval will have a long action potential duration. If a beat then occurs at a short cycle length immediately following the long cycle length, this will encounter a prolonged action potential duration that may not be completely repolarized. If this incompletely repolarized structure is, for example, the right bundle branch, the early beat will conduct with right bundle branch block aberration (Fig. 12-16).

In practice, it may be quite difficult to distinguish between aberrant conduction of atrial flutter or atrial fibrillation and premature ventricular contractions on the surface electrocardiogram (Fig. 12-16). With intracardiac electrophysiologic study, the differentiation can be made. We have resorted to such study in two patients and have found that each patient had both aberrantly conducted beats and premature ventricular contractions.

In describing premature beats, it is important to note their morphology, whether they occur in patterns, and their coupling interval.

Morphology of Premature Beats:
Uniform versus Multiform

Premature P waves that have the same shape in the same graphic lead are said to be "uniform" premature atrial contractions; if more than one morphology of premature P wave occurs, these are multiform premature atrial contractions (Fig. 12-17A). Similarly, premature abnormal QRS complexes with the same shape are uniform premature ventricular contractions, and if there are different shapes, these are multiform premature ventricular contractions (Fig. 12-17B). Until recently, the terms unifocal and multifocal were used, implying that if, for example, premature ventricular contractions had the same morphology, they originated in the same location. However, it has been demonstrated with intracardiac recordings that premature ventricular contractions with the same morphology can originate at different sites and those with different morphologies can originate at the same site.[12] Therefore, it is best to describe premature beats only in terms of their "form" rather than implying their "focality."

Patterns of Premature Beats:
Bigeminy, Trigeminy, and Couplets

Bigeminy is a regular alternation of premature and normal beats. Therefore, the pattern of atrial bigeminy is alternating sinus, premature atrial contraction, sinus, premature atrial contraction. Junctional

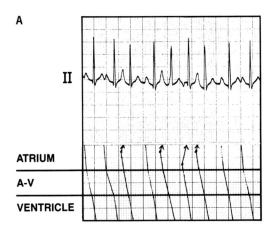

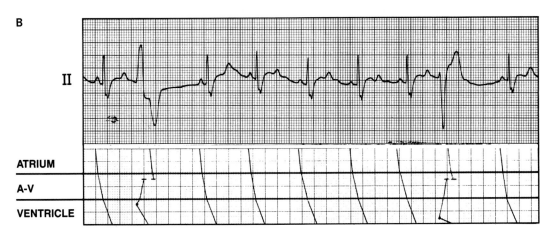

FIG. 12-17. Multiform premature contractions. A, Multiform premature atrial contractions. This tracing was taken from a 3-week-old infant. The third, fifth, and seventh P waves have the same morphology, causing a similar positive deformation of the previous T wave. The QRS complex following the fifth P wave is slightly aberrant since it occurs approximately 5 msec earlier than any of the other QRSs. The sixth P wave is negative in this lead, indicating a separate form. These atrial beats are diagrammed as originating from a different site, although they may have a common site with different conduction. B, Multiform premature ventricular contractions. In this 14-year-old, note that the basic sinus QRS complex is prolonged and has a slurred terminal component, indicating complete right bundle branch block. Nonetheless, multiform premature ventricular contractions can be recognized by their different morphology.

bigeminy is alternating sinus, premature junctional contraction, sinus, premature junctional contraction. The pattern of ventricular bigeminy is alternating sinus, premature ventricular contraction, sinus, premature ventricular contraction (Fig. 12-18). Bigeminy tends to be a very stable and self-sustaining rhythm. Langendorf explained this as the "rule of bigeminy,"[17] which begins with the observation that premature beats are more common when the prevailing rhythm is slow (long cycle length). If a premature beat (which, by definition, has a relatively short cycle length) is followed by a compensatory pause (longer cycle length), the long cycle length of the compensatory pause will favor a premature beat. The premature beat then generates another compensatory pause and the rhythm continues as bigeminy.

Trigeminy is a regular pattern of premature beats in which every third beat is premature. Thus, the pattern in atrial trigeminy is sinus,

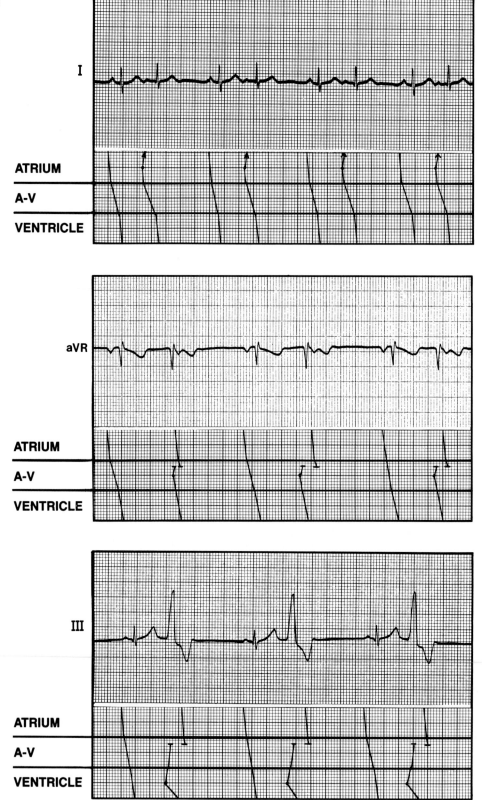

FIG. 12-18. Bigeminy. **Top**, Atrial bigeminy. **Middle**, Junctional bigeminy. Note that in lead aV$_R$, normal sinus P waves are inverted. **Bottom**, Ventricular bigeminy.

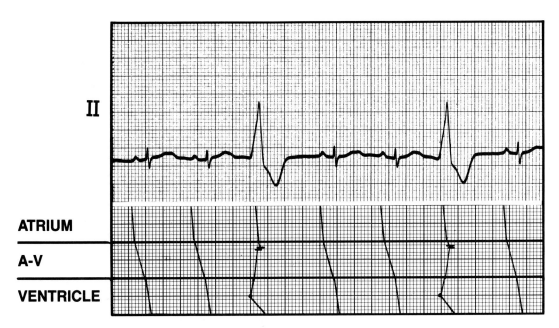

FIG. 12-19. Ventricular trigeminy.

sinus, premature atrial contraction. The patterns of junctional trigeminy and ventricular trigeminy are also observed (Fig. 12-19).

A couplet is defined as two premature beats in a row without an intervening normal beat. The pattern of atrial couplet is sinus, premature atrial contraction, premature atrial contraction. Junctional couplets and ventricular couplets are also observed (Fig. 12-20).

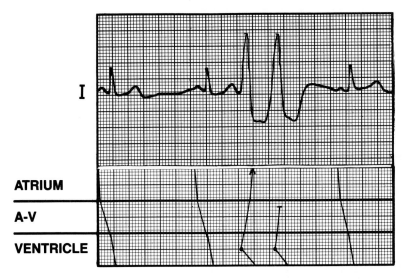

FIG. 12-20. Ventricular uniform couplet. Two premature ventricular contractions occur in the third and fourth beats. It is assumed that the first premature ventricular contraction conducted retrogradely to the atrium. It is also possible that no atrial activity occurred during the couplet.

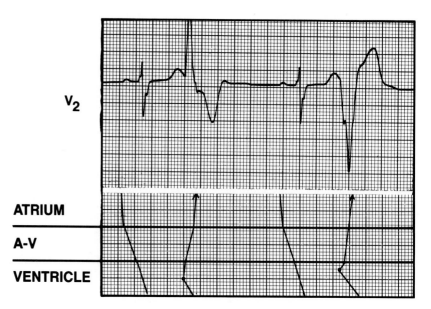

FIG. 12-21. Ventricular multiform bigeminy. Electrocardiogram showing a bigeminal rhythm with sinus beats alternating with premature ventricular contractions. The premature ventricular contractions are multiform, and therefore this is termed multiform bigeminy. A retrograde P wave can be seen on the downslope of the first premature ventricular contraction. Atrial activity is not seen following the second premature ventricular contraction but is assumed to conduct retrogradely to the atrium.

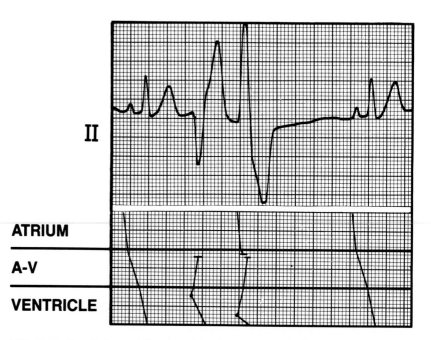

FIG. 12-22. Ventricular multiform couplet. Two premature ventricular contractions in a row, but with different morphologies. Atrial activity is not seen during the couplet and, for the purpose of this diagram, it is assumed that a sinus P wave occurred during the second QRS complex and was not conducted to the ventricles.

Bigeminy, trigeminy, and couplets may occur with uniform premature beats or multiform premature beats. For example, bigeminy with multiform premature ventricular contractions is termed "multiform bigeminy" (Figs. 12-21 and 12-22).

Coupling Interval:
Parasystole

The coupling interval is defined as the interval from the onset of the last depolarization in that chamber to the onset of the premature beat. For a premature atrial contraction, the coupling interval is from the last P wave to the premature P wave; for a premature junctional contraction and a premature ventricular contraction, the coupling interval is from the last QRS complex to the premature QRS complex (Fig. 12-23).

The coupling interval may be either fixed or variable. Variable coupling is defined as a difference in coupling interval of more than .08 sec for uniform premature beats.[6] With multiform premature beats, each morphology may have its own coupling interval which differs from other morphologies. However, if the coupling interval is the same for each beat of the same morphology, then this is fixed coupling.

If there is variable coupling with the same morphology of premature beat, the interectopic intervals (time between each premature beat) should be measured. If the interval can be factored so that each interval is a multiple of a single basic interval (within .08 sec) then parasystole is diagnosed. Parasystole is defined as an area that is constantly depolarizing and is largely unaffected by the predominant rhythm. In practice, if each interectopic interval is not a multiple of the shortest interectopic interval, then the shortest interectopic interval should be divided by two, three, or four and then all the interectopic intervals remeasured using the smaller factor. The electrocardiogram in Figure 12-24 shows premature ventricular contractions with variable coupling (.56, .42, .50, .48, and .58 sec). The interectopic intervals are: 2.99, 4.37, 2.92, and 2.98 sec. The common factor is 1.47 sec. With ventricular parasystole, we infer that a small area of the ventricle is depolarizing every 1.47 sec (41 times/min). There is variable "exit block" from this area. This means that some of the impulses are blocked on their way out of the area. For example, if the interectopic interval is 4.37 sec, the area depolarized three times but only one impulse "exited" the area to cause a QRS complex. In parasystole, there is also "entrance block." This means that this area of the ventricle is "protected" from being depolarized by the predominant rhythm.[18] For example, the sinus beats do not invade this area or affect the parasystolic rhythm. The constancy of the interectopic intervals proves that the parasystolic rhythm is unaffected regardless of changes in the predominant rhythm. Atrial and junctional parasystole also occur (Fig. 12-25).

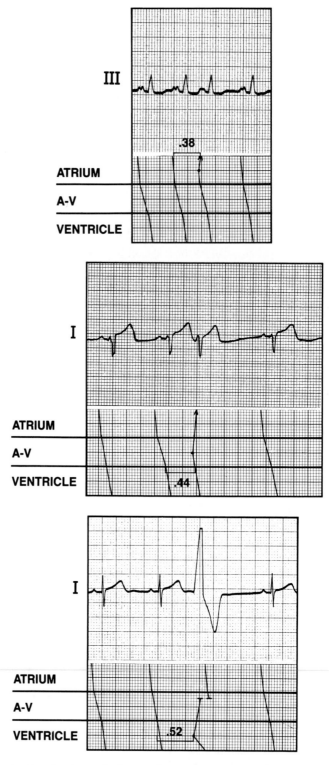

FIG. 12-23. Coupling interval. The coupling interval is measured from the preceding depolarization in that chamber. **Top,** Premature atrial contraction. The coupling interval is measured from the last sinus P wave to the premature P wave. In this example it is .38 sec. **Middle,** Premature junctional contraction. The coupling interval is measured from the last sinus QRS complex to the premature QRS complex. In this example it is .44 sec. **Bottom,** Premature ventricular contraction. The coupling interval is measured from the preceding QRS complex to the premature QRS. In this example it is .52 sec.

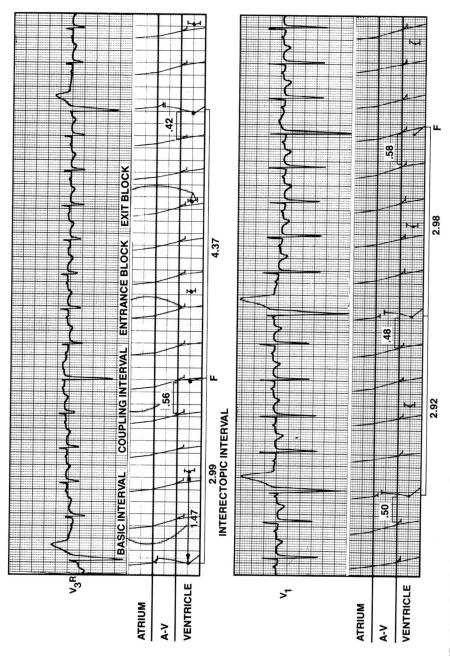

FIG. 12-24. Ventricular parasystole. The parasystolic focus in the ventricles is shown in the ladder diagram as regularly spaced dots in the ventricles at an interval of 1.47 sec corresponding to a rate of 41/min. Entrance block into the parasystolic focus is designated for each of the supraventricular impulses. Exit block is designated by both antegrade and retrograde block of the majority of the impulses originating in the ventricles. Top tracing, The first complex originates from the ventricles. This is followed by four sinus beats and then a fusion beat labelled F; 2.99 sec (approximately twice 1.47) has elapsed between the first and second ventricular complex. There are seven more supraventricular complexes followed by another ventricular complex. The interval between the second and third ventricular complexes is 4.37 sec (approximately three times 1.47). The coupling interval of the second and third ventricular complexes is markedly different. The coupling interval of the first complex is .56 sec and of the second complex is .42 sec. Bottom tracing, The interectopic intervals are relatively constant at 2.92 and 2.98 sec. The coupling intervals are variable at .50 sec, .48 sec, and .58 sec. Therefore, the diagnosis of parasystole is established.

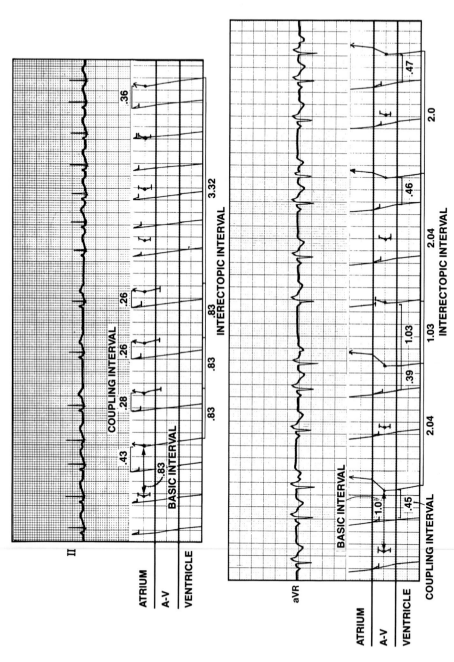

FIG. 12-25. Parasystole. Top tracing, Atrial parasystole. The atrial parasystolic focus is assumed to be firing every .83 sec (equivalent to a rate of 72/min). The coupling intervals vary from .26 to .43. The interectopic intervals are all .83 sec except for the last one, which is 3.32 sec. This is four times the basic interval of .83 sec. Therefore the diagnosis of atrial parasystole is made. Bottom tracing, Junctional parasystole. In lead aV_R, the sinus P waves are inverted. The basic cycle length of the parasystolic focus is 1.0 sec (equivalent to a heart rate of 60/min). The coupling intervals vary from .39 to 1.03 sec. The interectopic intervals are all multiples of approximately 1.0 sec. Thus, the diagnosis of junctional parasystole is made.

Capture
Beats

A capture beat is defined as conduction of an atrial impulse to the ventricles when the predominant rhythm originates in either the AV junction or the ventricles. The P wave temporarily "captures" the ventricles away from the predominant rhythm, shortening the RR interval. A capture beat is, therefore, a variety of premature beat, although, in a sense, the roles are reversed from the usual premature beat. In the usual premature beat, there is a normal predominant rhythm (i.e., sinus) which is interrupted by an abnormal premature beat (i.e., premature atrial contraction). In a capture beat, there is an abnormal predominant rhythm (i.e., junctional) which is interrupted by a normal "premature" beat (i.e., sinus) (Fig. 12-26).

Capture beats usually occur when the atria and ventricles are beating independently (i.e., during AV dissociation). The most common rhythm with capture beats is sinus bradycardia with junctional escape rhythm which does not have any retrograde conduction to the atria (Fig. 12-26B). In this rhythm, a QRS complex can be caused either by a junctional escape beat or by a sinus P wave which conducts antegradely from atria to ventricles. Therefore, in junctional rhythm, the regular RR intervals are caused by the junctional escape beats and the short RR intervals are caused by the sinus beats conducting to the ventricles. Junctional rhythm is usually extremely regular, so that any shortening of the RR interval by .04 sec or more that is preceded by a P wave should be taken as evidence of an atrial capture beat. It would be possible for a P wave to be conducted to the ventricles and not shorten the RR interval if the timing was so perfect that the escape beat and the conducted beat occurred at the same time. However, this could not be ascertained on the surface electrocardiogram and therefore, unless the RR interval is shortened, capture beats cannot be diagnosed.

Even in the presence of normal AV conduction, in junctional rhythm, not all P waves can be conducted from atria to ventricles. This is because when the junctional beat occurs, the AV node, His-Purkinje system, and ventricles are depolarized and it takes a certain amount of time (the "refractory period," which lasts about .3 to .4 sec) for these structures to be able to depolarize again.[19] Therefore, if a P wave occurs within .3 to .4 sec of the preceding QRS complex, it will not conduct to the ventricles. This is a normal phenomenon and does not imply any abnormality of AV conduction. It so happens that the normal T wave ends .3 to .4 sec after the preceding QRS complex, so it is a good "rule of thumb" that a P wave that occurs before the end of the T wave may not conduct to the ventricles, and P waves that fall beyond the T waves should conduct and cause a QRS complex. These are, of course, not electrophysiologically related since the P wave occurs in the atrium and the T wave occurs in the ventricle, but the timing can still be helpful.

Capture beats also occur in high-grade AV block where most P waves are not conducted to the ventricles. In this case, P waves occur

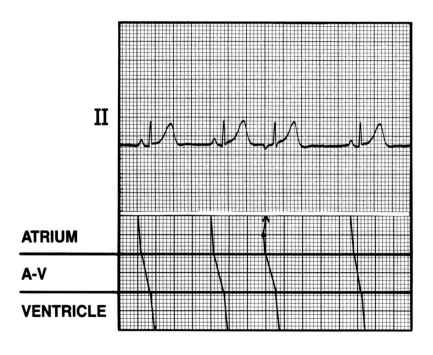

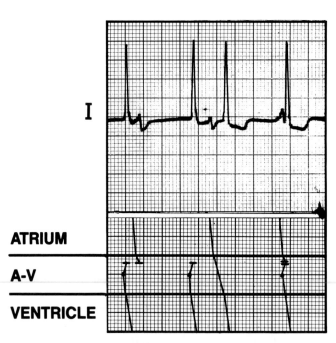

FIG. 12-26. "Premature" beats of different origin. **Top,** Sinus rhythm with premature atrial contraction. A premature P wave follows the preceding sinus P wave with a coupling interval of .58 sec. This results in a premature QRS complex which is also .58 sec after the preceding QRS. **Bottom,** Sinus capture beat. The basic underlying rhythm is a junctional rhythm with AV dissociation. There is no retrograde capture of the atria. A P wave falls at the appropriate interval so that it conducts to the ventricles, resulting in a QRS complex, that is premature for the prevailing rhythm. This occurs .36 sec after the preceding QRS complex.

beyond the T waves and are still not conducted to the ventricles. A regular junctional escape rhythm results, but when intermittent AV conduction does occur, the RR interval is shortened and these are called capture beats (Fig. 12-27).

Finally, capture beats may also occur during junctional or ventricular tachycardia with AV dissociation. A P wave may occur at just the right time to be conducted to the ventricles, thus shortening the RR interval with a capture beat (Fig. 12-28).

TACHYARRYTHMIAS

Tachyarrhythmias are those rhythm disturbances in which an area of the heart depolarizes at a rate faster than normal for at least three successive beats. Since the range of normal rates varies with both the age of the patient and the site of origin of the rhythm, the definition of tachycardia depends upon both of these factors. For example, a sinus rate of 95/min is abnormally slow for a newborn and abnormally fast for a teenager; a junctional rate of 95/min is abnormally fast at any age. One other way to envision tachycardia is as three successive premature beats: A pattern of three premature atrial contractions or premature junctional contractions in a row is called supraventricular tachycardia, and one of three premature ventricular contractions in a row is called ventricular tachycardia.

Sinus
Tachycardia

In sinus tachycardia, a P wave precedes each QRS complex and these P waves have the identical mean vector and morphology as the sinus P waves which had been recorded when the rate was slower. The rate exceeds the normal sinus rate for a child of a particular age (see Appendix, Table A-2). In children over the age of 1 year, we have not encountered sinus tachycardia at a rate over 220/min. In infants under the age of 1 year, it is rare for sinus tachycardia to have a rate over 230/min but we have encountered three infants in this age group, each severely ill with sepsis, with sinus tachycardia at rates up to 260/min (Fig. 12-29).[20]

Sinus tachycardia may occur with aberrancy. In the vast majority of children with sinus tachycardia and aberrancy, the QRS complex is similar to that found in sinus rhythm at a slower rate (i.e., the bundle branch block or Wolff-Parkinson-White was preexisting) (Figs. 12-30 and 12-31).

Causes of Sinus Tachycardia. In sinus tachycardia, a cause can usually be found for the rapid sinus rate (Table 12-5). Usually, sinus tachycardia varies in rate, with an increase in rate in response to a worsening clinical condition of the patient and a decrease in rate response to improvement of the patient's condition. For example, in the patient with hypovolemia and sinus tachycardia, the sinus rate decreases in response to volume infusion.

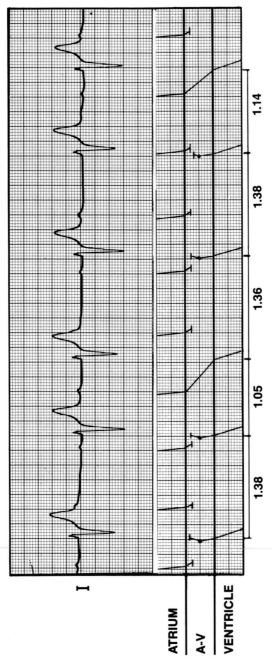

FIG. 12-27. Sinus capture beats. High-grade AV block. Almost none of the atrial impulses are conducted to the ventricles. The regular rhythm causing the QRS complexes is of junctional origin with a cycle length of 1.38 sec. There are two short RR intervals (1.05 sec and 1.14 sec). These are caused by conduction of the supraventricular P waves to the ventricles. Note that after the first sinus capture beat, the junctional rate is "reset." This means that after the junction is depolarized by the conducted supraventricular beat, it begins counting again and 1.36 sec later, when it has not found another conducted supraventricular impulse, it again fires off. We can infer that the basic underlying rhythm originates from the AV junction since the conducted QRS complex has the same morphology as the escape QRS complex.

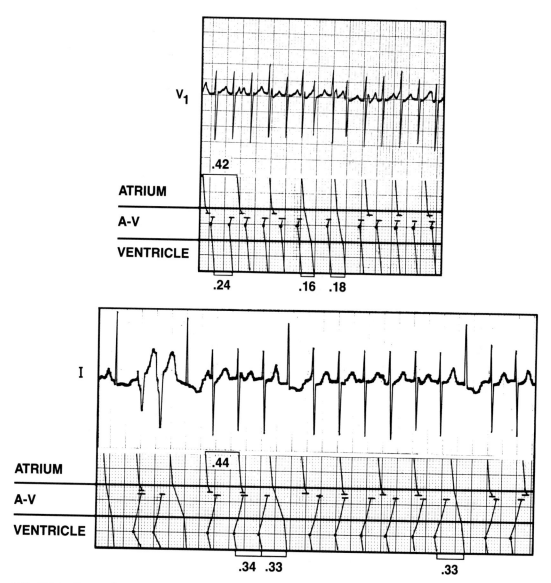

FIG. 12-28. Capture beats in tachyarrhythmias. **Top,** The basic underlying rhythm is junctional tachycardia with AV dissociation. The junctional cycle length is .24 sec, which corresponds to a rate of 250/min. The atrial cycle length is .42 sec, which corresponds to an atrial rate of 143/min. The atria and ventricles are almost completely unrelated or "dissociated." There are two short RR intervals of .16 and .18 sec. These represent sinus capture beats. Note that the QRS complex of the capture beats is similar to the QRS complex of the tachycardia, thus confirming the origin of the tachycardia as supraventricular. **Bottom,** The first beat in the tracing is a sinus beat, followed by a ventricular uniform couplet, which is followed by another sinus beat, and then ventricular tachycardia begins. The morphology of the ventricular tachycardia is similar to that of the ventricular couplet except that the two beats in the couplet are slightly wider. The QRS complexes, which are of supraventricular origin, are completely upright. During the established ventricular tachycardia, the ventricular cycle length is regular at .34 sec. The atria are dissociated with a cycle length of approximately .44 sec. There are two slightly short RR intervals of .33 sec. These are sinus capture beats. The difference in QRS morphology between the sinus capture beats and the tachycardia confirms that the tachycardia is of ventricular origin.

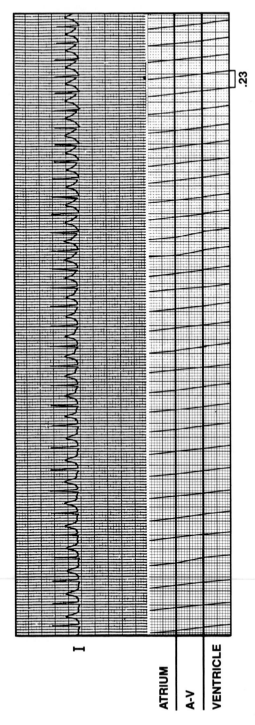

FIG. 12-29. Sinus tachycardia. This is a continuous tracing. P waves are seen between the T wave and the QRS complex to the left of the strip. The P waves "climb up" the descending limb of the T wave as the rate increases. The shortest RR interval is .23 sec, which corresponds to a rate of 260/min.

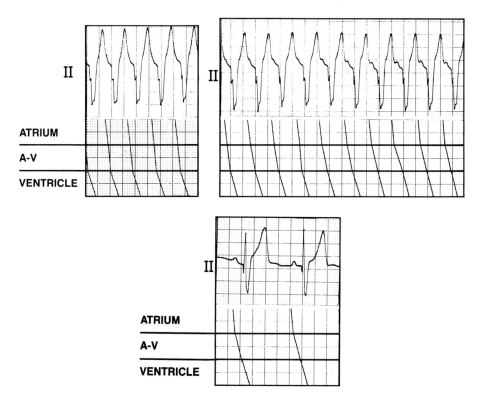

FIG. 12-30. Sinus tachycardia with aberrancy. These three tracings were taken from the same individual at different times during a 24-hour electrocardiogram. **Top left,** Tracing taken during exercise. There is a wide QRS tachycardia at a rate of approximately 170/min. In retrospect, the T wave following the second and fifth complex shows a suggestion of a P wave. However, this tracing, without the others, should be interpreted as a wide QRS tachycardia of uncertain origin. **Top right,** As the rate slows slightly, the P waves become more apparent. **Bottom,** With the patient asleep, the normal P and QRS complex can be seen. The patient has complete right bundle branch block. The QRS complexes in the top left and right tracings are slightly different from the QRS in the bottom tracing in that there is no R wave in the first two tracings. This could be due to either slight further aberration of the QRS or the limited frequency response of the electrocardiograph (see Chapter 3).

Supraventricular Tachycardia

Supraventricular tachycardia is a rapid regular tachyarrhythmia which results from an abnormal mechanism which originates proximal to the bifurcation to the bundle of His and which does not have the morphology of atrial flutter.[21] This definition of supraventricular tachycardia as "due to an abnormal mechanism" specifically excludes sinus tachycardia. Supraventricular tachycardia is generally defined as an abnormally rapid atrial rate for age and not necessarily the ventricular rate because in certain kinds of supraventricular tachycardia confined to the atrium, AV block may occur and the ventricular rate will be less than the atrial rate. Two difficulties are encountered with this definition. Firstly, P waves are not always visible on the surface electrocardiogram during supraventricular tachycardia. In these cases, if the QRS complex is normal and the ventricular rate is abnormally rapid, we infer that the diagnosis is supraventricular tachycardia. Secondly,

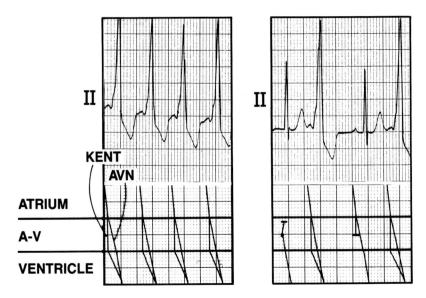

FIG. 12-31. Sinus rhythm with aberration due to Wolff-Parkinson-White. **Left,** P waves are seen preceding each QRS complex. There is a short PR interval of .08 sec. There is also a delta wave indicating conduction through both a Kent bundle and the AV node. This tracing, without the others, should be interpreted as a wide QRS tachycardia of uncertain origin. **Right,** There is no visible P wave preceding the first QRS complex, and the morphology of the QRS complex is normal. This is typical for patients with Wolff-Parkinson-White who have a junctional escape beat. In these patients, junctional escape beats and junctional rhythm have a normal, narrow QRS complex with the ventricles activated entirely by the His bundle and bundle branch system. Even if there were retrograde conduction to the atria from the junctional impulse, the ventricles would be largely depolarized by the normal pathway before the impulse could conduct retrogradely through the AV node and atrium and antegradely through the Kent bundle. In this example, the second beat is a fusion complex with a short PR interval and a delta wave similar to that found during the sinus tachycardia. The third complex has a normal QRS complex with a normal PR interval. This indicates block in the Kent bundle and conduction through the normal AV node. The fourth complex is similar to the second complex and has a short PR interval with a delta wave. The true nature of the wide QRS in the left panel is apparent from examining the electrocardiogram in the right panel when the rate is slower and there may be more conduction through the AV node.

the ventricular rate may exceed the atrial rate in supraventricular tachycardia that has its origin in the AV junction. This situation will exist if there is partial or complete retrograde block in the AV node of impulses that arise in the AV junction. This is the second cause for AV dissociation. The ventricles will be depolarized once for each impulse, but the atria may be completely dissociated and producing P waves

TABLE 12-5. *Causes of Sinus Tachycardia*

Any condition requiring increased cardiac output (thyrotoxicosis, postprandial, exercise, fever, infection, anemia, anxiety, hypovolemia), congestive heart failure, myocarditis, acute rheumatic fever

Hypocalcemia

Drugs: decongestants, sympathomimetic amines, vasodilators

---

that originate from the sinus node. Again, in this case, if the QRS complex is narrow and the ventricular rate is abnormally rapid, we infer that the diagnosis is supraventricular tachycardia. Finally, the distinction between supraventricular tachycardia and atrial flutter depends upon the morphology of atrial depolarization on the surface electrocardiogram. In atrial flutter, there are wide atrial depolarizations called "flutter waves." In a patient with an abnormally rapid ventricular rate and a narrow QRS complex, if there are no flutter waves, the diagnosis is supraventricular tachycardia.

The majority of supraventricular and ventricular tachycardias are caused either by reentry or by an ectopic focus.[21] Although an intracardiac electrophysiologic study is generally required to diagnose the mechanism of a particular tachycardia, it is more common for reentry tachycardias to be paroxysmal while ectopic focus tachycardias are nonparoxysmal and occur almost continuously. Other distinguishing features are presented in detail elsewhere.[21]

We have reviewed the records of 217 children with supraventricular tachycardia whose first episode occurred under the age of 18 years.[22] In 124 patients, the electrocardiogram during the first episode of supraventricular tachycardia was available. The mean heart rate was 240/min with a maximum of 325. In over 60%, the heart rate was 230/min or greater. P waves were visible on the surface electrocardiogram in 70/124 patients (56%) during supraventricular tachycardia. We inferred the presence of a P wave if part of the T wave was abnormally pointed (Figs. 6-14 and 12-32). The presence and location of P waves were confirmed by intracardiac electrophysiologic study. The P wave mean vector could be estimated in 60/70 patients (Table 12-6). The most common P wave vector was −1 to −90° indicating a low right atrial site of origin.[22]

The QRS complex during supraventricular tachycardia had a normal duration and configuration in 114/124 patients (92%). In 10 patients, the QRS duration was prolonged, with a right bundle block morphology in 8 and a left bundle branch morphology in 2. In 7 of the 10 patients with a prolonged QRS duration, the morphology was identical to that recorded during normal sinus rhythm. In only 3 of the 124 patients (2.4%) the QRS complex during supraventricular tachycardia was prolonged and of different morphology, indicating a rate-dependent change in conduction. Only 1 patient had a rate-dependent complete bundle branch block; in the other 2, there was an incomplete bundle branch block pattern. *Therefore, aberration of supraventricular tachycardia is so rare in children that if rate-dependent complete bundle branch block is observed with tachycardia, ventricular tachycardia should be strongly suspected.* This discussion applies to patients whose supraventricular tachycardia is sustained for more than a few beats. Occasionally, the first few beats of supraventricular tachycardia are aberrant but the QRS complex virtually always normalizes.

Second-degree AV block was found before treatment of supraventricular tachycardia in 8/124 of patients (6%). In 4 the block was type I and in 4 it was 2:1 (see section on AV block in this chapter). Complete AV dissociation (no relation of P waves to QRS complexes with QRS rate

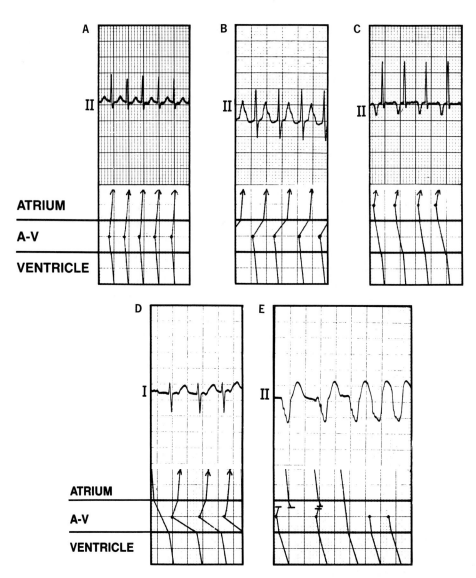

FIG. 12-32. Supraventricular tachycardia: P wave morphology. A, Supraventricular tachycardia at a rate of 290/min. There are no visible P waves. It is assumed that there is 1:1 retrograde capture of the atria and that the P wave falls within the QRS complex. The dot in the AV junction does not indicate that this is necessarily the site of origin of the tachycardia nor does it indicate that the mechanism is due to either an ectopic focus or reentry. This particular patient had supraventricular tachycardia due to reentry entirely within the AV node. B, Supraventricular tachycardia with normal P waves. The P wave is the pointed part of the T wave. These P waves were positive in leads I and aV$_F$, indicating a high right atrial origin of the P wave. This patient had supraventricular tachycardia due to a bundle of Kent located in the right anterior AV groove. This resulted in atrial activation with the earliest site of onset in the right atrial appendage. This actually produces normal appearing P waves during tachycardia. C, Atrial ectopic tachycardia located in the low right atrium. In this ladder diagram, the tachycardia is shown with its origin in the atrium. The P waves are the large negative deflections preceding the QRS complexes. D, Onset of supraventricular tachycardia with inverted P waves following the QRS complexes. Following the sinus beat with a long PR interval there is a QRS complex which is then followed by a P wave, which is inverted in lead I. The P waves continue to be inverted in lead I. This is most suggestive of supraventricular tachycardia due to a left Kent bundle since the atria begin activation from the left atrium, causing the negative P wave in lead I. E, Supraventricular tachycardia with a wide QRS complex. The first two QRS complexes are of junctional origin and there is AV dissociation. The third QRS is caused by a conducted sinus P wave. Supraventricular tachycardia results. Note that the QRS complex in the supraventricular tachycardia is identical to that found with a sinus capture beat. If the sinus capture beat had not been seen, this would have been mistakenly diagnosed as ventricular tachycardia. In most patients (see the four prior tracings in this figure), the QRS during supraventricular tachycardia is normal.

TABLE 12-6. *P Waves During Supraventricular Tachycardia*

	N	%
P wave not visible	54	44
P wave mean vector 0° to +90° (HRA)	22	18
P wave mean vector +91° to −91° (LA)	8	6
P wave mean vector −1° to −90° (LRA)	30	24
P wave visible, mean vector undetermined	10	8
	124	100

Abbreviations: HRA—high right atrial origin; LA—left atrial origin; LRA—low right atrium; N—number of patients

more rapid than the P wave rate) occurred in 4/124 patients (Fig. 12-33). While the mechanism of supraventricular tachycardia can rarely be inferred from the surface electrocardiogram, the presence of a narrow QRS tachycardia with AV dissociation is so characteristic of junctional ectopic tachycardia due to an automatic ectopic focus in the His bundle that the diagnosis can be made on this basis (Fig. 12-33, bottom).[23–24]

CAUSES OF SUPRAVENTRICULAR TACHYCARDIA. About half of the children with supraventricular tachycardia had an otherwise completely normal heart. In our series of 217 patients, 42% had a normal heart and 58% had a factor that might predispose to supraventricular tachycardia (Table 12-7).

Accelerated Atrial Rhythm
and Accelerated Junctional Rhythm

Although these arrhythmias are strictly defined as types of supraventricular tachycardia, it is helpful to identify them separately since they have different implications. These are the "slow supraventricular tachycardias." They are abnormally rapid for their site of origin but do not result in a rate faster than the maximum sinus rate for age.

Accelerated atrial rhythm is defined as a rhythm with an abnormal P wave mean vector at a rate faster than the normal atrial escape rate (Table 12-1) but not exceeding the maximum normal sinus rate for age. In infants less than 3 years old, this is approximately 160/min, and over 3 years old approximately 130/min (see Appendix, Table A-2). For example, in a 2-year-old, accelerated atrial rhythm has a rate between 100 and 160/min (Figs. 12-34 and 12-35).

Accelerated junctional rhythm has a normal QRS and either no visible P waves, a retrograde P wave following each QRS complex, or AV dissociation with a QRS rate faster than the normal junctional escape rate (Table 12-1) but not exceeding the maximum normal sinus rate for age (Fig. 12-34). This has also been called "nonparoxysmal junctional tachycardia."[6] For example, in a 6-year-old, accelerated junctional rhythm has a rate between 60 and 130/min (Fig. 12-36).

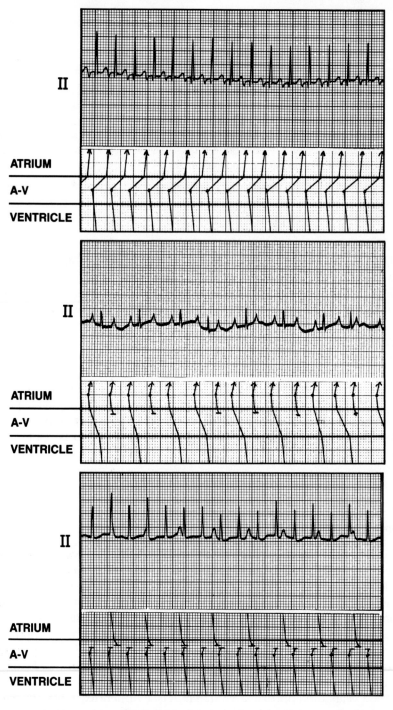

FIG. 12-33. P-QRS relationship during supraventricular tachycardia (see also Fig. 6-14). Top, 1:1 relationship between P waves and QRS complexes. The P wave is the inverted, pointed wave immediately preceding the QRS complex. This patient was shown to have reentry entirely within the AV node. Middle, Variable AV block. There are more P waves than QRS complexes, but each QRS complex is preceded by a P wave with a similar PR interval. This tachycardia was due to an ectopic focus high in the left atrium. The P waves are positive in lead II, which is shown here, but were negative in lead I. The atrial rate is irregular, varying from 150 to 270/min. It is more typical of ectopic focus tachycardias to vary in their rate. Bottom, Supraventricular tachycardia with AV dissociation. The junctional rate is constant at 230/min and the atrial rate is also constant at 125/min. Note that the P waves are upright in lead II suggesting sinus origin. There is complete AV dissociation. An electrocardiogram similar to this is virtually diagnostic of junctional ectopic focus supraventricular tachycardia.

TABLE 12-7. *Causes of Supraventricular Tachycardia in 217 Children*

ACUTE	N	(%)
Fever, sepsis, myocarditis, encephalitis, chest trauma, acidosis, hypoglycemia, RDS, hypotension during exchange transfusion	18	(8)
Drugs: sympathomimetic	7	(3)
caffeine (cola)	1	(1)
Total acute	26	(12)
CHRONIC		
CHD—SVT appeared pre-op	19	(9)
CHD—SVT appeared post-op	19	(9)
Cardiomyopathy	9	(4)
Hyperthyroidism	2	(1)
WPW*	47	(21)
LGL	4	(2)
Total chronic abnormal heart	100	(46)
Otherwise normal heart	91	(42)
Total	217	(100)

*Includes patients who also had CHD. These are not counted in CHD group.
Abbreviations: CHD—congenital heart disease; LGL—Lown-Ganong-Levine; N—number of patients; pre-op—preoperative; post-op—postoperative; RDS—respiratory distress syndrome; SVT—supraventricular tachycardia; WPW—Wolff-Parkinson-White

CAUSES OF ACCELERATED RHYTHMS. Accelerated atrial and junctional escape rhythms are probably due to a type of increased automaticity.[25] This can be due either to a focal reason for increased automaticity (e.g., trauma from a suture near the His bundle causing accelerated junctional rhythm in the immediate postoperative period after tetralogy of Fallot repair) or to a generalized increase in automaticity due to catecholamines with focal suppression of the sinus node (e.g., the sinus node and atria may be injured during a Mustard operation but in the immediate postoperative period, because of increased demands and an increase in catecholamines, an accelerated rhythm develops from a normal AV junction).

Atrial Flutter

Atrial flutter is characterized by a rapid, regular form of atrial depolarization: the "flutter wave" (Fig. 12-37). The characteristic electrocardiographic feature is a sawtooth or "picket fence" appearance; this results from merging of the P waves without an isoelectric interval and usually appears most prominently in leads II, III, aV$_F$, and V$_1$. Frequently, flutter waves are absent in lead V$_6$.[26] The morphology of atrial flutter (with flutter waves of .09 to .18 sec in duration) is the only diagnostic feature of this arrhythmia on the electrocardiogram and defines its presence. In our series of 24 pediatric patients, the atrial rate in atrial flutter was most commonly 300/min, but ranging from 280 to

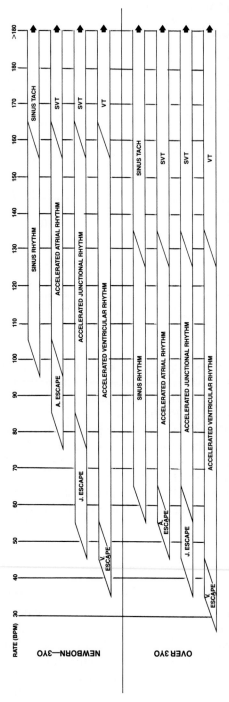

FIG. 12-34.   Distinction between normal escape rhythms, accelerated escape rhythms, and tachycardia. The border zones of the rates between these entities are inexact. BPM, beats per minute; A., atrial; J., junctional; SVT, supraventricular tachycardia; TACH, tachycardia; V., ventricular; VT, ventricular tachycardia; YO, years old.

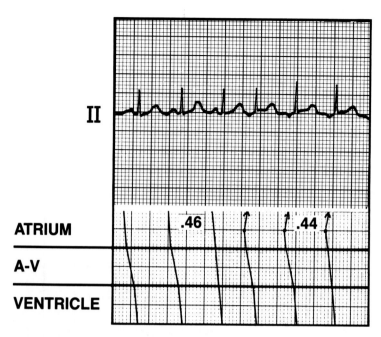

FIG. 12-35. Accelerated atrial rhythm. This tracing was taken from a 3-month-old infant. Following three sinus beats with a PP interval of .46 sec (corresponding to a rate of 130/min), an accelerated atrial rhythm develops with a PP interval of .44 sec (corresponding to a rate of 136/min). The P waves in the accelerated atrial rhythm are inverted in lead II, indicating a site of origin in the low atrium.

450/min.[27] Because of this variation in rate, we define atrial flutter in children only by morphology and not by rate.

AV conduction in atrial flutter is usually variable and therefore atrial flutter usually has an irregular ventricular rate. The most common AV conduction ratio is 2:1, yielding a ventricular rate of 150/min. In young infants with normal rapid conduction through the AV node and in children with AV node bypass tracts (i.e., James fibers or Kent bundles), periods of rapid 1:1 conduction of atrial flutter to the ventricles frequently occur.[28] In these situations, there is frequently ventricular aberration, causing a rapid wide QRS tachycardia (Figs. 12-37 and 12-38).

CAUSES OF ATRIAL FLUTTER. Atrial flutter occurs in the following three groups of patients. (1) In the hydropic newborn with intrauterine tachyarrhythmia, frequently supraventricular tachycardia and atrial flutter alternate in the same patient. This is associated with Wolff-Parkinson-White. (2) In the infant under 6 months of age, the heart is usually otherwise normal; most infants in this group had frequent premature atrial contractions as newborns (more than 20/hour). (3) In the older child, the heart is usually abnormal and atrial flutter results from chronic atrial dilation and pressure overload.[27] The other causes of atrial flutter in our group of children are shown in Table 12-8.

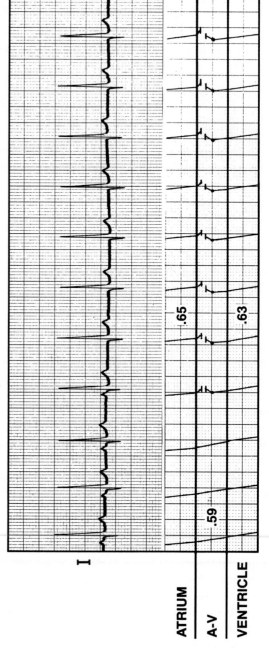

FIG. 12-36. Top. Legend on facing page.

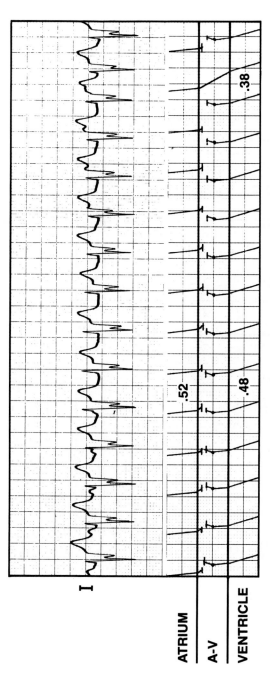

I

ATRIUM

A-V .52

VENTRICLE .48 .38

FIG. 12-36. Accelerated junctional rhythm. **Top.** Tracing taken from a 6-year-old boy. Following three sinus beats with a PP interval of .59 sec (rate 100/min), the sinus rhythm slows slightly (PP interval of .65 sec) and an accelerated junctional rhythm develops with an RR interval of .63 sec (corresponding to a rate of 95 min). The sinus and the junctional QRS complexes are identical and are both normal. **Bottom.** Tracing taken from an 11-year-old. The tracing shows a wide QRS rhythm with an RR interval of .48 sec (corresponding to a rate of 125/min) and AV dissociation with an atrial cycle length of .52 sec (corresponding to a rate of 115/min). On the far right of the tracing, there is a short RR interval of .38 sec. This is preceded by a P wave and indicates a sinus capture beat. The fact that the QRS complex with the capture beat is the same as that during the accelerated rhythm indicates that the rhythm is an accelerated junctional rhythm rather than an accelerated ventricular rhythm. In this latter case, the sinus capture beat would have a narrower QRS with a different morphology. This accelerated junctional escape rhythm with right bundle branch block is frequently seen in patients immediately after repair of tetralogy of Fallot.

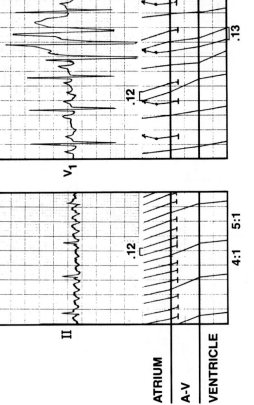

FIG. 12-37.   Top. Legend on facing page.

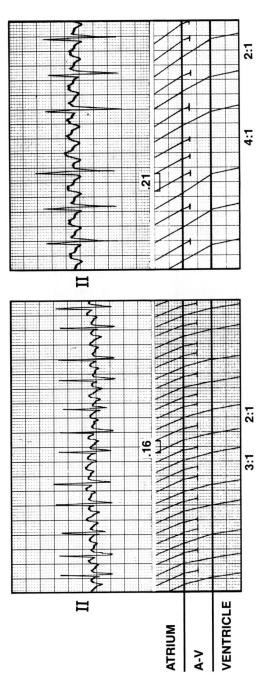

FIG. 12-37. Atrial flutter. **Top tracings.** Both the left and the right tracing were taken from infants less than 1-week-old. In the left tracing, classic flutter waves are seen with a cycle length of .12 sec. This corresponds to an atrial rate of 500/min. 4:1 and 5:1 AV block occur, resulting in the characteristically irregular ventricular rate in atrial flutter in infants. In these ladder diagrams, atrial flutter is shown as prolonged intraatrial conduction. The time from the onset to the end of the atrial depolarization is equal to the cycle length. That is, the bottom of the preceding atrial diagonal line corresponds to the top of the next one. In the right tracing, the rapid ventricular response of atrial flutter in the newborn infant is demonstrated. The first sinus beat is followed by a blocked premature atrial contraction. This sequence is repeated except that following the premature atrial contraction are two beats of atrial flutter at a cycle length of .12 sec. The first of these beats of flutter is conducted to the ventricles. The flutter stops spontaneously and another sequence of a sinus beat takes place, followed by a premature atrial contraction. This premature atrial contraction, which occurs with a slightly longer coupling interval and conducts to the ventricle. This premature atrial contraction initiates the same two beats of atrial flutter as were initiated by the prior premature atrial contraction. Also similarly, the first beat of the atrial flutter conducts to the ventricle with a cycle length of .13 sec (corresponding to a ventricular rate of 460/min). The second beat of atrial flutter is not conducted. This is followed again by a sinus beat and a blocked premature atrial contraction. **Bottom tracings.** The left tracing is taken from a 3-month-old in atrial flutter. Note again the characteristic flutter morphology. The atrial cycle length is .16 sec, which corresponds to an atrial rate of 375/min. Again, there is variable AV block from 2:1 to 3:1, resulting in an irregular ventricular rate. The right tracing is taken from a 16-year-old. The flutter cycle length is .21 sec. This corresponds to an atrial rate of 285/min. Varying 4:1 and 2:1 AV block occurs, resulting in an irregular ventricular rate.

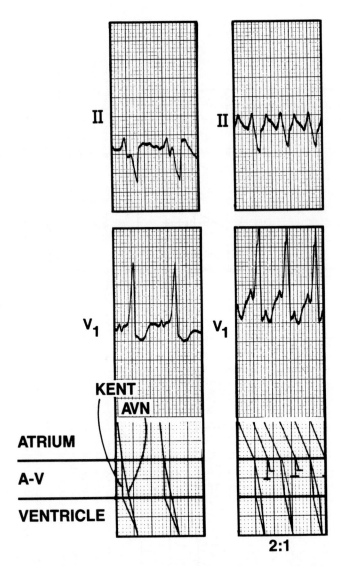

FIG. 12-38. Atrial flutter with Wolff-Parkinson-White. Left, In sinus rhythm, a P wave precedes each QRS. There is a short PR interval with a delta wave. The ladder diagram refers to lead V_1. Atrial flutter develops. Note the sawtooth pattern in lead II. In lead V_1, there are two atrial depolarizations for each ventricular depolarization. As can be seen in the ladder diagram, 2:1 block exists in both the AV node and Kent bundle. The conducted beats are similar to the beats found during sinus rhythm with Wolff-Parkinson-White, which are shown in the left tracings.

TABLE 12-8. *Causes of Atrial Flutter in 24 Children*

	N	(%)
Otherwise normal heart	8	(33)
CHD—flutter appeared pre-op	5	(21)
CHD—flutter appeared post-op	7	(29)
Cardiomyopathy	4	(17)
	24	(100)

Abbreviations: Same as Table 12-7

Atrial
Fibrillation

Atrial fibrillation is characterized by an extremely rapid and irregular form of continuous atrial activation. Atrial depolarization is bizarre and chaotic. Two types are recognized. The first is "coarse atrial fibrillation" with prominent irregular atrial depolarizations and the second is "fine atrial fibrillation" with small, unprominent atrial depolarizations that only distort the baseline minimally (Fig. 12-39). These two types may alternate in the same patient.[26]

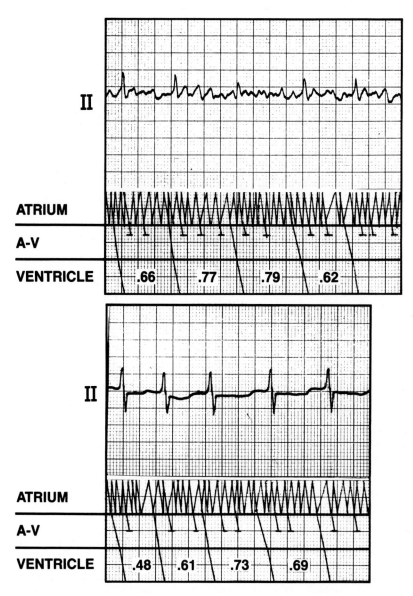

FIG. 12-39. Atrial fibrillation. **Top,** The atrial depolarizations are extremely prominent and irregular. This is "coarse" atrial fibrillation. The ventricular response is irregularly irregular. None of the RR intervals is the same. **Bottom,** The atrial depolarizations are not seen. This is "fine" atrial fibrillation. The ventricular response is irregularly irregular and thus the diagnosis of atrial fibrillation can still be made.

In atrial fibrillation, over 600 atrial impulses bombard the AV node per minute. All cannot be transmitted, and an extremely variable AV block results. Therefore, in a rhythm strip, it is rare for two RR intervals to be identical in atrial fibrillation. Very rapid ventricular responses may occur in patients with AV node bypass tracts. These patients may present with a rapid wide QRS tachycardia but in atrial fibrillation, unlike the other dysrhythmias, the ventricular rate is still extremely variable (Fig. 12-40).

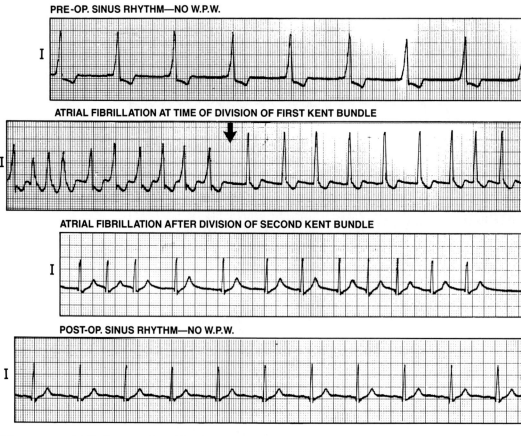

PRE-OP. SINUS RHYTHM—NO W.P.W.

ATRIAL FIBRILLATION AT TIME OF DIVISION OF FIRST KENT BUNDLE

ATRIAL FIBRILLATION AFTER DIVISION OF SECOND KENT BUNDLE

POST-OP. SINUS RHYTHM—NO W.P.W.

FIG. 12-40. Atrial fibrillation with Wolff-Parkinson-White. These are all tracings taken from a 16-year-old boy. He had two Kent bundles which were divided surgically. **Top tracing,** This tracing was taken before operation. There is sinus rhythm with a P wave preceding each QRS complex. There is a short PR interval and a delta wave. **Second tracing,** This tracing was taken during the operation exactly at the time that the first Kent bundle was surgically divided (arrow). On the left, note the irregularly irregular rhythm with a wide QRS. This is characteristic of atrial fibrillation with Wolff-Parkinson-White. Although the QRS complex is wide, ventricular tachycardia would not be this irregular. Immediately after the surgical interruption of the first Kent bundle, at the arrow, the rhythm remains irregularly irregular and the QRS morphology has changed. However, the QRS morphology is still not normal. Note the QRS-T discordance. The QRS rate also changes considerably after division of the first Kent bundle. The shortest RR interval before division of the Kent bundle was .24 sec. In the 3 seconds before division of the Kent bundle, the average ventricular rate was 180/min. In the 5 seconds immediately after division of the first Kent bundle, the mean ventricular rate was 132/min. This indicates that the first Kent bundle had a shorter refractory period (allowed more atrial impulses to pass to the ventricles) than the second bundle. **Third tracing,** After the second Kent bundle was divided, the QRS complex is completely normal. No atrial activity is seen, and the ventricular response is irregularly irregular. This is diagnostic of continuing atrial fibrillation. After division of the second Kent bundle, the ventricular rate again decreases. In the 8 seconds of this tracing, the mean ventricular rate is 98/min. **Bottom tracing,** After the operation, sinus rhythm has returned. The RR interval is regular. A P wave precedes each QRS complex, and the QRS complexes are all normal. W.P.W., Wolff-Parkinson-White.

TABLE 12-9. *Causes of Atrial Fibrillation in 8 Children*

	N	(%)
Otherwise normal heart	3	(37)
Cardiomyopathy	1	(13)
CHD—atrial fib appeared pre-op	3	(37)
WPW	1	(13)
	8	(100)

Abbreviations: WPW—Wolff-Parkinson-White; remainder same as Table 12-7

CAUSES OF ATRIAL FIBRILLATION. Atrial fibrillation is rare in pediatric patients and is extremely uncommon before adolescence.[29] Patients usually have either a structurally abnormal heart or Wolff-Parkinson-White (Table 12-9).[26]

Ventricular
Tachycardia

Ventricular tachycardia is a series of 3 or more repetitive excitations that originate from the ventricles. The complexes are therefore different from the patient's normal QRS; usually, the QRS duration is prolonged for the age of the patient (greater than .09 sec up to age 4 years and greater than .10 sec from 4 years to 16 years). It is therefore usually a "wide QRS" tachycardia. Ventricular tachycardia usually has a uniform morphology with one type of QRS complex (Fig. 12-41). In our series of 46 children under 18 years of age, 67% had left bundle branch block, 26% had right bundle branch block, and 7% had an indeterminant morphology.

The following characteristics of ventricular tachycardia are helpful in the diagnosis, if present. (1) AV dissociation (Fig. 12-42). Since 1:1 retrograde conduction to the atria is common in children, the absence of AV dissociation is not helpful.[30,31] (2) Intermittent sinus capture or fusion beats (Fig. 12-43). These prove that the QRS causing the tachycardia is not of supraventricular origin (see section on Premature ventricular contractions). (3) The morphology of ventricular tachycardia is similar to the morphology of single premature ventricular contractions (Fig. 12-44). If the patient had other electrocardiograms and premature ventricular contractions were noted, the morphology of the ventricular tachycardia should be compared to that of the premature ventricular contractions. This is helpful only if the morphology is similar. If the morphology is not identical, the tachycardia still could be of ventricular origin but from a different area of the ventricles than the single premature ventricular contractions.

In our series, the mean rate of ventricular tachycardia was 195/min with 93% of the patients having a rate less than 300/min. Although the majority were under 300/min, we did find individuals with more rapid rates. In fact, we have found that the rate of ventricular tachycardia may be as high as 428/min (Fig. 12-45).[32]

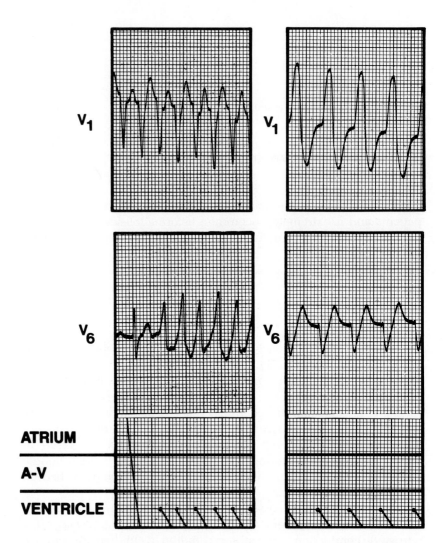

FIG. 12-41. Ventricular tachycardia. **Left,** Tracings from an 11-month-old infant. The tracings are not simultaneous but are taken from the same patient. In the *bottom* tracing, a sinus beat is followed by ventricular tachycardia. The ladder diagram reflects ventricular tachycardia at a rate of approximately 300/min. Atrial activity cannot be seen. This ventricular tachycardia has the morphology of left bundle branch block. **Right,** Ventricular tachycardia in a 15-year-old. The ventricular tachycardia has a right bundle branch block morphology. The rate is approximately 180/min. Atrial activity is not seen.

Occasionally, the QRS morphology changes from one type to another type and back again with almost normal looking QRS complexes at the point where the morphology changes. This is called "torsade de pointes" (Fig. 12-46A) and is associated with a prolonged QT interval either from drugs or on a congenital basis (see Chapter 11).[33] Another rare morphology of ventricular tachycardia is called "bidirectional tachycardia." It characteristically has constant right bundle branch block with alternating right axis deviation and left axis deviation (Fig. 12-46B). This type of ventricular tachycardia is associated with digitalis intoxication, hypokalemia, or end-stage myocardial failure.[34]

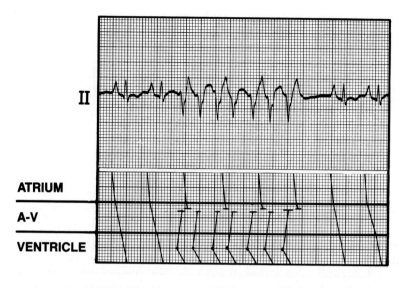

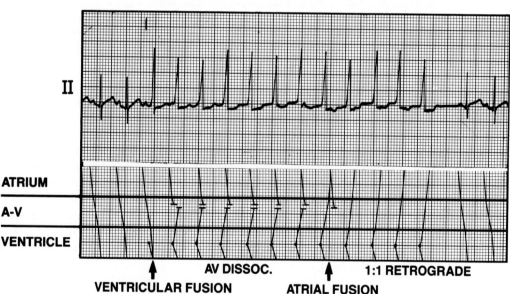

FIG. 12-42. Ventricular tachycardia with AV dissociation. **Top,** After two sinus beats, ventricular tachycardia begins. The rate is slightly irregular but approximately 270/min. The large P waves are seen to "walk through" the ventricular tachycardia. There is no conduction from atria to ventricles nor from ventricles to atria. Two sinus beats end the tracing. Note that the QRS duration of the ventricular tachycardia is .09 sec. The sinus QRS has an entirely different morphology with a shorter duration of .07 sec. **Bottom,** Ventricular tachycardia in a 2-day-old infant. After two sinus beats, a fusion complex begins the ventricular tachycardia. The QRS complexes during the tachycardia are only .05 sec in duration. The sinus QRS is .04 sec. The presence of the fusion beat, nonetheless, proves that this is ventricular tachycardia. For the six beats of ventricular tachycardia that follow the fusion complex, there is AV dissociation. There is neither atrioventricular nor ventriculoatrial conduction. On the seventh beat, a fusion P wave appears. This results both from antegrade conduction of the sinus impulse and retrograde conduction of the impulse which originates from the ventricular tachycardia. This P wave is biphasic. The P waves following the last four beats of the ventricular tachycardia are inverted and result from 1:1 retrograde capture of the atria by the ventricular tachycardia. This stops spontaneously and the tracing ends with two sinus beats.

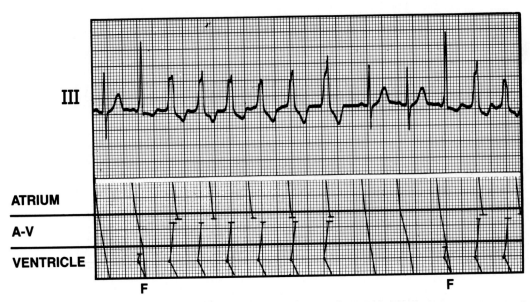

III

ATRIUM

A-V

VENTRICLE

F · F

FIG. 12-43. Ventricular tachycardia—fusion. In this tracing from an 11-year-old, fusion complexes (F) are clearly seen between the sinus QRS and the QRS from the ventricular tachycardia. There is also AV dissociation.

CAUSES OF VENTRICULAR TACHYCARDIA. Unlike patients with premature ventricular contractions, the majority of our patients with chronic ventricular tachycardia had an abnormal heart.[35] We originally had referred to us 27 children with ventricular tachycardia who were thought to have a normal heart. After extensive evaluation, which included cardiac catheterization in most, 12 of the 27 (44%) were found not to have a normal heart but rather a predisposing factor to ventricular tachycardia and only 15 truly had a normal heart (Table 12-10). No child with ventricular tachycardia under the age of 2 years had a normal heart. Therefore, in a patient with ventricular tachycardia, anatomic cardiac catheterization is indicated to be certain the heart is truly normal.

*Ventricular
Fibrillation*

Ventricular fibrillation is a series of uncoordinated ventricular depolarizations associated with no cardiac output. On the electrocardiogram, ventricular fibrillation is a series of low amplitude, rapid irregular depolarizations without identifiable QRS complexes (Fig. 12-47). In ventricular fibrillation, two types of onset are observed. The first type (type A) is characterized by a rapid initiation of fibrillation following one or two premature beats, whereas in the second variety (type B), the excitation process becomes gradually disorganized after relatively long periods of ventricular tachycardia.[15] The morphology of ventricular fibrillation is not unlike that of electrical interference or that observed when an electrocardiographic electrode has lost contact with

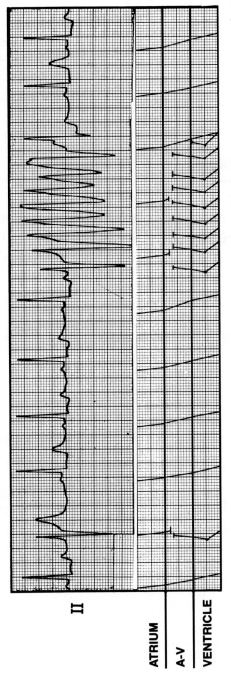

FIG. 12-44. Ventricular tachycardia with morphology similar to single premature ventricular contraction. In the right side of this tracing, there is a rapid, wide QRS tachycardia which could result either from aberration of a supraventricular rhythm or from ventricular tachycardia. The last complex in the tachycardia is probably a fusion complex. The ventricular origin is substantiated by the observation of a single premature ventricular contraction four beats before the onset of the tachycardia with a similar morphology.

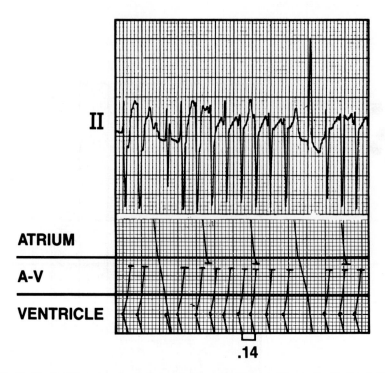

FIG. 12-45. Rapid ventricular tachycardia. Recorded from a 20-month-old, this is the most rapid ventricular tachycardia that we have encountered. The shortest RR interval is .14 sec. This corresponds to a ventricular rate of 428/min. The presence of AV dissociation, and a fusion beat (3rd QRS) and a capture beat (12th QRS) substantiates the ventricular origin.

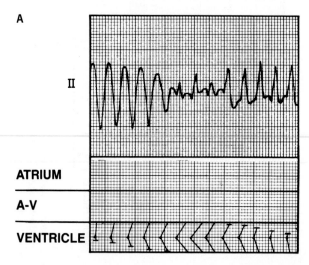

FIG. 12-46. A, Torsade de pointes. This is a multiform ventricular tachycardia with changing morphology and an almost isoelectric segment between different morphologies. The ladder diagram reflects a possible mechanism whereby there is continuously changing exit block from a single area of ventricular tachycardia.

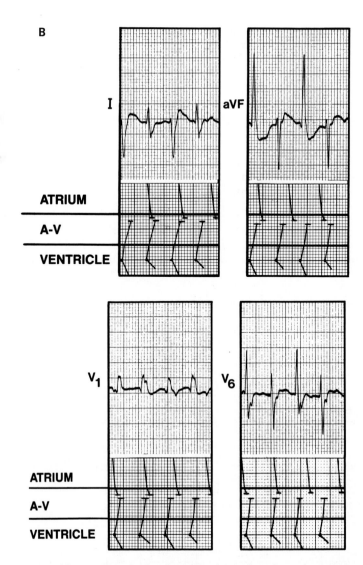

FIG. 12-46. Cont'd   B, Bidirectional tachycardia. This is also a form of ventricular tachycardia which characteristically has complete right bundle branch block in all complexes but alternating right axis deviation and left axis deviation. This is thought to be a single area of ventricular tachycardia with an alternating exit pathway. At first glance, in all leads except for lead V_1, this appears to be ventricular bigeminy. However, the RR interval is exactly the same in all complexes. This would not be the case with bigeminy, which would have alternating long and short cycles. In addition, this example of bidirectional tachycardia contains AV dissociation.

the patient. Therefore, when ventricular fibrillation is suspected, the electrocardiographic electrodes should be rapidly checked for patient contact, and the loss of pulse in the patient should be confirmed.

Ventricular fibrillation is rare in children. In a review of the terminal electrical activity of 100 children under 18 years of age, only six (6%) had ventricular fibrillation as the terminal event. In all the others, the terminal event was bradycardia followed by asystole.[15]

TABLE 12-10. *Causes of Ventricular Tachycardia in 46 Children*

Final DX	INITIAL DX	
	Referred as "normal"	Known abnormal
ARVD	4	0
CM	3	6
Long QT	3	1
Tumor	2	0
CHD—VT appeared pre-op	0	9
CHD—VT appeared post-op	0	2
Mitral prolapse	0	1
Normal	15	0
Total	27	19

Abbreviations: ARVD—arrhythmogenic right ventricular dysplasia; CM—cardiomyopathy; DX—diagnosis; Long QT—prolonged QT interval; CHD—congenital heart disease; VT—ventricular tachycardia

Simultaneous

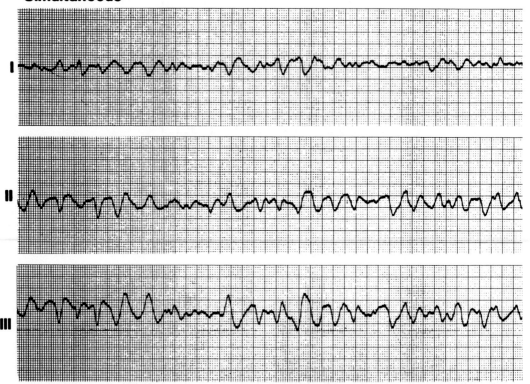

FIG. 12-47.   Ventricular fibrillation. The depolarizations are disorganized and resemble electrical interference or loss of electrode contact with the patient.

Accelerated
Ventricular Rhythm

Although this arrhythmia is strictly defined as ventricular tachy-cardia, it is helpful to identify it separately since it has a different implication. This is "slow ventricular tachycardia." It is abnormally rapid for idioventricular rhythm but does not result in a rate faster than the maximum sinus rate for age.[36] Accelerated ventricular rhythm has an abnormal QRS and either no visible P waves, a retro-grade P wave following each QRS complex, or AV dissociation with a QRS rate faster than the normal ventricular escape rate but not ex-ceeding the maximum normal sinus rate for age (Table 12-1 and Fig. 12-34). For example, in an 11-year-old, accelerated ventricular rhythm has rates between 40 and 130/min (Fig. 12-48).

Unlike accelerated atrial and junctional rhythm, accelerated ven-tricular rhythm usually occurs in children with an otherwise normal heart and is benign.[37]

Differential Diagnosis
of Tachyarrhythmias

The most common and most difficult differential diagnosis is in the patient with a regular, narrow QRS tachycardia. This is basically the distinction between sinus tachycardia and supraventricular tachycar-dia. Atrial fibrillation always has an irregular ventricular rate and atrial flutter usually has an irregular rate with visible flutter waves. These can therefore be eliminated from consideration. In distinguishing sinus tachycardia from supraventricular tachycardia, the rate may be helpful. In all but a few infants, the rate of sinus tachycardia is below 230/min, whereas over 60% of infants and children with supraventricu-lar tachycardia have QRS rates of 230/min or more. In the vast majority of patients with sinus tachycardia, P waves are visible with a normal (0 to +90°) mean vector. P waves with a normal mean vector were found in only 15% of our cases with supraventricular tachycardia. Therefore, the presence of P waves with a normal mean vector is a strong point in favor of sinus tachycardia. The absence of visible P waves is in favor of supraventricular tachycardia.

If the patient's history is available, certain clinical clues may be helpful. The four most common clinical situations in which marked sinus tachycardia is found are hypovolemia, sepsis, fever of any cause, and iatrogenic overdose with isoproterenol, epinephrine, or theophyl-line. While any of these conditions can predispose to supraventricular tachycardia, sinus tachycardia is much more common in such situa-tions. It is rare to observe the initiation of tachycardia, but observation of the cessation of tachycardia can be planned. If in response to an intervention such as phenylephrine or vagal maneuvers, the heart rate changes abruptly, the problem is most likely supraventricular tachy-cardia. If the heart rate slows gradually in response to an intervention, the diagnosis is more than likely sinus tachycardia. If the heart rate is unaffected, it could be either sinus tachycardia or supraventricular

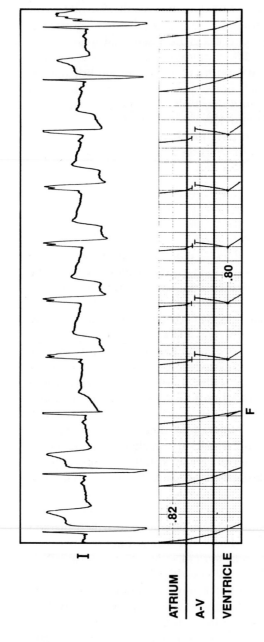

FIG. 12-48. Accelerated ventricular rhythm. Tracing from an 11-year-old. The first beat is a sinus beat followed by a fusion complex. The sinus PP interval is .82 sec. This corresponds to a rate of 73/min. An accelerated ventricular rhythm then occurs with an RR interval of .80 sec (corresponding to a rate of 75/min). The tracing ends with two sinus beats. The ventricular origin is substantiated by the fusion beat, by the different morphology of the QRS complexes, and by the AV dissociation.

tachycardia. The final method of establishing the diagnosis is by observing the response to specific treatment for supraventricular tachycardia. If the rhythm abruptly converts to a slower sinus rhythm after cardioversion, the patient had supraventricular tachycardia. If the rhythm continues unchanged, it could have been supraventricular tachycardia but is most likely sinus tachycardia, and the search for the cause of sinus tachycardia should be continued.

A less common but equally challenging differential diagnosis is the patient with a regular wide QRS tachycardia. The three major arrhythmias are ventricular tachycardia, supraventricular tachycardia with aberration, and atrial flutter with aberration. Ventricular tachycardia is virtually always a wide QRS tachycardia; by contrast, only 10% of sustained supraventricular tachycardia is associated with a wide QRS complex in children.[22] In 7 of the 10 cases of supraventricular tachycardia with a wide QRS that we found in children, the QRS complex was wide before the supraventricular tachycardia started. Therefore, in making the diagnosis in a patient with a wide QRS complex tachycardia, it is helpful to examine prior tracings taken when the patient was in sinus rhythm. From our data, if the QRS complex was narrow before the tachycardia began and was wide during tachycardia, there is only a 2.4% chance that this was supraventricular tachycardia. Similar data are available for atrial flutter (which would most likely be more irregular with varying amounts of aberration). The concept is clear: In any child with a regular wide QRS tachycardia, ventricular tachycardia should be suspected.

The presence of fusion beats, capture beats, and AV dissociation with a wide QRS tachycardia is diagnostic of ventricular tachycardia, but not helpful if absent. The morphology of the wide QRS (right bundle branch block or left bundle branch block pattern) is not helpful in children with one exception: If the wide QRS is mainly positive and has a similar morphology in all the precordial leads, this could represent conduction of a supraventricular tachycardia antegradely through a bundle of Kent (Fig. 12-49).[38] In this case, the QRS in sinus rhythm usually shows Wolff-Parkinson-White with a morphology similar to that found in tachycardia. Finally, although the rate of supraventricular tachycardia is generally faster than the rate of ventricular tachycardia in children,[30,39] since we have found rates up to 428/min for ventricular tachycardia, in the individual child the rate is not a good differentiating point between supraventricular tachycardia and ventricular tachycardia.

In many wide QRS tachycardias, the diagnosis cannot be made with certainty. These tracings should not be overread. A perfectly acceptable interpretation of such an arrhythmia might be: "Wide QRS tachycardia, uncertain origin. Suggest electrophysiology study."

AV
BLOCK

AV block is defined as either delay in conduction or lack of conduction of impulses from atria to ventricles. AV block may occur within the atrium, AV node, or bundle of His. In order for AV block to occur in the

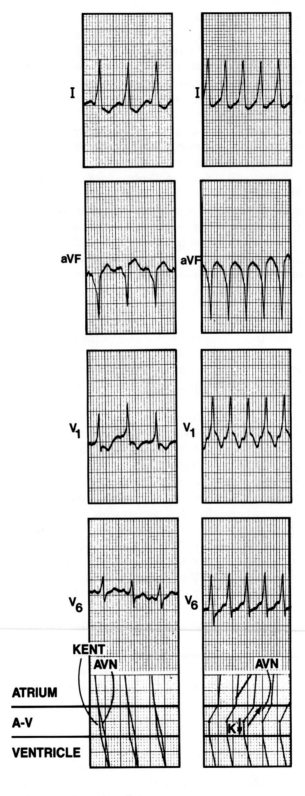

FIG. 12-49.   Legend on facing page.

bundle branches, both the right and the left bundle branch must block simultaneously. Each of these structures requires a certain amount of time before it can conduct again, namely, the refractory period. If an impulse arrives at a structure within the relative refractory period, the impulse will conduct through that structure slowly, but if the impulse arrives at a structure within the absolute refractory period, it will not conduct at all (see Chapter 2). In children, most AV conduction block occurs within the AV node.[40] The normal AV node in a child should conduct atrial impulses to the ventricles at rates of at least 180/min.[19] In some infants and children it is possible to have 1:1 conduction through the normal AV node at rates over 300/min. If there is an AV node bypass tract, it is common to conduct atrial impulses to the ventricles at rates over 300/min.[28] If the AV node or bundle of His is diseased, or if there is heightened vagal tone such as that found when the patient is asleep, AV block may occur at atrial rates lower than 180/min.

First-Degree
AV Block

First-degree AV block is defined as prolongation of the atrioventricular conduction time, with conduction of all impulses. This is manifest on the electrocardiogram as prolongation of the PR interval (Fig. 12-50). The normal PR interval correlates both with age and heart rate.[41] The increase in PR interval with decreased heart rate can be accounted for by the fact that heart rate decreases normally with increasing age. Therefore, in Table A-3 of the Appendix, the PR interval is correlated with age and not heart rate.

CAUSES OF FIRST-DEGREE AV BLOCK. The causes of AV block in children are listed in Table 12-11. First-degree AV block occurs in 8% of normal children while asleep.[4] It is otherwise most often due to associated unoperated congenital heart disease. A prolonged PR interval occurs in 10 to 25% of those with patent ductus arteriosus, ostium primum atrial septal defect, Ebstein's anomaly of the tricuspid valve, severe pulmonary stenosis, double outlet right ventricle, ventricular septal defect, and coarctation of the aorta.[42,43] Shortening of the PR interval

FIG. 12-49. Supraventricular tachycardia due to antegrade conduction over a Kent bundle simulating ventricular tachycardia. **Left column,** Sinus rhythm. The short PR interval and delta wave are visible. The ladder diagram refers to lead V_6. There is antegrade conduction over both the Kent bundle and the AV node forming a fusion complex of Wolff-Parkinson-White. **Right column,** Supraventricular tachycardia. The reentry circuit for this tachycardia travels antegradely over the Kent bundle and retrogradely through the AV node. This is the unusual type of supraventricular tachycardia due to Wolff-Parkinson-White. Usually, in the supraventricular tachycardia of Wolff-Parkinson-White, the QRS complex is narrow. This tachycardia has a rate of 270/min with a morphology identical to that found during sinus rhythm. Retrograde P waves occur following each QRS complex. These tracings were taken from a 13-month-old. If the tracings in sinus rhythm had not been available, this would have been diagnosed as a wide QRS tachycardia of undetermined origin with 1:1 retrograde atrial capture, although the positive QRS complexes in leads V_1 and V_6 might suggest antegrade conduction via a bundle of Kent.

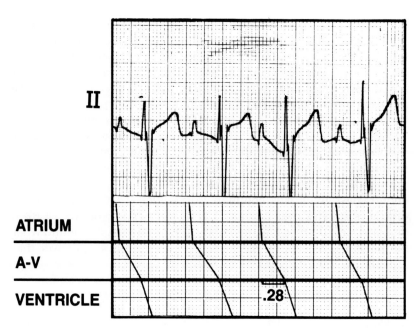

FIG. 12-50.   First-degree AV block. The PR interval is .28 sec.

after correction of some of the defects implies that abnormal hemodynamics (especially stretch of the right atrium or right fibrous trigone) may be partially responsible for the AV block.[44] In other patients with surgery near the AV junction, PR prolongation may develop due to injury to the AV node or bundle of His. PR prolongation is also common in rheumatic fever and myocarditis and usually occurs with digitalis or propranolol effect (Table 12-11).

TABLE 12-11. *Causes of AV Block*

ACUTE

Abnormally increased vagal tone (increased intracranial pressure, increased blood pressure, pharyngeal stimulation, ocular pressure, abdominal distention, idiopathic)

Myocarditis, acute rheumatic fever, endocarditis

Hyperkalemia, hypokalemia, hypercalcemia, hypocalcemia, hypoglycemia, hypoxia, hypothermia

Drugs: digoxin, quinidine, propranolol, verapamil

CHRONIC

Normal variant (first-degree and second-degree, type I only)

Congenital defect in conduction tissue, surgically uncorrected congenital heart disease, postoperative congenital heart disease

Cardiomyopathy, myocardial infarction

Uremia, hyperthyroidism, sarcoid

Second-Degree
AV Block

Second-degree AV block is defined as failure of conduction of some, but not all, of the impulses from the atria to the ventricles. The number of atrial beats that are conducted to the ventricles is expressed as the AV conduction ratio. A ratio of 5:4 implies that of every five atrial impulses, four are conducted to the ventricles.

TYPE I SECOND-DEGREE AV BLOCK. Wenckebach originally described this type of AV block on physical examination and it still bears his name.[45] Mobitz correlated these findings with the electrocardiogram.[46] This is variously referred to as "Wenckebach," "Mobitz type I," or "type I." There is progressive prolongation of the PR interval prior to a nonconducted ("blocked" or "dropped") P wave. "Typical Wenckebach periodicity" also includes the following characteristics. (1) The maximum increase in the PR interval occurs between the first and second conducted beats in a series; thereafter, the increase in the PR interval becomes less with each successive beat. (2) Since each PR interval lengthens by less each time, the RR intervals progressively shorten (Fig. 12-51). (3) The pause created by the blocked P wave is less than twice the preceding RR interval.[47,48] These typical findings may

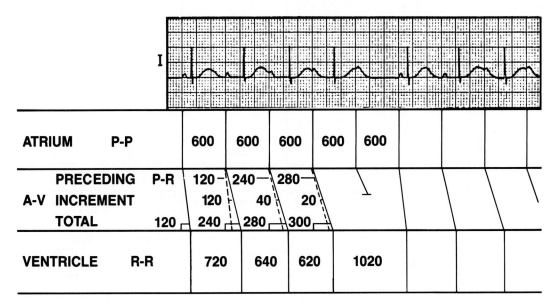

ATRIUM	P-P	600	600	600	600	600			
PRECEDING	P-R	120	240	280					
A-V INCREMENT		120	40	20					
TOTAL	120	240	280	300					
VENTRICLE	R-R		720	640	620	1020			

FIG. 12-51. Mobitz type I ("Wenckebach") AV block. The reason for the shortening RR interval in Wenckebach is demonstrated. The numbers are in milliseconds (100 msec equals .1 sec). In this tracing, the atrial rate (P-P) is constant at 600 msec. The first PR interval is 120 msec. The second PR interval is 240 msec. Thus, the increment from the first to the second PR interval is 120 msec. The third PR interval is 280 msec. The increment from the second PR interval to the third PR interval is 40 msec. The fourth PR interval is 300 msec. The increment is 20 msec between the third and the fourth interval. Therefore, although the PR interval is increasing with each beat, the increment is decreasing. It is the decreasing increment in the PR interval that is responsible for the decrease in the RR interval. In the ladder diagram, the solid lines indicate the measured AV interval. The dotted lines indicate the preceding AV interval. Thus, the increment is represented by the difference in time between the dotted line and the solid line for the AV interval. The fifth P wave does not conduct to the ventricles. Following this, the cycle begins again.

not occur in each patient. The most common variation is a sudden further prolongation of the RR interval prior to the blocked P wave.[49] The important part in the diagnosis of type I second-degree AV block is that the PR interval changes during the sequence of conducted beats. The pause created by the blocked P wave creates groups of QRS complexes and this has been referred to as "grouped beating."[6] Type I

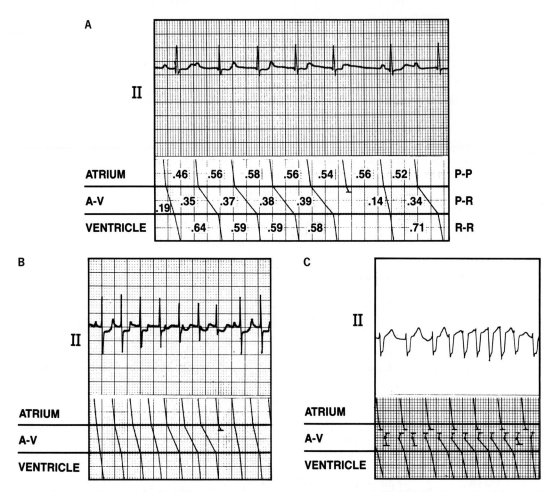

FIG. 12-52. Type I second-degree AV block with various rhythms. A, Wenckebach with sinus arrhythmia. The PP intervals vary from .46 to .58. Nonetheless, the PR intervals progressively lengthen and the RR intervals progressively shorten. Some of the shortening in the RR interval is slightly disturbed by the variation in the PP interval. B, Wenckebach with atrial ectopic supraventricular tachycardia. The atrial rate is slightly variable and approximately 240/min. The PR interval progressively lengthens and is followed by a nonconducted P wave. Then the cycle begins again. C, Wenckebach with junctional ectopic focus tachycardia in a 1-week-old infant. Despite the normal QRS duration, this has the pattern of complete right bundle branch block. The basic junctional cycle length is .20 sec (corresponding to a rate of 300/min). The first three QRS complexes result from 2:1 conduction out of the junctional ectopic focus. Then there is a Wenckebach sequence with longer and longer conduction from the junctional focus to the ventricles. This is not manifest on the surface electrocardiogram; however, the decreasing RR interval is manifest. Conduction then fails from the junction to the ventricles, giving a pause, and then the sequence begins again. There is complete AV dissociation. On other tracings from the same patient, sinus capture beats with a similar morphology demonstrated that this was a supraventricular rhythm.

second-degree AV block can occur with any supraventricular rhythm (sinus tachycardia, supraventricular tachycardia, atrial flutter) and should be suspected whenever groups of QRS complexes occur with either a progressive lengthening of the PR interval or a progressive shortening of the RR interval (Fig. 12-52). In children, type I second-degree AV block usually indicates block within the AV node.[50]

Causes of Type I Second-Degree AV Block. The caues of AV block are listed in Table 12-11. Type I second-degree AV block has been reported to occur in 11% of normal children while asleep without progression to complete AV block.[3–6,51] In patients who have had surgery near the AV junction, rheumatic fever, or myocarditis, type I second-degree AV block is abnormal. Digitalis, propranolol, or verapamil toxicity is diagnosed if type I second-degree AV block occurs in sinus rhythm at rates below 180/min; in the patient with a faster atrial rate (e.g., in atrial flutter), AV block may be the desired effect and should not be considered as evidence of toxicity.

TYPE II SECOND-DEGREE AV BLOCK. In type II block, there is a sudden failure of AV conduction without prolongation of the PR interval before the blocked P wave. If a nonconducted P wave follows several conducted P waves, the diagnosis of type II second-degree AV block is readily made by the constant PR interval (Fig. 12-53). If every other P wave is conducted, this is referred to as 2:1 block. It is not possible to determine if 2:1 block is type I or type II since there is only one PR interval preceding the dropped P wave and therefore progressive prolongation cannot be identified. Frequently, in the patient with 2:1

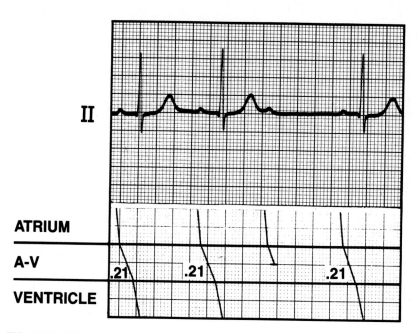

FIG. 12-53. Mobitz type II second-degree AV block. The PR intervals before and after the nonconducted P wave are identical at .21 sec.

block, if a 24-hour electrocardiogram is examined, the underlying type of block can be found. With an increase or decrease in atrial rate, the conduction ratio may change. For example, with a reduction in atrial rate, 4:3 Wenckebach (type I) may be observed and it can be inferred that the underlying cause of the 2:1 block was type I (Fig. 12-54).

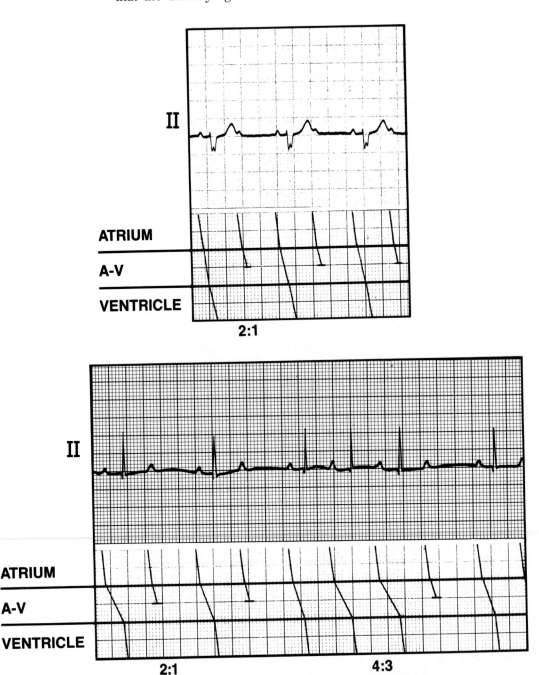

FIG. 12-54. 2:1 block. Top, Tracing taken from a 9-month-old. There is sinus rhythm and every other P wave is not conducted. It is impossible on this tracing to determine if the mechanism for the 2:1 block is type I or type II. Bottom, The tracing begins with 2:1 block but then, due to a variability in the atrial rate, there is an episode of 4:3 Wenckebach conduction. This indicates that the 2:1 block was probably due to a type I mechanism.

"Advanced" type II second-degree AV block is defined as any conduction ratio greater than 2:1 (i.e., 3:1 or 4:1). In this case, several atrial impulses in a row are not conducted to the ventricles (Fig. 12-55). The majority of type II second-degree AV block is localized to the bundle of His or simultaneous block in both bundle branches and is not due to block within the AV node.[52]

Causes of Type II Second-Degree AV Block. Since type II block is generally associated with disease in both the bundle of His and bundle branches, the conducted QRS complexes may have bundle branch block.[53] Type II second-degree AV block was not found in any normal child on 24-hour electrocardiogram.[3-5] It is therefore always abnormal in a child at atrial rates below 180/min and is associated with congenital heart disease, infectious processes, or cardiac surgery. If type II block occurs during sinus rhythm, it more commonly progresses to complete AV block than does type I.[54,55] Type II second-degree AV block normally occurs in rapid atrial rhythms such as atrial flutter, which is frequently conducted with 2:1 or 3:1 block.

AV DISSOCIATION DUE TO SECOND-DEGREE AV BLOCK. The third cause of AV dissociation is AV block. In either type I or type II second-degree AV block, if the pause created by conduction block is sufficiently long, a junctional escape beat or junctional escape rhythm will occur. This will continue until the next atrial beat conducts through the AV junction, thus resetting the timing of the junctional escape pacemaker (Fig. 12-56).

Third-Degree ("Complete") AV Block

Third-degree AV block is defined as a complete lack of transmission of atrial impulses to the ventricles. Long rhythm strips must be examined to be certain that atrial impulses occur that could be conducted to the ventricles (Fig. 12-57). If even occasional atrial impulses conduct to the ventricles, this is classified as "advanced" second-degree AV block.

Complete AV block is the paradigm of complete AV dissociation: The atria and the ventricles are beating completely independently. In complete AV block, any atrial rhythm can coexist with any ventricular rhythm; therefore, both atrial and ventricular rhythms should be specified in the interpretation of the electrocardiogram. In the usual case of congenital complete AV block, the patient has sinus rhythm with a junctional escape rhythm and the atria are beating faster than the ventricles. However, complete AV block may also occur in, for example, a patient with atrial flutter and a junctional escape rhythm (atria faster than ventricles) (Fig. 12-58), or in a patient with sinus bradycardia and accelerated junctional rhythm (ventricles faster than atria). In the latter case, it is important to determine if P waves occur that should conduct to the ventricles: If the atrial rate is less than 180/min and a P wave occurs beyond the preceding T wave and does not conduct to the ventricles, AV block is diagnosed. If, in addition to the sinus brady-

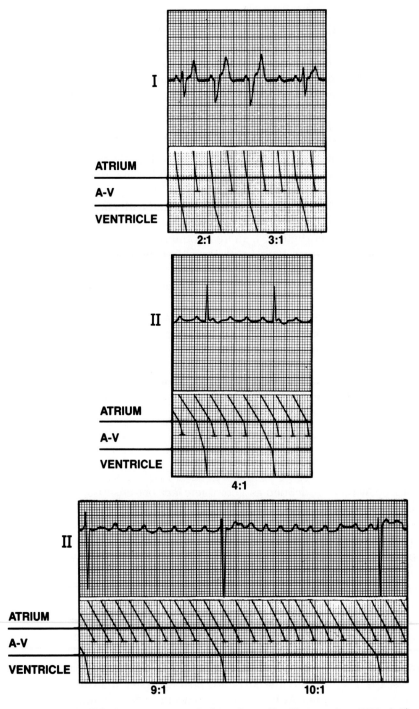

FIG. 12-55. Advanced type II AV block. **Top,** Supraventricular tachycardia with 2:1 and 3:1 AV block. The atrial cycle length is constant at .26 sec. The PR interval is slightly variable. **Middle,** Atrial flutter with 4:1 block. The atrial cycle length is constant at 240 msec. There is 4:1 AV conduction. **Bottom,** Atrial flutter with 9:1 block and 10:1 block. The "PR" interval is variable. It is possible that the atria and ventricles are completely unrelated and that the ventricular depolarization is actually caused by junctional rhythm. In this case, however, this is doubtful because the ventricular rate is variable, thus indicating at least some capture of the ventricles by the atria. Were there no ventricular capture, the ventricular rate would be absolutely regular. In this 3-year-old patient, there is also a suppression of junctional automaticity since there is a 2.1 sec pause without a junctional escape beat.

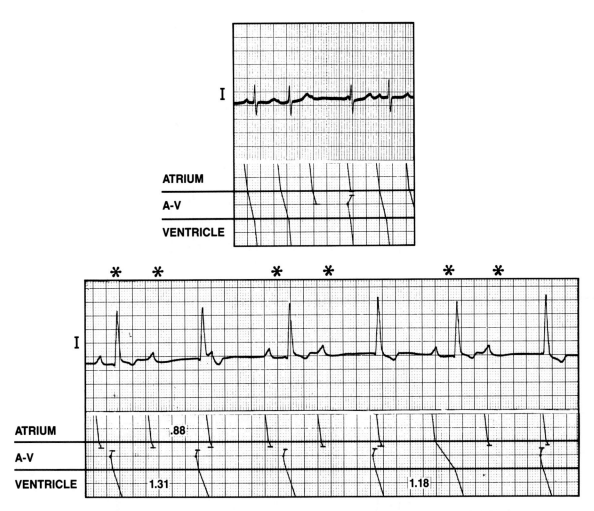

FIG. 12-56. AV dissociation with AV block. **Top,** Type I second-degree AV block. A typical Wenckebach sequence occurs in the first three beats with a prolongation of the PR interval and a nonconducted P wave. The pause is ended by the almost simultaneous appearance of a P wave and a QRS complex. The PR interval is too short to be conducted normally and this is a junctional escape beat. This frequently occurs at the end of Wenckebach cycles. **Bottom,** AV dissociation with advanced type II second degree AV block and intermittent sinus capture. No constant relationship exists between the P waves and the QRS complexes. The ventricles are controlled by a junctional rhythm with a cycle length of 1.31 sec (corresponding to a rate of 46/min). The atrial cycle length is .88 sec (corresponding to a rate of 68/min). There is one conducted P wave which is demonstrated by the shortened RR interval to 1.18 sec. The cause for this AV dissociation is AV block. Those P waves marked by asterisks should conduct to the ventricles since they occur beyond the end of the T wave.

cardia and accelerated junctional rhythm, additional AV block is diagnosed, the patient has all three causes for AV dissociation at the same time (Fig. 12-59).

CAUSES OF THIRD-DEGREE AV BLOCK. Complete AV block in children may be congenital or acquired. Approximately 1/20,000 infants are born with congenital complete AV block.[1,56] In those infants with congenital complete AV block, there may be a relationship to connective tissue disease in their mothers.[57] The majority of congenital complete AV block occurs because of a lack of continuity between the atria and

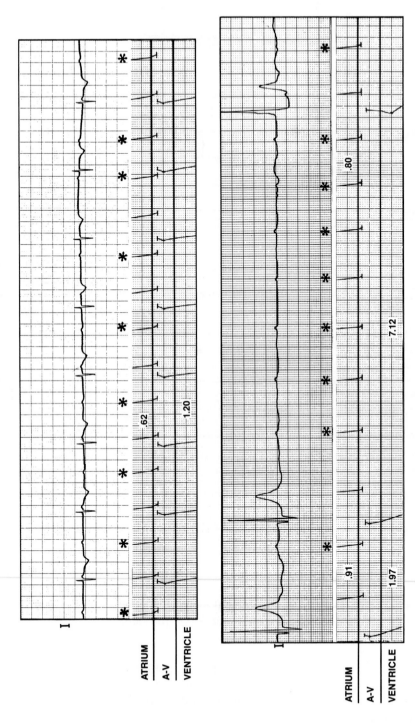

FIG. 12-57. Complete AV block: complete AV dissociation. Top, Complete AV block in a 1-month-old child. The atrial cycle length is .62 sec (corresponding to an atrial rate of 97/min) and the ventricles are controlled by a junctional, narrow QRS-rhythm with a cycle length of 1.2 sec (ventricular rate of 50/min). The P waves with asterisks should conduct to the ventricles. The reason for the complete AV dissociation is complete AV block. Bottom, Complete AV block with a slow junctional rhythm. The atrial cycle length originally is .91 sec but increases as the period of asystole lengthens. The original junctional cycle length is 1.97 sec (corresponding to a rate of 30/min) and this is followed by a period of asystole which lasts for 7.12 sec (corresponding to a ventricular rate of 8/min) and is ended by an idioventricular escape beat. P waves that should have conducted are marked by asterisks.

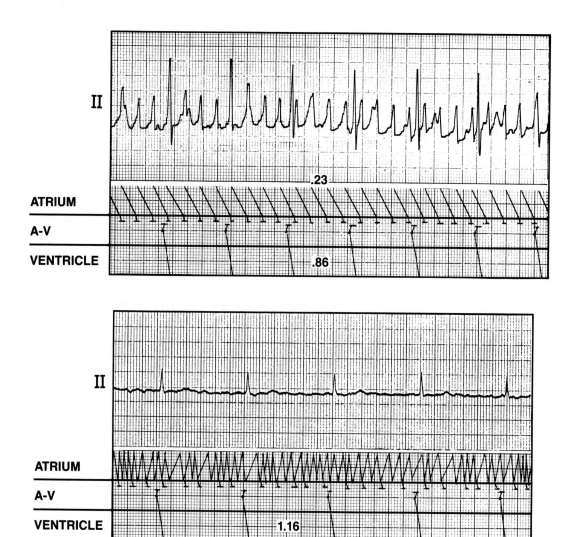

FIG. 12-58. Complete AV block with rapid supraventricular rhythms. **Top,** Atrial flutter with complete AV block. The atrial cycle length is constant at .23 sec. This corresponds to an atrial rate of 260/min. The junctional rate is constant at a cycle length of .86 sec. This corresponds to a ventricular rate of 70/min. There is complete AV dissociation with no relationship between the P waves and the QRS complexes, and the ventricular rate is regular. This suggests complete AV block. **Bottom,** Atrial fibrillation with complete AV block. The ventricular cycle length is absolutely regular at 1.16 sec (corresponding to a rate of 52/min). The hallmark of atrial fibrillation is an irregularly irregular ventricular rate. When the ventricular rate is absolutely regular in atrial fibrillation this indicates complete AV block.

the AV node.[58] About one third of infants with congenital complete AV block have associated congenital heart disease, mostly L-transposition of the great arteries with ventricular inversion.[59] Patients with ventricular inversion have an abnormally situated anterior AV node and nonbranching portion of the bundle of His. This abnormally situated AV node and bundle may not connect with the normal conduction system. In patients with congenital complete AV block, the escape rhythm usually has a narrow QRS, indicating a junctional origin. If the QRS is wide, it indicates a ventricular origin. Ventricular escape rhythms in congenital complete AV block may be irregular and slow, leading to long pauses in ventricular activity.[59]

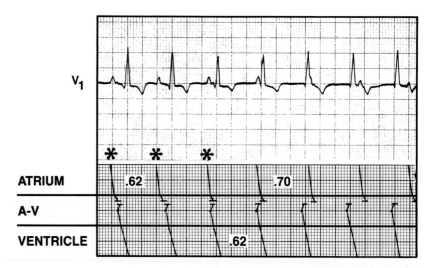

FIG. 12-59. AV dissociation due to all three causes. Tracing taken from a 1-month-old. There is complete AV dissociation without any relationship of the P waves to the QRS complexes. There is sinus bradycardia. The atrial cycle length varies from .62 to .70 corresponding to rates from 86 to 97/min. There is an accelerated junctional rhythm with a cycle length of .62 sec (corresponding to a junctional rate of 97/min). In addition, the pattern has AV block, since the P waves that are asterisked should have conducted and shortened the RR interval. Therefore, in this patient, simply stating that the diagnosis is AV dissociation is not helpful because all three possible causes are contributing: sinus bradycardia, accelerated junctional rhythm, and AV block.

The most common causes of acquired complete AV block are: (1) surgery near the AV junction (AV canal, ventricular septal defect, tetralogy of Fallot, aortic stenosis) in patients with normally related ventricles, or repair of pulmonary stenosis or ventricular septal defect in patients with ventricular inversion;[59,60] and (2) myocarditis, especially due to diphtheria[51] (see Table 12-11). Acquired AV block in children may occur within the AV node or bundle of His, or below the bundle of His with injury to both bundle branches. Because the majority of patients with surgically acquired AV block have additional bundle branch block acquired at the time of surgery, the location of the escape rhythm (junctional or ventricular) cannot be ascertained on the surface electrocardiogram if there is a wide QRS complex.[60] If there is a narrow QRS complex, this is a junctional escape rhythm. Acquired AV block may be reversible, but the patient should be closely observed for the later development of sudden complete AV block.

The Morphologic Approach

INTRODUCTION TO THE SYSTEMATIC INTERPRETATION OF CARDIAC ARRHYTHMIAS IN CHILDREN

Certain principles are helpful in the analysis of the cardiac rhythm in children. We have developed a step-by-step method of diagnosis which, while not including every possible arrhythmia, will place most rhythm disturbances in a single category. In an analysis of the electrocardiogram, certain questions must be answered sequentially (Fig. 12-60).

This method differs from most others in that it begins with the QRS complex. The QRS is the most obvious feature of the electrocardiogram and, in actual practice, the first determination made is usually the regularity of the QRS complexes. We have used hand-drawn electrocardiographic tracings in the teaching of this method. This has several advantages. First, it allows us to vary one part of the electrocardiogram at a time, while keeping all other parts constant; for example, we can keep the QRS rate and P rate exactly the same while varying only the P mean vector. In this way, focus is directed at the important teaching point rather than the unimportant slight change in rate or QRS morphology. The second advantage is that the tracings are easy to read, without wandering baselines or electrical interference.

The use of this method requires no expertise with the electrophysiologic principles that underlie the electrocardiogram. This is a stepwise deductive method used by pediatric cardiologists. It can be learned by anyone who knows the basics of the electrocardiogram in

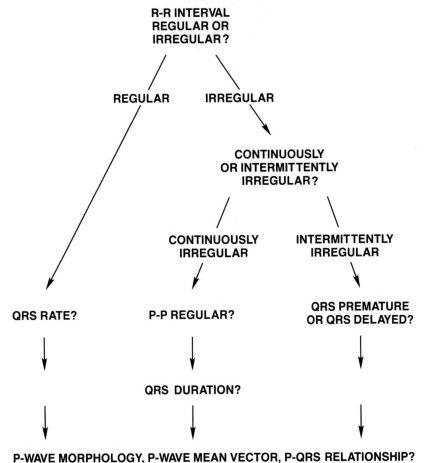

FIG. 12-60. Schema for interpretation of arrhythmias.

adults or children: morphology, rate, mean vector, and duration of both the P wave and QRS complex. Once learned, it is a method that may be easily and quickly reviewed by those who encounter arrhythmias infrequently in children. When the questions in Figure 12-60 are answered, the arrhythmias will be identified.

The first step is to decide whether the ventricular rate (RR interval) is regular. We consider a rhythm to be regular if the RR intervals in the electrocardiogram vary by less than 0.08 sec (Figs. 12-61 and 12-62). The examples shown in the figures are idealized drawings taken from the electrocardiograms of different 4-year-old patients. For patients in the 3- to 4-year age range, the normal QRS rate ranges from 70 to 140/min, the normal PR interval is .09 to .16 sec, and the normal QRS duration is .04 to .10 sec.

If the ventricular rate is regular, the answers to three further questions will categorize the rhythm. The first question is whether the ventricular rate is decreased, normal, or increased for a child of the

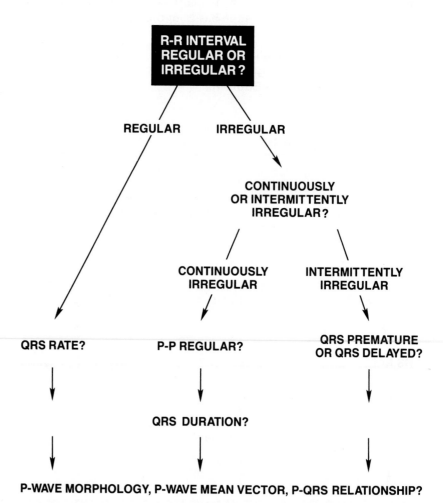

FIG. 12-61. Regular versus irregular RR interval.

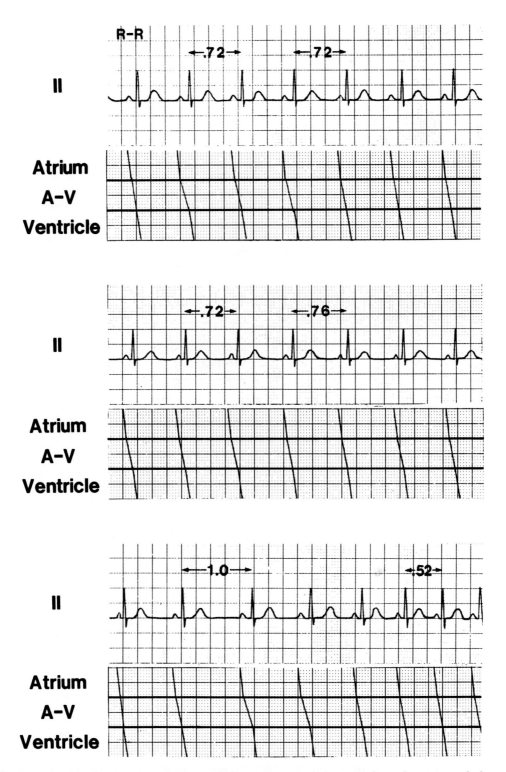

FIG. 12-62. Regular versus irregular rhythm. **Top tracing,** Sinus rhythm; absolutely regular RR interval of .72 sec (QRS rate = 85/min). **Middle tracing,** Sinus rhythm; first three RR intervals are .72 sec, followed by three RR intervals of .76 sec. Since the RR intervals vary by .08 sec or less, this is considered a regular rhythm. **Bottom tracing,** Sinus arrhythmia; the RR intervals vary from .52 to 1.0 sec. This is a markedly irregular rhythm.

patient's age (Fig. 12-63). For example, Figure 12-64 shows three sample electrocardiograms, each taken from a 4-year-old patient. The ventricular rates are 50/min, 85/min, and 180/min. For a 4-year-old child, a ventricular rate of 50/min indicates bradycardia and 180/min indicates tachycardia.

The second question to be answered is whether the QRS duration is normal or prolonged (Fig. 12-65). If the QRS duration is prolonged, the specific morphology must be determined. In a 4-year-old, the upper limit of normal for QRS duration is .10 sec. Any QRS complex that is longer than .10 sec is prolonged. An abnormally long QRS complex may have one of four distinct morphologies (Fig. 12-66A and B). It is most helpful to distinguish among these different morphologies by looking at leads V$_1$ and V$_6$. In complete right bundle branch block, the initial .04 sec shows a rapid, normal deflection and the terminal forces are inscribed slowly (wide QRS). These terminal forces are directed anteriorly and to the right (positive in V$_1$ and negative in V$_6$) because the right ventricle has delayed activation. Therefore, in complete right

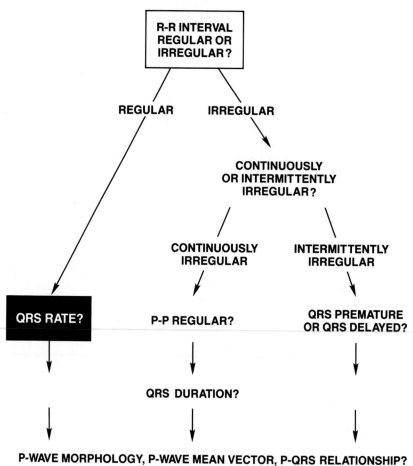

FIG. 12-63.   Regular RR interval: variation in QRS rate.

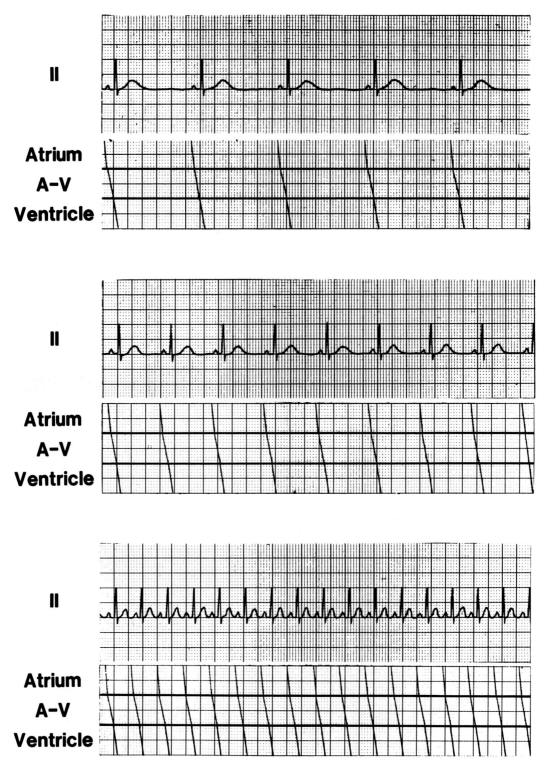

FIG. 12-64. Variation in QRS rate. **Top tracing,** Sinus bradycardia; QRS rate is 50/min. **Middle tracing,** Sinus rhythm; QRS rate is 85/min. **Bottom tracing,** Sinus tachycardia; QRS rate is 180/min.

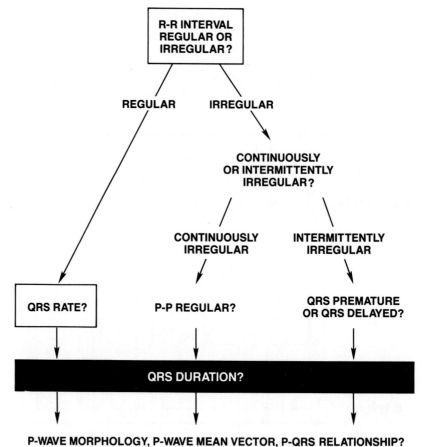

FIG. 12-65. Regular RR interval: QRS duration.

bundle branch block, in V_1 the complex is mainly positive with an RSR' morphology. In complete left bundle branch block, the delayed terminal forces are directed posteriorly and to the left, because the left ventricle has delayed activation; in complete left bundle branch block in V_1 the complex is mainly negative, and in V_6 it is mainly positive with an RR' morphology (Fig. 12-66A).

In the Wolff-Parkinson-White syndrome, the PR interval is short and the abnormally prolonged QRS complex is inscribed slowly in the initial .02 to .04 sec. This slow initial deflection is called the "delta" wave. The remainder of the QRS complex is inscribed rapidly and normally.

The QRS complex of diffuse intraventricular conduction delay found in quinidine toxicity, myocarditis, hypoglycemia, myocardial ischemia, and hyperkalemia involves delay in all phases of depolarization and the inscription of the entire QRS complex is prolonged (Fig. 12-66B).

The third question to be answered concerns atrial activity (Fig. 12-67). When the atria depolarize, one of three patterns is observed in the

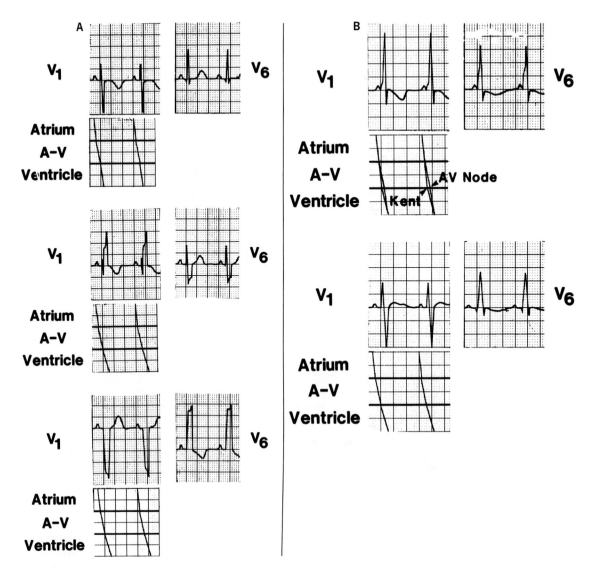

FIG. 12-66. Types of ventricular aberration. A, **Top tracing,** Normal duration (.08 sec) QRS complex. **Middle tracing,** Prolonged duration (.12 sec) QRS complex with complete right bundle branch block morphology. Note the terminal slowing which is positive in V₁. **Bottom tracing,** Prolonged duration (.12 sec) QRS complex with complete left bundle branch block morphology. Note the M-shaped complex with an absent Q wave in V₆. B, **Top tracing,** Prolonged duration (.12 sec) QRS complex with Wolff-Parkinson-White morphology. The PR interval is short (.08 sec). The initial .04 sec of the QRS has a slurred upstroke—the "delta" wave. The latter part of the QRS is normal. **Bottom tracing,** Prolonged duration (.12 sec) QRS complex with morphology of diffuse intraventricular conduction delay. This is a wide QRS complex without the specific morphology of complete right bundle branch block, complete left bundle branch block, or Wolff-Parkinson-White.

electrocardiogram (Fig. 12-68):

  (1) P waves—distinct depolarizations, normally .03 to .08 sec in
      duration and more pointed than T waves.
  (2) Flutter waves—.09 to .18 sec in duration and occurring in suc-
      cession, giving the impression of a "sawtooth" baseline. Flutter

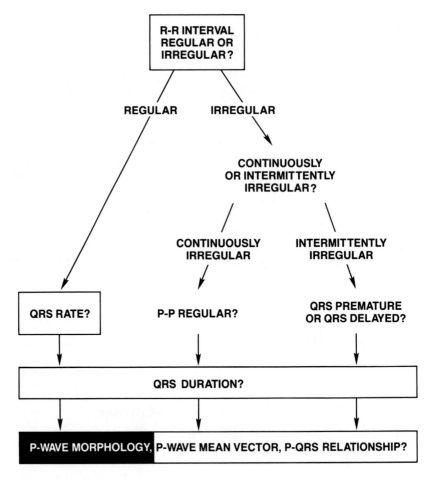

FIG. 12-67. Regular RR interval: P wave morphology.

waves may not be visible in all electrocardiographic leads; the most likely leads to show flutter waves are II, III, aV$_F$, and V$_1$

(3) Fibrillation—coarse or fine irregular oscillations of the baseline without other demonstrable atrial activity.

If P waves are visible, the P wave mean vector must be determined (Figs. 12-69 and 12-70A and B) (see Chapter 5, "P Wave Mean Vector").

Finally, the relationship of the atrial depolarizations to the QRS complexes must be determined (Fig. 12-71). Either the atrial depolarizations are related in a regular way to the QRS complexes or the atrial depolarizations are unrelated to the QRS complexes (AV dissociation). If an atrial depolarization precedes each QRS complex with a constant PR interval, we assume that the atrial depolarization conducted through the His bundle and caused the ventricular depolarization (Fig. 12-72). See the discussion on "Isochronic Dissociation" in the following paragraphs. If an atrial depolarization follows each QRS complex with a constant RP interval (and a mean vector of −1 to −90°), we assume that the AV junction or ventricle initiated the depolarization

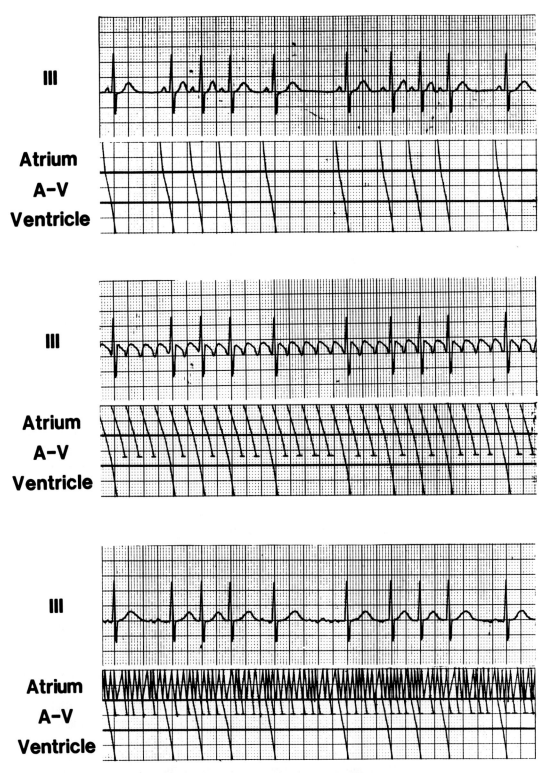

FIG. 12-68. Morphology of atrial depolarization. **Top tracing,** Sinus arrhythmia; a P wave precedes each QRS complex. **Middle tracing,** Atrial flutter with varying type II second-degree AV block; flutter waves are visible throughout the tracing. **Bottom tracing,** Atrial fibrillation; note the fine oscillations in the baseline.

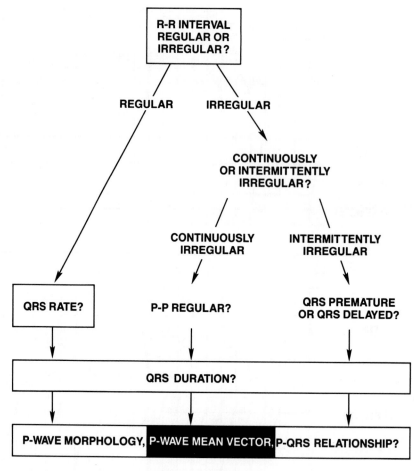

FIG. 12-69.   Regular RR interval: P wave mean vector.

and the impulse conducted retrogradely through the AV node and depolarized the atrium. One other type of P-QRS relationship occurs if there are more P waves than QRS complexes; if the RR interval is regular and the PP interval (atrial rate) is a constant multiple of the ventricular rate (every second, third, or fourth atrial depolarization is followed by a QRS complex), the diagnosis is second-degree AV block. In this case, each ventricular depolarization is caused by an atrial depolarization.

If the atrial and ventricular depolarizations are unrelated, the diagnosis is AV dissociation. Atrioventricular dissociation occurs in several arrhythmias of entirely different mechanisms. Therefore, AV dissociation should never be the only diagnosis in the interpretation of an electrocardiogram. The following are the three major causes for AV dissociation (Fig. 12-73A and B).

(1) Slowing of sinus or atrial rhythm with junctional rhythm occurring at a normal junctional rate. If retrograde conduction to the atria does not occur during junctional rhythm, AV dissociation may occur, with the slow sinus beats continuing to depolarize

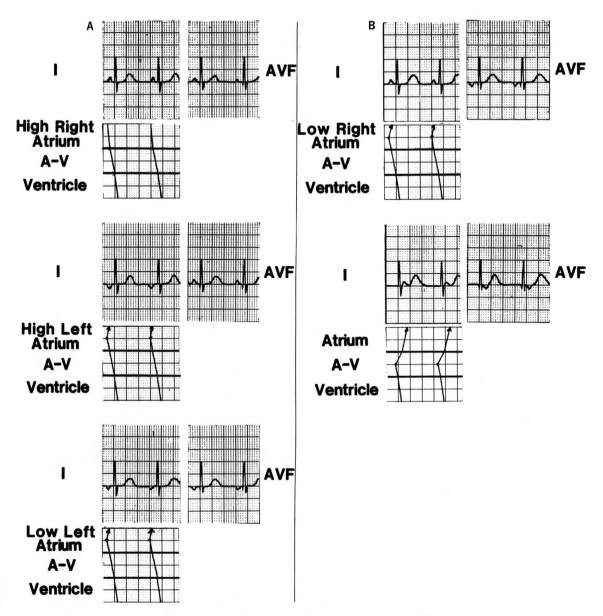

FIG. 12-70. P wave mean vector. A, **Top tracing,** Sinus rhythm; P wave mean vector 0° to +90°. **Middle tracing,** High left atrial rhythm; P wave mean vector +91° to 180°. **Bottom tracing,** Low left atrial rhythm; P wave mean vector −179° to −91°. B, **Top tracing,** Low right atrial rhythm; P wave mean vector −1° to −90°. **Bottom tracing,** Junctional rhythm; P wave mean vector −1° to −90° with P wave following QRS complex.

the atria while the impulses arising in the junction depolarize the ventricles. (Fig. 12-73A).

(2) An accelerated junctional or a ventricular rhythm without retrograde conduction results in an abnormally rapid ventricular rate with a normal sinus rate (Fig. 12-73A).

(3) Complete AV block is the best example of AV dissociation because, by definition, the atria and ventricles are unrelated (Fig. 12-73B).

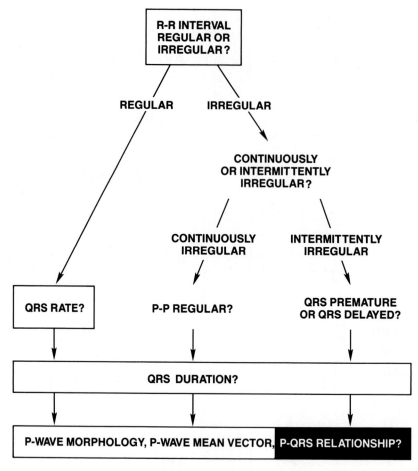

FIG. 12-71.   Regular RR interval: P-QRS relationship.

It is possible to have the atria and ventricles beating at exactly the same rate and have a constant PR interval with no conduction from atria to ventricles. This is called "isorhythmic" or "isochronic" dissociation. (Fig. 12-73B). The only way to prove the existence of isochronic dissociation is to find, in a long rhythm strip, that one of the two rates changes (atria or ventricles) and the other stays the same. For example, if the PP interval lengthens and the PR interval remains constant, AV dissociation will then become evident.

If the RR intervals are irregular, they can either be irregular continuously or there can be a basic, regular RR interval into which an irregular RR interval is intermittently introduced (Figs. 12-74 and 12-75).

If the RR interval varies continuously, the next question to be answered is whether the PP intervals are regular. Next, the QRS duration should be ascertained and, finally, if the QRS is continuously irregular, the P wave mean vector, P morphology, and P-QRS relationship should be determined (Figs. 12-76 and 12-77). In pediatrics, if the PP intervals vary, generally the atrial and ventricular depolarizations are related and, therefore, the RR interval will also vary. The two most common

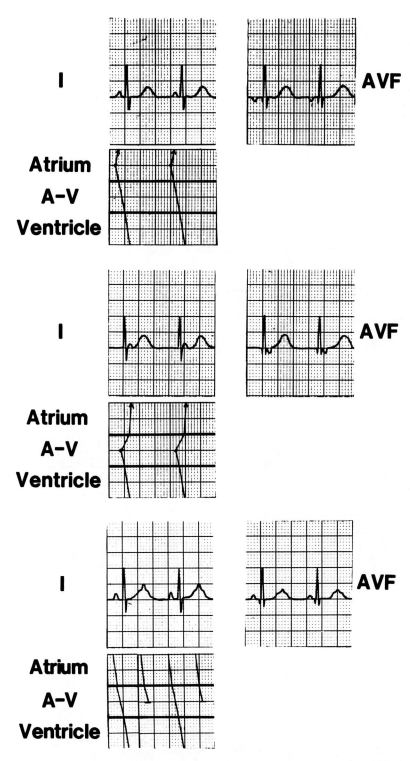

FIG. 12-72. P-QRS relationship. **Top tracing:** Low right atrial rhythm; P wave precedes each QRS complex. **Middle tracing:** Junctional rhythm; P wave follows each QRS complex. **Bottom tracing:** Sinus tachycardia with fixed type II second-degree AV block; a QRS complex follows every other P wave; QRS rate is 85/min and P rate is 170/min.

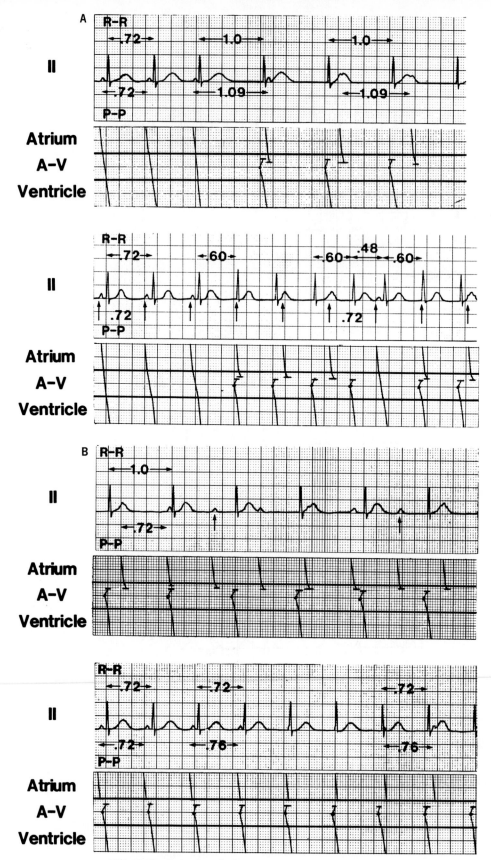

FIG. 12-73. Legend on facing page.

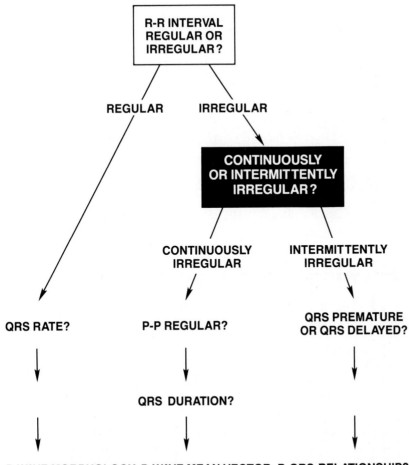

FIG. 12-74. Irregular RR interval: continuously versus intermittently irregular.

FIG. 12-73. AV dissociation. A, Top tracing, Sinus rhythm followed by junctional rhythm with AV dissociation; the first three complexes are sinus rhythm at a rate of 85/min. The sinus rate then slows to 55/min (PP interval = 1.09 sec). The patient's normal junctional rate of 60/min (RR interval = .72 sec) is usually suppressed by the faster sinus rate. However, at this time, the junctional rate is faster than the sinus rate and the junction assumes the function of the pacemaker. The sinus P waves continue dissociated through the tracing because in this patient there is no retrograde conduction to the atrium from the junction, so sinus rhythm is not disturbed. Bottom tracing, Sinus rhythm followed by accelerated junctional rhythm with AV dissociation. The first three complexes are sinus rhythm at a rate of 85/min. The sinus rate remains at 85/min (sinus P waves marked by arrows every .72 sec), but the AV junction develops an abnormally rapid rate of 100/min (RR interval .60 sec) and assumes the pacemaker function. The P waves and QRS complexes are dissociated because there is no retrograde conduction from the junction to the atria; however, conduction is intact from atria to ventricles. A short RR interval (.48 sec) is found when a sinus P wave occurs sufficiently after the preceding QRS complex that the AV node is not refractory and AV conduction can occur. This is a sinus "capture" beat; accelerated junctional rhythm resumes after the capture beat. B, Top tracing, Complete AV block; the junctional rate is 60/min (RR interval 1.0 sec); the atrial rate is 85/min (PP interval .72 sec); the P waves and QRS complexes are dissociated because there is no conduction through the AV node in either antegrade or retrograde direction. If antegrade conduction was intact, two P waves (arrows) should have changed the RR interval (see Fig. 12-73A, bottom). The RR interval was not influenced by the intervening P waves and therefore the P waves probably did not conduct to the ventricles. Bottom tracing, Complete AV block with isochronic dissociation; the RR intervals remain absolutely constant at .72 sec; the PP intervals begin at .72 sec. However, the PP intervals lengthen to .76 sec, with a shortening PR interval, and the RR interval is unaffected. The change in atrial rate without a corresponding change in ventricular rate is the clue that, most likely, the first three P waves were not conducted to the ventricles but only appeared to be because the atria and ventricles were beating independently at exactly the same rate ("isochronic" dissociation).

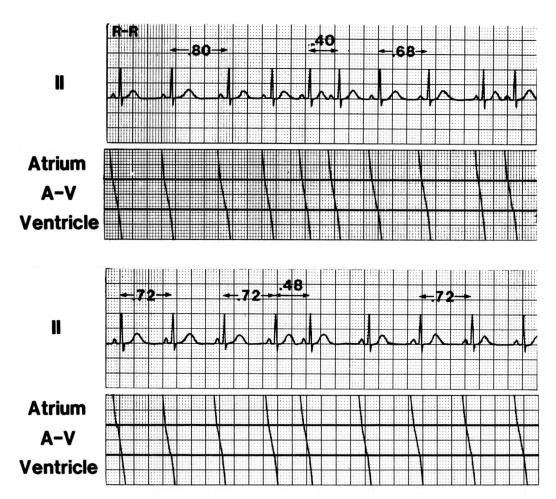

FIG. 12-75. Continuously irregular versus intermittently irregular. **Top tracing,** Sinus arrhythmia; the RR intervals vary throughout the tracing; this is "continuously irregular." **Bottom tracing,** Sinus rhythm with premature atrial contraction; the RR intervals are basically constant but are interrupted by an irregular RR interval; this is "intermittently irregular."

causes of irregular PP and RR intervals are sinus arrhythmia and wandering pacemaker. In sinus arrhythmia, the P wave mean vector varies between 0 and +90°. In wandering pacemaker, P waves are not always present; when P waves are present in wandering pacemaker, the P wave mean vector may vary throughout the four quadrants. Of course, atrial fibrillation is "irregularly irregular" (no two RR intervals the same) and falls into the category of irregular RR intervals.

If the RR interval is irregular but the PP interval is regular, the most likely diagnosis is second-degree AV block of a type in which the RR intervals vary. In typical type I second-degree AV block (Wenckebach), the PR intervals progressively lengthen and the RR intervals progressively shorten until an atrial depolarization occurs without a following QRS complex and the cycle begins again. In type II second-degree AV

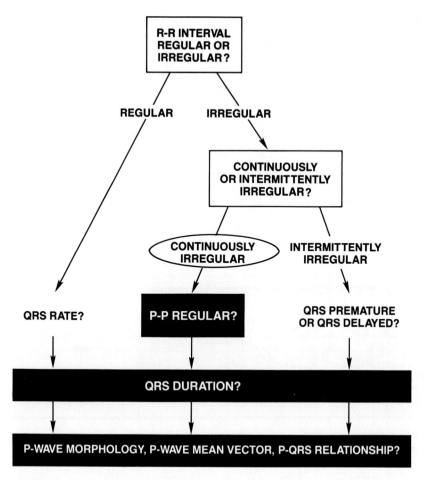

FIG. 12-76. Continuously irregular: PP interval, QRS duration, and atrial activity.

block, the PR intervals remain constant but the RR intervals may vary if the number of atrial depolarizations that are conducted to the ventricles varies (Fig. 12-77). Each type of AV block can occur with any type of supraventricular rhythm: either sinus or ectopic atrial rhythm, supraventricular tachycardia, or atrial flutter.

If there is a basic, regular RR interval that is interrupted intermittently, the initial question to be answered is whether the first irregular RR interval is shorter or longer than the basic, regular RR interval (Figs. 12-78 and 12-79). To be considered irregular, the RR interval must vary from the basic RR interval by at least .04 to .08 sec, depending on the regularity of the predominant rhythm.

If the QRS is premature, the RR interval that follows the premature QRS may be prolonged (Fig. 12-80). The degree of prolongation has been used to distinguish among types of premature beats. In children, any type of premature beat may be followed by a "compensatory pause," so that the degree of prolongation is of little value.

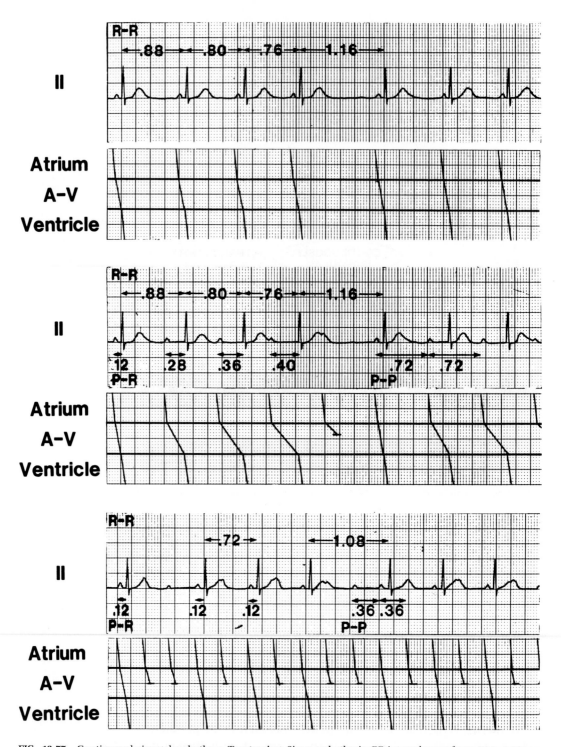

FIG. 12-77. Continuously irregular rhythms. **Top tracing,** Sinus arrhythmia; RR intervals vary from .76 to 1.16 sec; each QRS complex is preceded by a P wave with a constant PR interval. **Middle tracing,** Sinus rhythm with type I second-degree AV block (Wenckebach); the RR intervals are identical to those in the top tracing; the PR interval lengthens until a P wave is not followed by a QRS. **Bottom tracing,** Sinus tachycardia with varying type II second-degree AV block; the atrial rate is 167 (PP interval = .36 sec); the RR interval varies from .72 with 2:1 block to 1.08 with 4:1 block.

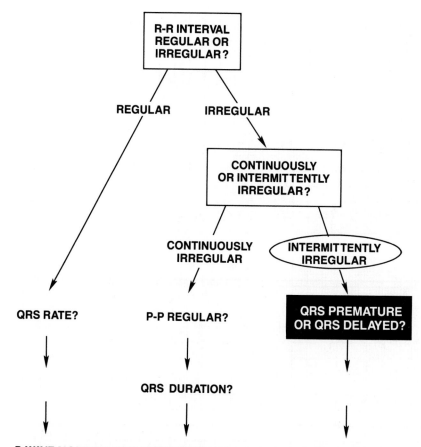

FIG. 12-78. Intermittently irregular: premature versus delayed QRS.

The QRS duration is determined next. If the QRS duration is normal, the premature QRS can have one of three causes (Fig. 12-81):

(1) Intermittent conduction of a sinus beat. In the presence of atrial or junctional rhythm, the sinus node continues to depolarize. If the early QRS is preceded by a P wave with a normal mean vector (0 to $+90°$), the sinus node depolarization has conducted to the atria, causing the P wave, and the atrial impulse has conducted to the ventricles (so-called "sinus capture").

(2) In either sinus, atrial, or junctional rhythm, if the early QRS is preceded by a premature P wave, this is a premature atrial contraction.

(3) If the QRS is not preceded by a premature P wave, this is a premature junctional contraction.

If the premature QRS has a prolonged duration (Fig. 12-82), there are three possible causes which are similar to those for a normal duration QRS:

(1) Sinus capture with aberration

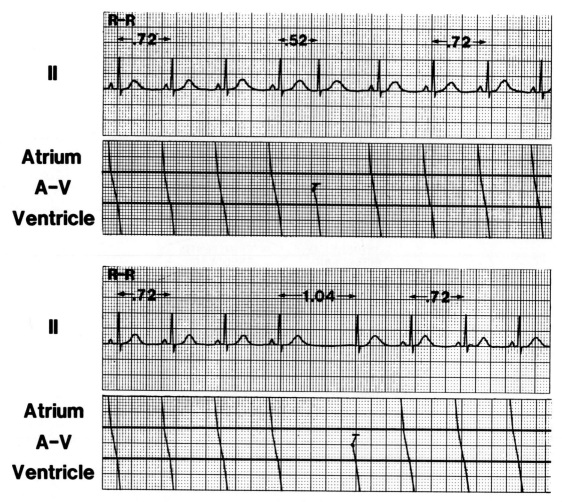

FIG. 12-79. Intermittently irregular: premature versus delayed QRS. **Top tracing,** Sinus rhythm with premature junctional contraction; basic RR interval is regular at .72 sec; it is interrupted by a premature QRS with an RR interval of .52 sec. **Bottom tracing,** Sinus rhythm with sinus pause and junctional escape beat; basic RR interval is regular at .72 sec; it is interrupted by a delayed QRS with an RR interval of 1.04 sec.

(2) Premature atrial contraction with aberration

(3) Premature ventricular contraction

It is possible to have a premature QRS complex without a preceding P wave due to a premature junctional contraction with aberration; but it is impossible on the surface electrocardiogram in children to distinguish a premature junctional contraction with aberration from a premature ventricular contraction (Fig. 12-83). Therefore, we have chosen to classify all QRS complexes that are premature and have a prolonged duration without preceding P waves as premature ventricular contractions.

If the QRS is not premature, but rather delayed by 0.04 to .08 sec or more, then the QRS duration should be determined (Fig. 12-84). If the QRS duration is normal, the answers to three questions will classify the rhythm. The first question concerns the basic supraventricular

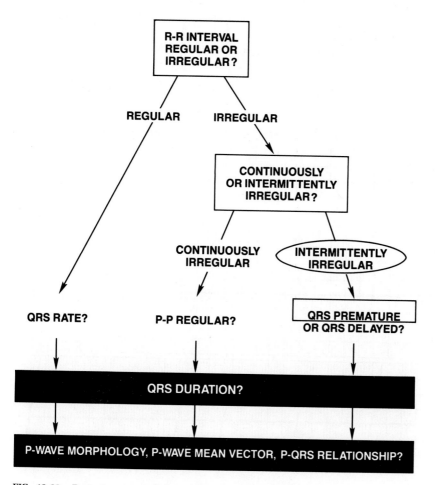

FIG. 12-80. Premature normal duration QRS: atrial activity.

rhythm: (a) In second-degree AV block, the supraventricular rhythm continues uninterrupted; (b) in a nonconducted premature atrial contraction, a different morphology P wave is introduced prematurely; and (c) with a "pause" in the supraventricular rhythm, no atrial activity is observed (Fig. 12-85A and B).

Second, what is the RR interval from the delayed QRS complex back to the immediately preceding QRS? In type II second-degree AV block, the RR interval is twice the basic RR interval; in a nonconducted premature atrial contraction the RR interval is less than twice the basic RR interval. While most premature atrial contractions can be followed by either a compensatory or a noncompensatory pause, virtually all nonconducted premature atrial contractions have less than a fully compensatory pause. Therefore, both the PP and RR intervals should be less than twice the basic RR interval. In a "pause," the RR interval can be of any duration, but it is always longer than the basic RR interval (Fig. 12-85A and B).

The third question concerns the atrial activity immediately preceding the delayed QRS complex. In AV block, the delayed QRS is pre-

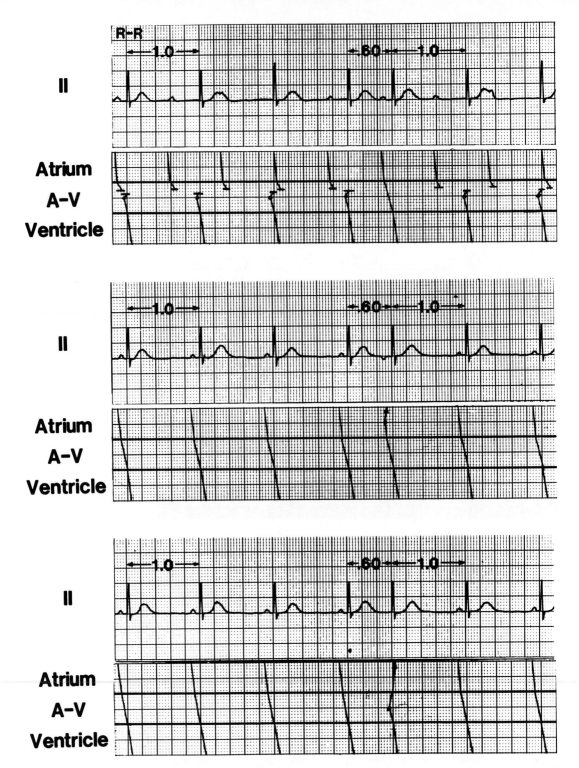

FIG. 12-81. Intermittently irregular: premature QRS. Top tracing, Sinus rhythm with advanced second-degree AV block and junctional escape rhythm; the basic RR interval is 1.0 sec (junctional rhythm at 60/min). The premature QRS is due to a sinus "capture" beat (see Fig. 12-73). This is the only P wave that conducts. All the other P waves are blocked. This is "advanced" second-degree AV block. Middle tracing, Sinus rhythm with premature atrial contraction; the basic RR interval is 1.0 sec (sinus rhythm at 60/min). The premature QRS is preceded by a P wave which is negative in lead II; this is a premature atrial contraction originating from an inferior location in the atria. Bottom tracing, Sinus rhythm with premature junctional contraction; the basic RR interval is 1.0 sec (sinus rhythm at 60/min). The premature QRS is not preceded by a P wave; this is a premature junctional contraction.

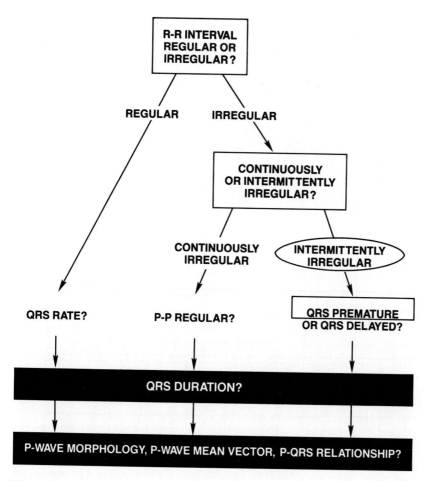

FIG. 12-82.   Premature prolonged duration QRS: atrial activity.

ceded by a supraventricular P wave that is identical to that seen in the basic rhythm. In a nonconducted premature atrial contraction, the delayed QRS is also preceded by a supraventricular P wave that is identical to that seen in the basic supraventricular rhythm. In a pause with atrial escape, the delayed QRS is preceded by a P wave with a different mean vector and morphology from the basic P wave. In a pause with junctional escape, the delayed QRS is not preceded by a P wave.

If the QRS complex is delayed and the QRS duration is prolonged, the most common rhythm is a pause with ventricular escape (Fig. 12-85B).

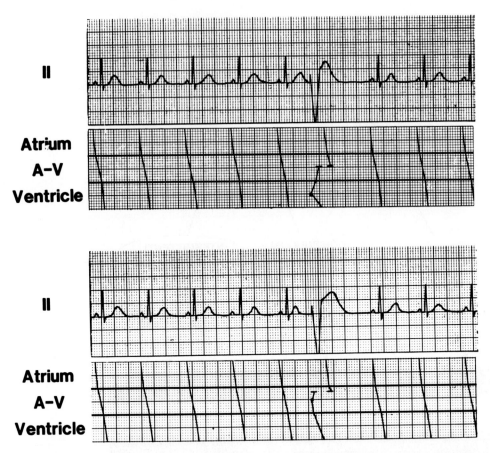

FIG. 12-83. Premature ventricular contraction versus premature junctional contraction with aberration. **Top tracing,** Sinus rhythm and premature ventricular contraction; basic RR interval interrupted by a premature QRS with prolonged duration. **Bottom tracing,** Sinus rhythm and premature junctional contraction with aberration; basic RR interval interrupted by a premature QRS with prolonged duration. These two arrhythmias are indistinguishable on the surface electrocardiogram.

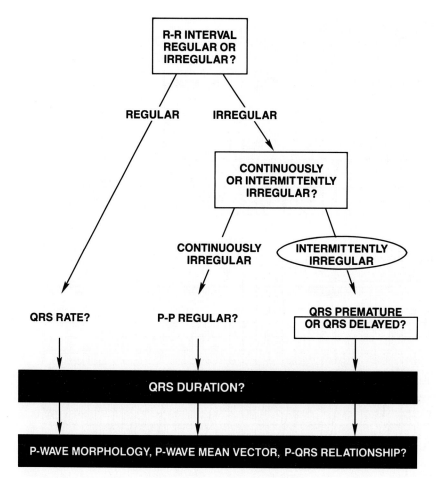

FIG. 12-84. Delayed QRS: QRS duration, atrial activity.

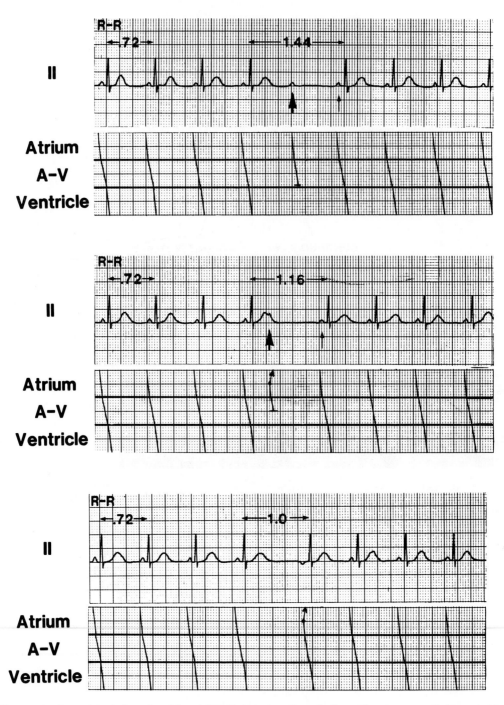

FIG. 12-85A. Intermittently irregular: delayed QRS. **Top tracing,** Sinus rhythm with type II second-degree AV block; the basic RR interval is interrupted by an irregular RR interval that is exactly twice the basic RR interval. Sinus rhythm continues after the last regular QRS (large arrow); sinus rhythm initiates the QRS, which is delayed (small arrow). **Middle tracing,** Sinus rhythm with nonconducted premature atrial contraction; the basic RR interval is interrupted by an irregular RR interval that is less than twice the basic RR interval. The last regular QRS complex is followed by a premature P wave (large arrow); sinus rhythm initiates the QRS, which is delayed (small arrow). **Bottom tracing,** Sinus rhythm with sinus pause and low atrial escape beat; the basic RR interval is interrupted by an irregular RR interval that is greater than the basic RR interval. The last regular QRS complex is not followed by a P wave. An inverted P wave (small arrow) precedes the delayed QRS, indicating that this is a low atrial escape beat.

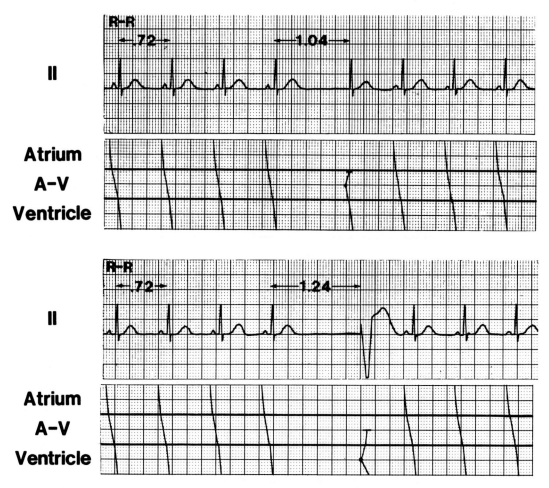

FIG. 12-85B. Intermittently irregular: delayed QRS. **Top tracing,** Sinus rhythm with sinus pause and junctional escape beat; the basic RR interval is interrupted by an irregular RR interval that is greater than the basic RR interval and also greater than the RR interval in low atrial escape (see Fig. 12-85A, bottom). This is because the junctional escape rate is slower than the atrial escape rate, the last regular QRS complex is not followed by a P wave, and no P wave precedes the delayed QRS, indicating that this is a junctional escape beat. **Bottom tracing,** Sinus rhythm with sinus pause and ventricular escape beat; the basic RR interval is interrupted by an irregular RR interval that is greater than the basic RR interval and also greater than the RR interval in either low atrial or junctional escape. The last regular QRS complex is not followed by a P wave. No P wave precedes the delayed QRS, which has prolonged duration, indicating that this is a ventricular escape beat. Strictly speaking, a ventricular escape beat should occur only at intervals longer than 1.5 sec. Therefore, this is an "accelerated ventricular escape beat" since it occurs 1.24 sec after the preceding QRS complex.

CATEGORIES
OF ARRHYTHMIAS

With this background, the major common cardiac rhythm disturbances in children can be better understood. The arrhythmias are discussed in 14 categories. Assignment to a category depends upon the following:

(1) Regularity of the RR interval
(2) QRS rate
(3) QRS duration

TABLE 12-12.

Dysrhythmias With a Regular R-R Interval

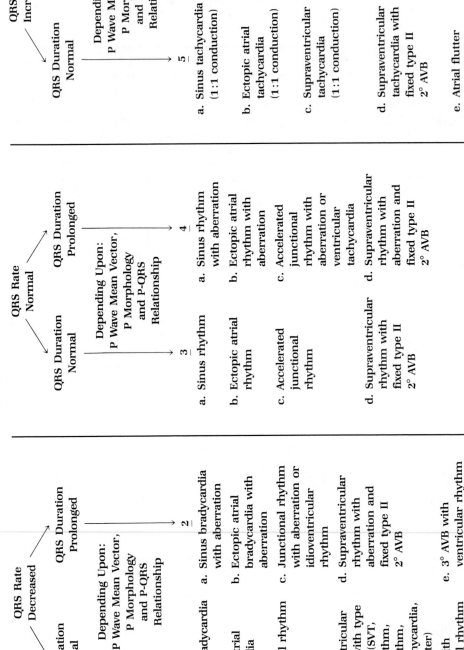

QRS Rate Decreased		QRS Rate Normal		QRS Rate Increased	
QRS Duration Normal	QRS Duration Prolonged	QRS Duration Normal	QRS Duration Prolonged	QRS Duration Normal	QRS Duration Prolonged
Depending Upon: P Wave Mean Vector, P Morphology and P-QRS Relationship		Depending Upon: P Wave Mean Vector, P Morphology and P-QRS Relationship		Depending Upon: P Wave Mean Vector, P Morphology and P-QRS Relationship	
1*	2	3	4	5	6
a. *Sinus bradycardia	a. Sinus bradycardia with aberration	a. Sinus rhythm	a. Sinus rhythm with aberration	a. Sinus tachycardia (1:1 conduction)	a. Sinus tachycardia (1:1 conduction) with aberration
b. Ectopic atrial bradycardia	b. Ectopic atrial bradycardia with aberration	b. Ectopic atrial rhythm	b. Ectopic atrial rhythm with aberration	b. Ectopic atrial tachycardia (1:1 conduction)	b. Ectopic atrial tachycardia (1:1 conduction) with aberration
c. Junctional rhythm	c. Junctional rhythm with aberration or idioventricular rhythm	c. Accelerated junctional rhythm	c. Accelerated junctional rhythm with aberration or ventricular tachycardia	c. Supraventricular tachycardia (1:1 conduction)	c. Supraventricular tachycardia with aberration or ventricular tachycardia
d. Supraventricular rhythm with type II 2° AVB (SVT, sinus rhythm, atrial rhythm, sinus tachycardia, atrial flutter)	d. Supraventricular rhythm with aberration and fixed type II 2° AVB	d. Supraventricular rhythm with fixed type II 2° AVB	d. Supraventricular rhythm with aberration and fixed type II 2° AVB	d. Supraventricular tachycardia with fixed type II 2° AVB	d. Supraventricular tachycardia with aberration and fixed type II 2° AVB
e. 3° AVB with junctional rhythm	e. 3° AVB with ventricular rhythm			e. Atrial flutter with fixed type II 2° AVB	e. Atrial flutter with aberration and fixed type II 2° AVB

*Numbers and letters refer to categories that follow in the text.

TABLE 12-13.

Dysrhythmias With an Irregular R-R Interval

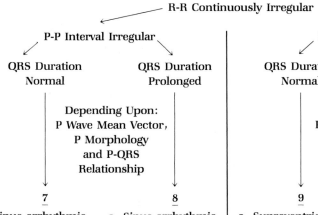

— R-R Continuously Irregular —

P-P Interval Irregular		P-P Interval Regular	
QRS Duration Normal	QRS Duration Prolonged	QRS Duration Normal	QRS Duration Prolonged
	Depending Upon: P Wave Mean Vector, P Morphology and P-QRS Relationship		Depending Upon: P Wave Mean Vector, P Morphology and P-QRS Relationship
7	**8**	**9**	**10**
a. Sinus arrhythmia	a. Sinus arrhythmia with aberration	a. Supraventricular rhythm with varying type II 2° AVB	a. Supraventricular rhythm with aberration and varying type II 2° AVB
b. Wandering pacemaker	b. Wandering pacemaker with aberration	b. Supraventricular rhythm with type I 2° AVB (Wenckebach)	b. Supraventricular rhythm with aberration and type I 2° AVB (Wenckebach)
c. Atrial fibrillation	c. Atrial fibrillation with aberration		

TABLE 12-14.

Dysrhythmias With an Irregular R-R Interval

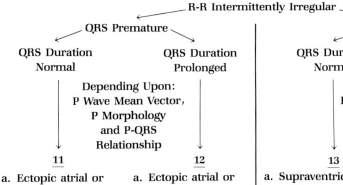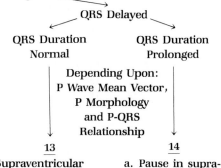

— R-R Intermittently Irregular —

QRS Premature		QRS Delayed	
QRS Duration Normal	QRS Duration Prolonged	QRS Duration Normal	QRS Duration Prolonged
	Depending Upon: P Wave Mean Vector, P Morphology and P-QRS Relationship		Depending Upon: P Wave Mean Vector, P Morphology and P-QRS Relationship
11	**12**	**13**	**14**
a. Ectopic atrial or junctional rhythm with sinus capture	a. Ectopic atrial or junctional rhythm with sinus capture and aberration	a. Supraventricular rhythm with intermittent type II 2° AVB	a. Pause in supraventricular rhythm with ventricular escape
b. Sinus, ectopic atrial or junctional rhythm with premature atrial contraction	b. Sinus, ectopic atrial or junctional rhythm with premature atrial contraction and aberration	b. Supraventricular rhythm with nonconducted premature atrial contraction	
c. Sinus, ectopic atrial or junctional rhythm with premature junctional contraction	c. Sinus, ectopic atrial or junctional rhythm with premature ventricular contraction	c. Pause in supraventricular rhythm with ectopic atrial escape	
		d. Pause in supraventricular rhythm with junctional escape	

In the following discussion, arrhythmia categories are grouped according to whether the RR interval is regular (categories 1 to 6, Table 12-12), continuously irregular (categories 7 to 10, Table 12-13), or intermittently irregular (categories 11 to 14, Table 12-14). Each category is then discussed separately with criteria provided for each of the arrhythmias in the category. Sample *hand drawn* electrocardiographic tracings are also included with each category to facilitate comparison between arrhythmias.

---

1. RR   INTERVAL —REGULAR
   QRS RATE   —DECREASED
   QRS DURATION—NORMAL

(See Fig. 12-86A, B, and C)

a. SINUS BRADYCARDIA. P wave precedes each QRS complex with normal P wave mean vector (0 to 90°).
b. ECTOPIC ATRIAL BRADYCARDIA. P wave precedes each QRS complex with abnormal P wave mean vector (−1 to 91°).
c. JUNCTIONAL RHYTHM.

(1) Sinus P rate less than QRS rate with AV dissociation, or
(2) "Retrograde" P wave (mean vector −1 to −90° follows some or all QRS complexes.

d. SUPRAVENTRICULAR RHYTHM WITH FIXED TYPE II SECOND-DEGREE AV BLOCK. P rate a multiple of QRS rate with fixed relationship of P waves to QRS complexes (every second, third, or fourth P wave precedes a QRS complex with the same PR interval). The supraventricular rhythm, which is blocked, must then be ascertained:

(1) SINUS RHYTHM WITH AV BLOCK. P mean vector and P rate are normal for age.
(2) ATRIAL RHYTHM WITH AV BLOCK. P mean vector is abnormal and P rate is normal.
(3) SINUS TACHYCARDIA WITH AV BLOCK. P mean vector is normal and P rate is increased (≤230/min).
(4) SUPRAVENTRICULAR TACHYCARDIA WITH AV BLOCK. P mean vector is abnormal and P rate is increased, *or* P mean vector is normal and P rate is >230 min.
(5) ATRIAL FLUTTER WITH AV BLOCK. P waves have flutter morphology with fixed relationship of flutter waves to QRS complexes.

Note: In any rhythm with fixed type II second-degree AV block, it is important to obtain long rhythm strips to demonstrate that, as the supraventricular rhythm changes, so does the ventricular response. A ventricular response that remains unchanged with a change in the supraventricular rhythm may be complete AV block with isochronic dissociation.

e. COMPLETE AV BLOCK WITH JUNCTIONAL RHYTHM. Sinus P rate equal to or greater than QRS rate with AV dissociation.

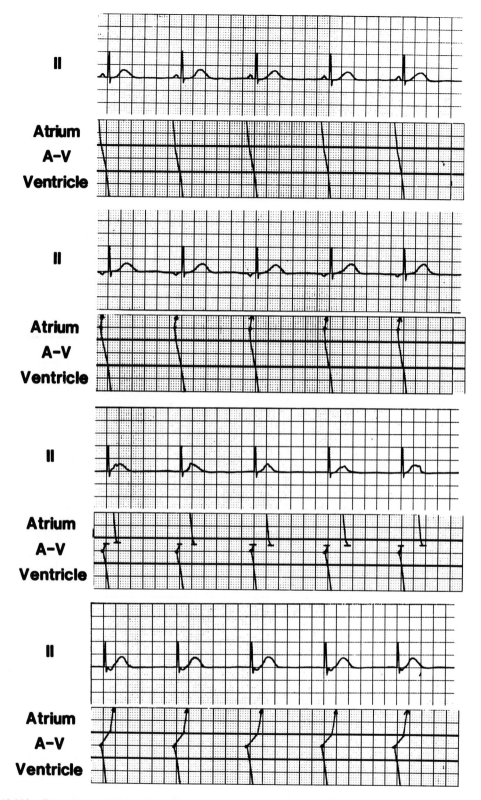

FIG. 12-86A. Category 1: RR interval—regular; QRS rate—decreased; QRS duration—normal. *Top tracing,* Sinus bradycardia. Ventricular rate = 50/min; atrial rate = 50/min. *Second tracing,* Ectopic atrial bradycardia. Ventricular rate = 50/min; atrial rate = 50/min. *Third tracing,* Junctional rhythm with AV dissociation. Ventricular rate = 50/min; atrial rate = 48/min. Conduction does not occur from ventricles to atria. *Bottom tracing,* Junctional rhythm. Ventricular rate = 50/min; atrial rate = 50/min; Retrograde conduction is intact with inverted P waves following each QRS complex.

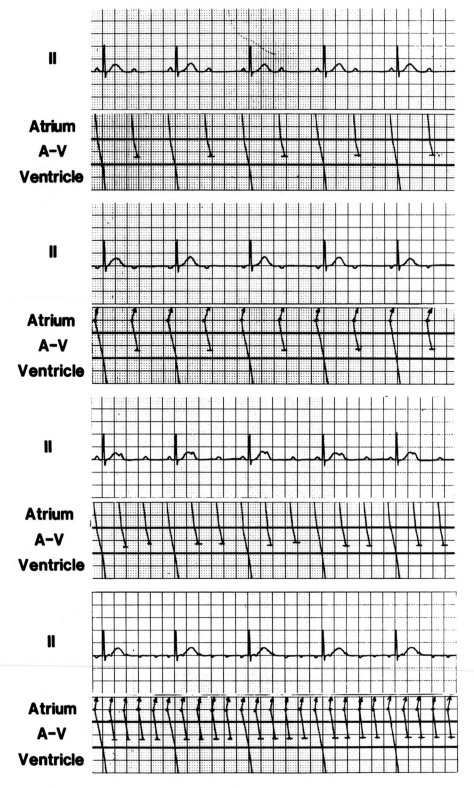

FIG. 12-86B. Category 1. *Top tracing,* Sinus rhythm with second-degree AV block (2:1). Ventricular rate = 50/min; atrial rate = 100/min. Every other P wave is followed by a QRS complex; when AV block is 2:1, it is not possible to determine whether this is type I or type II second-degree AV block. *Second tracing,* Atrial rhythm with second-degree AV block (2:1). Ventricular rate = 50/min; atrial rate = 100/min. *Third tracing,* Sinus rhythm (rapid rate) with fixed type II second-degree AV block (3:1). Ventricular rate = 50/min; atrial rate = 150/min. *Bottom tracing,* Supraventricular tachycardia with fixed type II second-degree AV block (5:1). Ventricular rate = 50/min; atrial rate = 250/min.

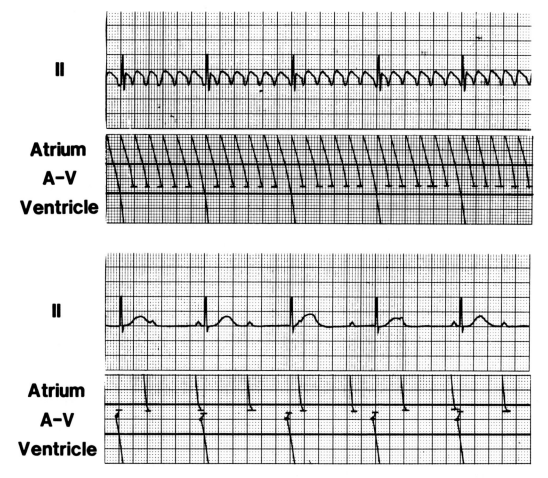

FIG. 12-86C. Category 1. *Top tracing,* Atrial flutter with fixed type II second-degree AV block (6:1). Ventricular rate = 50/min; atrial rate = 300/min. *Bottom tracing,* Complete AV block with AV dissociation and junctional rhythm. Ventricular rate = 50/min; atrial rate = 85/min.

---

2. RR   INTERVAL —REGULAR

QRS RATE   —DECREASED

QRS DURATION—PROLONGED

(See Fig. 12-87A, B, and C)

a. SINUS BRADYCARDIA WITH ABERRATION. P wave precedes each QRS complex with normal P wave mean vector.

b. ECTOPIC ATRIAL BRADYCARDIA WITH ABERRATION. P wave precedes each QRS complex with abnormal P wave mean vector.

c. JUNCTIONAL RHYTHM WITH ABERRATION OR IDIOVENTRICULAR RHYTHM.

(1) P rate less than QRS rate with AV dissociation, *or*

(2) "Retrograde" P wave follows some or all QRS complexes.

d. SUPRAVENTRICULAR RHYTHM WITH FIXED TYPE II SECOND-DEGREE AV BLOCK AND ABERRATION. P rate a multiple of QRS rate with fixed relationship of P waves to QRS complexes (see Category 1d).

e. COMPLETE AV BLOCK WITH VENTRICULAR RHYTHM. P rate equal to or greater than QRS rate with AV dissociation.

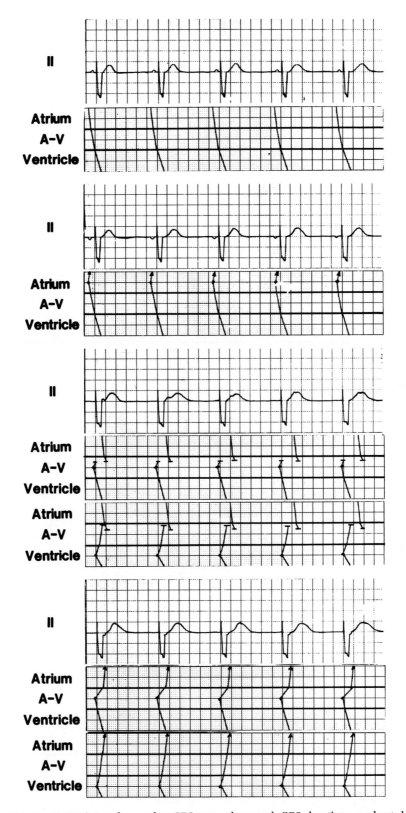

FIG. 12-87A. Category 2: RR interval—regular; QRS rate—decreased; QRS duration—prolonged. *Top tracing,* Sinus bradycardia with complete right bundle branch block. Ventricular rate = 50/min; atrial rate = 50/min. *Second tracing,* Ectopic atrial bradycardia with complete right bundle branch block. Ventricular rate = 50/min; atrial rate = 50/min. *Third tracing,* Junctional rhythm with complete right bundle branch block or idioventricular rhythm with AV dissociation (it is impossible to distinguish between these on surface electrocardiogram); a ladder diagram for each is shown. Ventricular rate = 50/min; atrial rate = 48/min. Conduction does not occur from ventricles to atria. *Bottom tracing,* Junctional rhythm with complete right bundle branch block or idioventricular rhythm (inverted P waves following each QRS complex); a ladder diagram for each is shown. Ventricular rate = 50/min; atrial rate = 50/min. Retrograde conduction is intact with inverted P waves following each QRS complex.

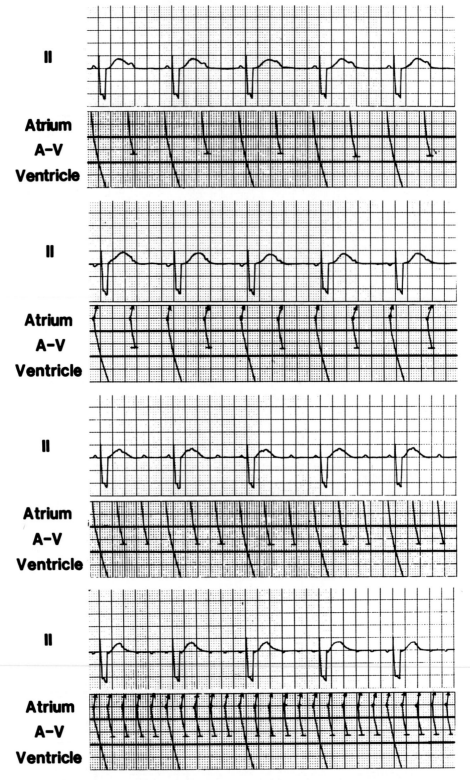

FIG. 12-87B. Category 2. *Top tracing,* Sinus rhythm with second-degree AV block (2:1) and complete right bundle branch block. Ventricular rate = 50/min; atrial rate = 100/min. Every other P wave is followed by a QRS complex; when AV block is 2:1, it is not possible to determine if this is type I or type II second-degree AV block. *Second tracing,* Atrial rhythm with second-degree AV block (2:1) and complete right bundle branch block. Ventricular rate = 50/min; atrial rate = 100/min. *Third tracing,* Sinus rhythm (rapid rate) with fixed type II second-degree AV block (3:1) and complete right bundle branch block. Ventricular rate = 50/min; atrial rate = 150/min. *Bottom tracing,* Supraventricular tachycardia with fixed type II second-degree AV block (5:1) and complete right bundle branch block. Ventricular rate = 50/min; atrial rate = 250/min.

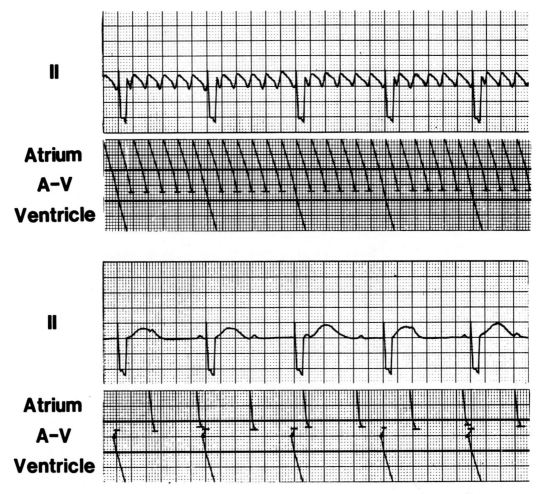

FIG. 12-87C. Category 2. *Top tracing,* Atrial flutter with fixed type II second-degree AV block (6:1) and complete right bundle branch block. Ventricular rate = 50/min; atrial rate = 300/min. *Bottom tracing,* Complete AV block with AV dissociation and junctional rhythm with complete right bundle branch block or idioventricular rhythm. Ventricular rate = 50/min; atrial rate = 85/min.

---

3. RR   INTERVAL —REGULAR
   QRS RATE   —NORMAL
   QRS DURATION—NORMAL

(See Fig. 12-88A, B, and C)

a. SINUS RHYTHM. P wave precedes each QRS complex with normal P wave mean vector.

b. ECTOPIC ATRIAL RHYTHM. P wave precedes each QRS complex with abnormal P wave mean vector.

c. ACCELERATED JUNCTIONAL RHYTHM.

   (1) Sinus P rate less than QRS rate with AV dissociation, *or*
   (2) No P waves visible, *or*
   (3) Retrograde P wave follows some or all QRS complexes.

d. SUPRAVENTRICULAR RHYTHM WITH FIXED TYPE II SECOND-DEGREE AV BLOCK. P rate a multiple of QRS rate with fixed relationship of P waves to QRS complexes (see Category 1d).

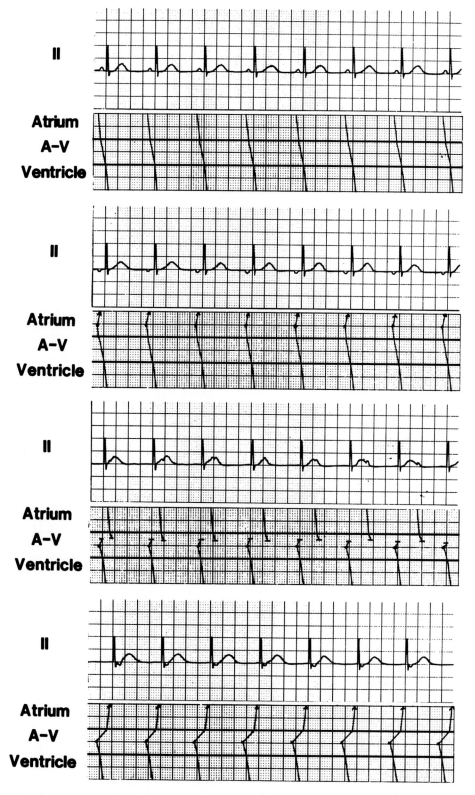

FIG. 12-88A. Category 3: RR interval—regular; QRS rate—normal; QRS duration—normal. *Top tracing,* Sinus rhythm. Ventricular rate = 75/min; atrial rate = 75/min. *Second tracing,* Ectopic atrial rhythm. Ventricular rate = 75/min; atrial rate = 75/min. *Third tracing,* Accelerated junctional rhythm with AV dissociation. Ventricular rate = 75/min; atrial rate = 71/min. Conduction does not occur from ventricles to atria. *Bottom tracing,* Accelerated junctional rhythm. Ventricular rate = 75/min; atrial rate = 75/min. Retrograde conduction is intact with inverted P waves following each QRS complex.

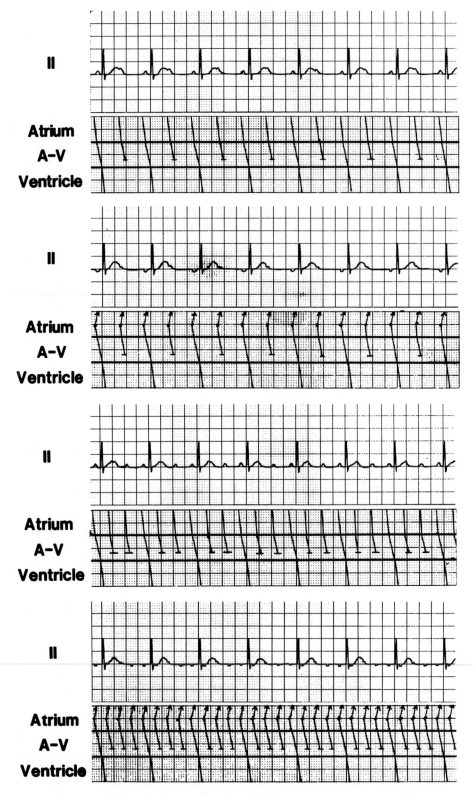

FIG. 12-88B. Category 3. *Top tracing,* Sinus rhythm with second-degree AV block (2:1). Ventricular rate = 75/min; atrial rate = 150/min. Every other P wave is followed by a QRS complex; when AV block is 2:1, it is not possible to determine if this is type I or type II second-degree AV block. *Second tracing,* Atrial rhythm with second-degree AV block (2:1). Ventricular rate = 75/min; atrial rate = 150/min. *Third tracing,* Sinus tachycardia with fixed type II second-degree AV block (3:1). Ventricular rate = 75/min; atrial rate = 225/min. *Bottom tracing,* Supraventricular tachycardia with fixed type II second-degree AV block (4:1). Ventricular rate = 75/min; atrial rate = 300/min.

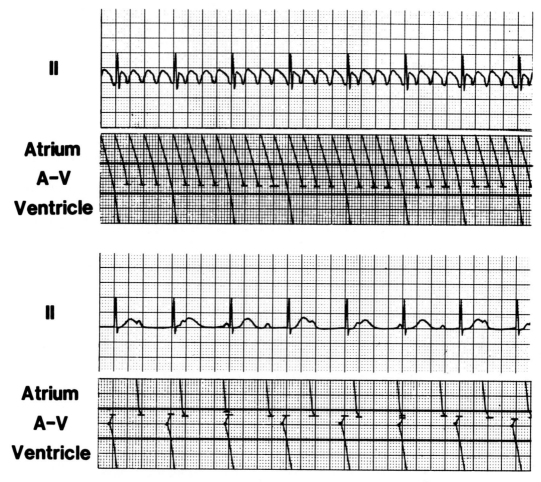

FIG. 12-88C.   Category 3. *Top tracing,* Atrial flutter with fixed type II second-degree AV block (4:1). Ventricular rate = 75/min; atrial rate = 300/min. *Bottom tracing,* Complete AV block with AV dissociation and accelerated junctional rhythm. Ventricular rate = 75/min; atrial rate = 100/min.

4. RR   INTERVAL —REGULAR
QRS RATE   —NORMAL
QRS DURATION—PROLONGED

(See Fig. 12-89A, B, and C)

a. SINUS RHYTHM WITH ABERRATION. P wave precedes each QRS complex with normal P wave mean vector.

b. ECTOPIC ATRIAL RHYTHM WITH ABERRATION. P wave precedes each QRS complex with abnormal P wave mean vector.

c. ACCELERATED JUNCTIONAL RHYTHM WITH ABERRATION OR VENTRICULAR TACHYCARDIA.

(1) Sinus P rate less than QRS rate with AV dissociation, *or*
(2) No P wave visible, *or*
(3) Retrograde P wave follows some or all QRS complexes.

d. SUPRAVENTRICULAR RHYTHM WITH ABERRATION AND FIXED TYPE II SECOND-DEGREE AV BLOCK. P rate a multiple of QRS rate with fixed relationship of P waves to QRS complexes (see Category 1d).

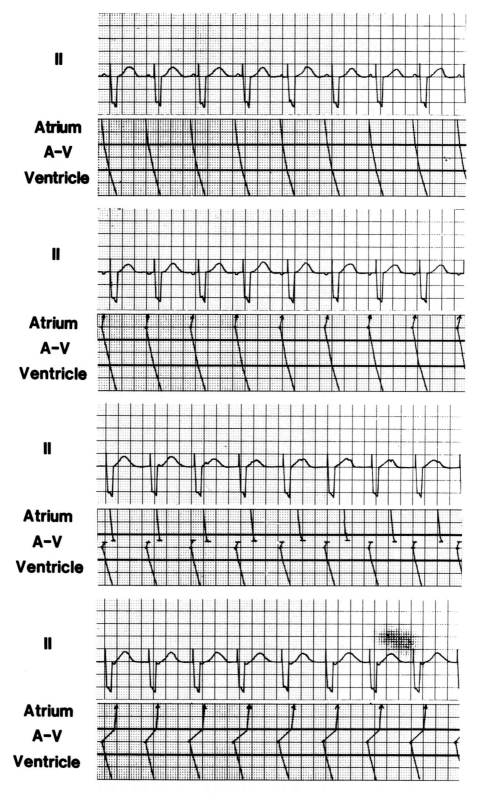

FIG. 12-89A. Category 4: RR interval—regular; QRS rate—normal; QRS duration—prolonged. *Top tracing,* Sinus rhythm with complete right bundle branch block. Ventricular rate = 85/min; atrial rate = 85/min. *Second tracing,* Ectopic atrial rhythm with complete right bundle branch block. Ventricular rate = 85/min; atrial rate = 85/min. *Third tracing,* Accelerated junctional rhythm with complete right bundle branch block or ventricular tachycardia with AV dissociation (it is impossible to distinguish between these on surface electrocardiogram). Ventricular rate = 85/min; atrial rate = 80/min. Conduction does not occur from ventricles to atria. *Bottom tracing,* Accelerated junctional rhythm with complete right bundle branch block or ventricular tachycardia. Ventricular rate = 85/min; atrial rate = 85/min. Retrograde conduction is intact with inverted P waves following each QRS complex.

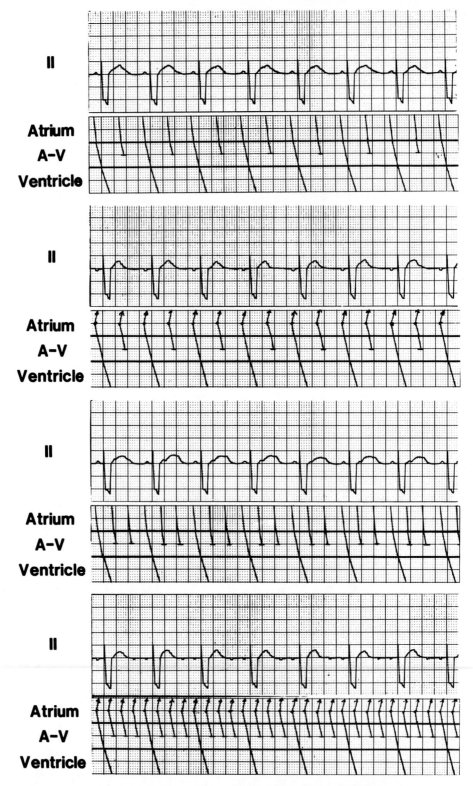

FIG. 12-89B. Category 4. *Top tracing,* Sinus rhythm with second-degree AV block (2:1) and complete right bundle branch block. Ventricular rate = 75/min; atrial rate = 150/min. Every other P wave is followed by a QRS complex; when AV block is 2:1, it is not possible to determine if this is type I or type II second-degree AV block. *Second tracing,* Atrial rhythm with second-degree AV block (2:1) and complete right bundle branch block. Ventricular rate = 75/min; atrial rate:150/min. *Third tracing,* Sinus tachycardia with fixed type II second-degree AV block (3:1) and complete right bundle branch block. Ventricular rate = 75/min; atrial rate = 225/min. *Bottom tracing,* Supraventricular tachycardia with fixed type II second-degree AV block (4:1) and complete right bundle branch block. Ventricular rate = 75/min; atrial rate = 300/min.

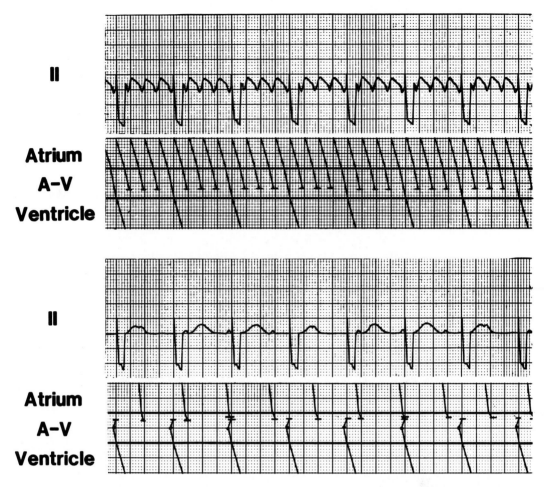

FIG. 12-89C. Category 4. *Top tracing,* Atrial flutter with fixed type II second-degree AV block (4:1) and complete right bundle branch block. Ventricular rate = 75/min; atrial rate = 300/min. *Bottom tracing,* Complete AV block with AV dissociation and accelerated junctional rhythm with complete right bundle branch block or ventricular tachycardia. Ventricular rate = 75/min; atrial rate = 100/min.

---

5. RR　INTERVAL —REGULAR
   QRS　RATE　　　—INCREASED
   QRS　DURATION—NORMAL

(See Fig. 12-90A, B, and C)

a. SINUS TACHYCARDIA (1:1 CONDUCTION). P wave precedes each QRS complex with normal P wave mean vector and P rate ≤230/min.
b. ECTOPIC ATRIAL TACHYCARDIA (1:1 CONDUCTION). P wave precedes each QRS complex with abnormal P wave mean vector.
c. SUPRAVENTRICULAR TACHYCARDIA (1:1 CONDUCTION).

   (1) P wave visible between some or all QRS complexes with constant PR interval, *or*
   (2) No P wave visible, *or*
   (3) Sinus P rate less than QRS rate with AV dissociation.

d. SUPRAVENTRICULAR TACHYCARDIA WITH FIXED TYPE II SECOND-DEGREE AV BLOCK. P rate a multiple of QRS rate with fixed relationship of P waves to QRS complexes.
e. ATRIAL FLUTTER WITH FIXED TYPE II SECOND-DEGREE AV BLOCK. P waves have flutter morphology with fixed relationship of flutter waves to QRS complexes.

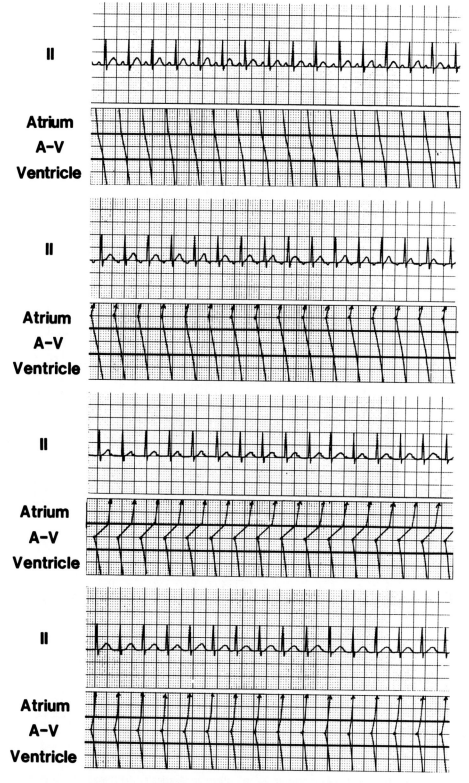

FIG. 12-90A. Category 5: RR interval—regular; QRS rate—increased; QRS duration—normal. *Top tracing,* Sinus tachycardia. Ventricular rate = 160/min; atrial rate = 160/min; P mean vector 0°–90°; PR interval .12 sec. *Second tracing,* Ectopic atrial tachycardia. (This is a type of supraventricular tachycardia. In supraventricular tachycardia, P waves may be present or absent and the PR interval may be normal or prolonged. In this and the next five tracings, some of the morphologies of supraventricular tachycardia are presented.) Ventricular rate = 160/min; atrial rate = 160/min; P mean vector −1°–90°; PR interval .12 sec. *Third tracing,* Supraventricular tachycardia. Ventricular rate = 160/min; atrial rate = 160/min; P mean vector −1° to −90°; PR interval .20 sec. *Bottom tracing,* Supraventricular tachycardia. Ventricular rate = 160/min. No P waves are visible.

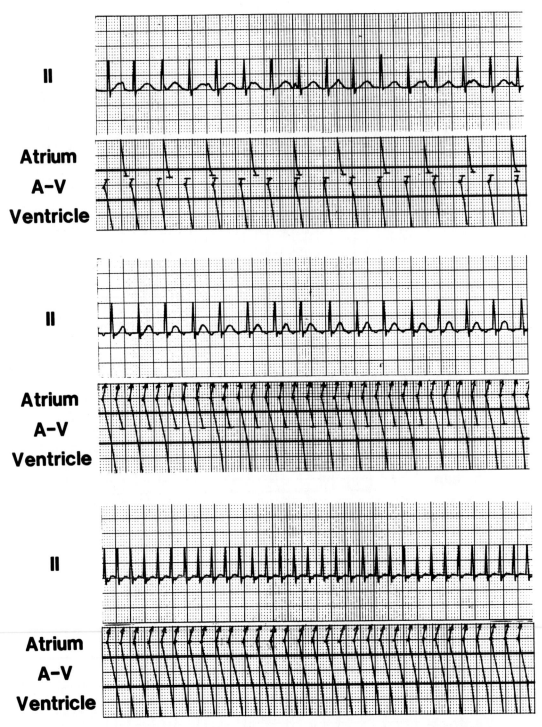

FIG. 12-90B.   Category 5. *Top tracing,* Supraventricular tachycardia with AV dissociation. Ventricular rate = 160/min; atrial rate = 100/min; P mean vector 0° to +90°; PR interval variable. The P waves are from the sinus node depolarizing the atria, and the QRS complexes are from the AV junction depolarizing the ventricles. *Middle tracing,* Supraventricular tachycardia with second-degree AV block (2:1). Ventricular rate = 160/min; atrial rate = 320/min; P mean vector −1° to −90°. There are two PR intervals: .12 sec and .33 sec. From the surface electrocardiogram it is not possible to determine which P wave causes the QRS. *Bottom tracing,* Supraventricular tachycardia. This is the same example shown in the middle tracing, but with 1:1 conduction. Ventricular rate = 320/min; atrial rate = 320/min; P mean vector −1° to −90°; PR interval .14 sec. Inverted P waves immediately follow each QRS.

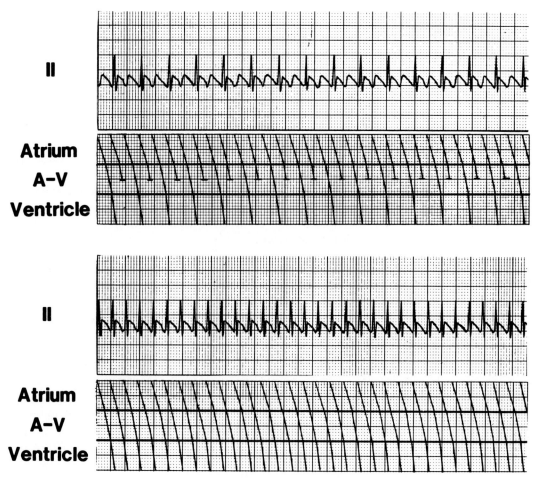

FIG. 12-90C. Category 5. *Top tracing,* Atrial flutter with second-degree AV block (2:1). Ventricular rate = 160/min; atrial rate = 320/min. *Bottom tracing,* Atrial flutter. This is the same example shown in the top tracing, but with 1:1 conduction. Ventricular rate = 320/min; atrial rate = 320/min.

---

6. RR   INTERVAL —REGULAR

QRS RATE   —INCREASED

QRS DURATION—PROLONGED

(See Fig. 12-91A, B, C, and D)

a. SINUS TACHYCARDIA (1:1 CONDUCTION) WITH ABERRATION. P wave precedes each QRS complex with normal P wave mean vector.

b. ECTOPIC ATRIAL TACHYCARDIA (1:1 CONDUCTION) WITH ABERRATION. P wave precedes each QRS complex with abnormal P wave mean vector.

c. SUPRAVENTRICULAR TACHYCARDIA (1:1 CONDUCTION) WITH ABERRATION OR VENTRICULAR TACHYCARDIA.

(1) P wave visible between some or all QRS complexes with constant PR interval, *or*

(2) No P wave visible, *or*

(3) Sinus P rate less than QRS rate with AV dissociation.

d. SUPRAVENTRICULAR TACHYCARDIA WITH ABERRATION AND FIXED TYPE II SECOND-DEGREE AV BLOCK. P rate a multiple of QRS rate with fixed relationship of P waves to QRS complexes.

e. ATRIAL FLUTTER WITH ABERRATION AND FIXED TYPE II SECOND-DEGREE AV BLOCK. P waves have flutter morphology with fixed relationship of flutter waves to QRS complexes.

FIG. 12-91A.   Category 6: RR interval—regular; QRS rate—increased; QRS duration—prolonged. *Top tracing*, Sinus tachycardia with complete right bundle branch block. Ventricular rate = 160/min; atrial rate = 160/min; P mean vector 0° to +90°; PR interval .12 sec. *Second tracing*, Sinus tachycardia with complete right bundle branch block. This tracing is the same as the top tracing, except that the T waves have greater amplitude and the P waves are on the downslope of the T waves. Ventricular rate = 160/min; atrial rate = 160/min; P mean vector 0° to +90°; PR interval .12 sec. This is unlikely to be ventricular tachycardia because the P waves are related to the QRS complexes and the P wave mean vector is normal. *Third tracing*, Ectopic atrial tachycardia with complete right bundle branch block or ventricular tachycardia with 1:1 retrograde conduction to the atria; a ladder diagram of each is shown below the fourth tracing. Ventricular rate = 160/min; atrial rate = 160/min; P mean vector −1° to −90°; PR interval .12 sec. The P waves could either originate in the low atrium (from ectopic supraventricular tachycardia) and conduct to the ventricles or could be conducted retrogradely from ventricular tachycardia. It is impossible to distinguish between the two on surface electrocardiogram. However, in children, supraventricular tachycardia with aberration is much less common than ventricular tachycardia. *Bottom tracing*, Ectopic atrial tachycardia with complete right bundle branch block or ventricular tachycardia; a ladder diagram of each is shown below the fourth tracing. This tracing is the same as the third tracing, except that the T waves have greater amplitude and the P waves are on the downslope of the T waves. Ventricular rate = 160/min; atrial rate = 160/min; P mean vector −1° to −90°; PR interval .12 sec.

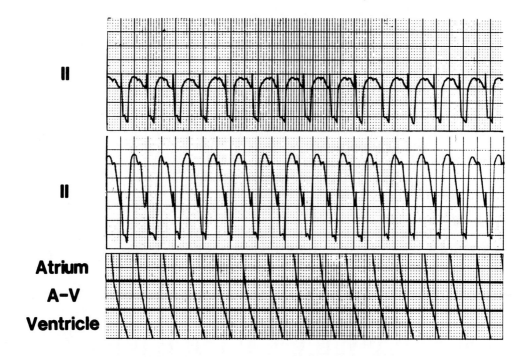

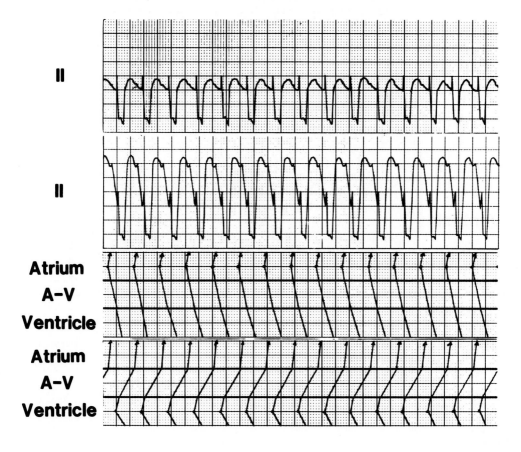

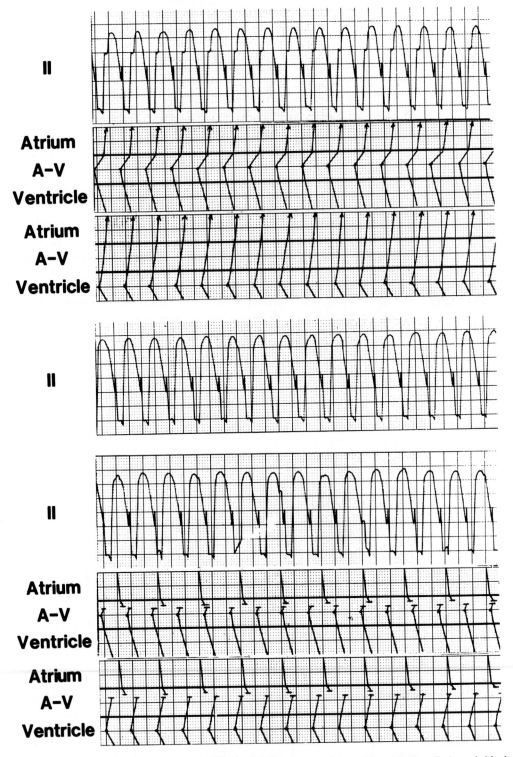

FIG. 12-91B. Category 6. *Top tracing,* Supraventricular tachycardia with complete right bundle branch block or ventricular tachycardia; a ladder diagram of each is shown below the top tracing. Ventricular rate = 160/min; atrial rate = 160/min. Inverted P waves are visible on the upstroke of the T waves. P mean vector −1° to −90°; PR interval .24 sec. *Second tracing,* Supraventricular tachycardia with complete right bundle branch block or ventricular tachycardia. Ventricular rate = 160/min. P waves are not visible consistently; no ladder diagram is shown because atrial activity cannot be discerned. *Bottom tracing,* Supraventricular tachycardia with complete right bundle branch block or ventricular tachycardia; a ladder diagram of each is shown below the bottom tracing. There is complete AV dissociation. Ventricular rate = 160/min; atrial rate = 100/min; P mean vector 0° to +90° (sinus P waves); PR interval variable.

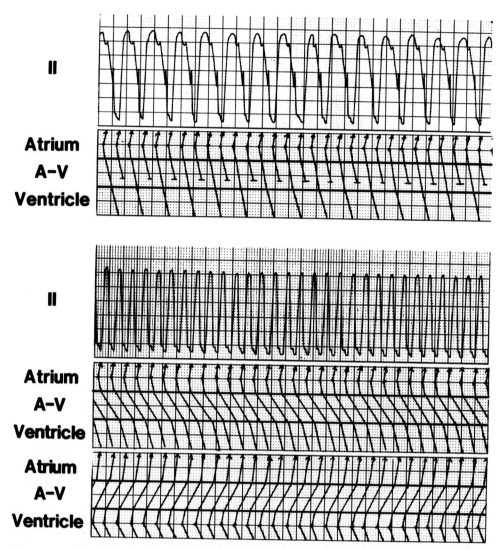

FIG. 12-91C. Category 6. *Top tracing,* Supraventricular tachycardia with complete right bundle branch block and second-degree AV block (2:1). Ventricular rate = 160/min; atrial rate = 320/min; P mean vector −1° to −90°. There are two PR intervals: .12 sec and .32 sec. (The P wave with the PR interval of .32 sec is concealed in the S wave of the bundle branch block pattern—compare with Fig. 12-90B.) Ventricular tachycardia would be an unlikely diagnosis because the P waves and QRS complexes are related, with two P waves for each QRS complex. *Bottom tracing,* Supraventricular tachycardia with complete right bundle branch block or ventricular tachycardia; a ladder diagram of each is shown. This is the same example as the top tracing, except with 1:1 conduction. Ventricular rate = 320/min; atrial rate = 320/min; P mean vector −1° to −90°; PR interval .32 sec. It is impossible to distinguish between the two on surface electrocardiogram, except that this is an uncommonly high rate for ventricular tachycardia.

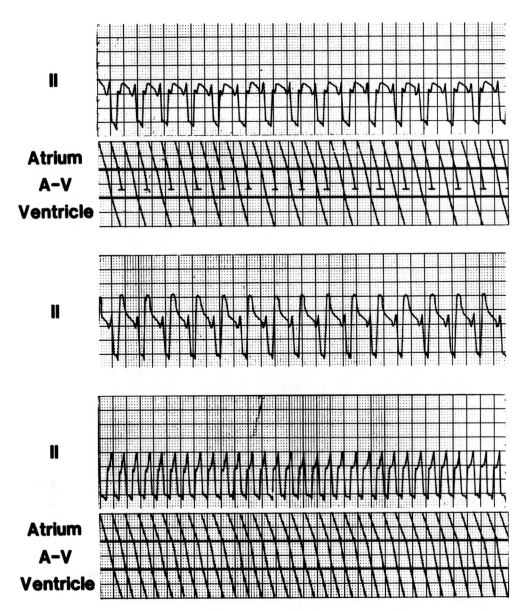

FIG. 12-91D. Category 6. *Top tracing,* Atrial flutter with second-degree AV block (2:1) and complete right bundle branch block. Ventricular rate = 160/min; atrial rate = 320/min; P mean vector −1° to −90°. The sawtooth baseline is partially concealed. This could be mistaken for supraventricular tachycardia with complete right bundle branch block or for ventricular tachycardia. *Middle tracing,* Atrial flutter with second-degree AV block (2:1) and complete right bundle branch block. This is the same example as the top tracing, except that the T waves have greater amplitude. Ventricular rate = 160/min; atrial rate = 320/min. The sawtooth baseline is concealed. This could be mistaken for supraventricular tachycardia with complete right bundle branch block or ventricular tachycardia. An esophageal lead showing two atrial depolarizations for each QRS complex would help with the diagnosis. *Bottom tracing,* Atrial flutter with complete right bundle branch block or ventricular tachycardia. This is the same example as the top and middle tracings, except with 1:1 conduction. Ventricular rate = 320/min; atrial rate = 320/min. The sawtooth appearance is apparent between QRS complexes, but this could be mistaken for ventricular tachycardia. This is a common rate for atrial flutter and an uncommon rate for ventricular tachycardia.

7. RR INTERVAL —IRREGULAR
   RR INTERVAL —VARIES CONTINUOUSLY
   PP INTERVAL —IRREGULAR
   QRS DURATION—NORMAL

(See Fig. 12-92)

a. SINUS ARRHYTHMIA.

(1) P wave mean vector may vary between 0 and $+90°$.
(2) P wave precedes each QRS complex with variation in PR interval ≤ 0.02 sec.
(3) RR interval prolongs and shortens cyclically with respiration. (Sinus, atrial, and junctional pacemakers are all under vagal influence, so the rate of rhythms originating from all these sites can vary cyclically. Therefore, sinus, atrial, and junctional rhythm can all have "sinus arrhythmias".)

b. WANDERING PACEMAKER.

(1) P wave mean vector continually changes—sinus, atrial, and junctional.
(2) QRS complexes related to all P waves—P wave either precedes QRS (sinus or atrial origin of P wave) or follows QRS (junctional origin of P wave); P waves may not be visible following junctional beats.

c. ATRIAL FIBRILLATION.

(1) Atrial depolarizations have fibrillation morphology.
(2) "Irregularly irregular"—RR intervals are all usually different.

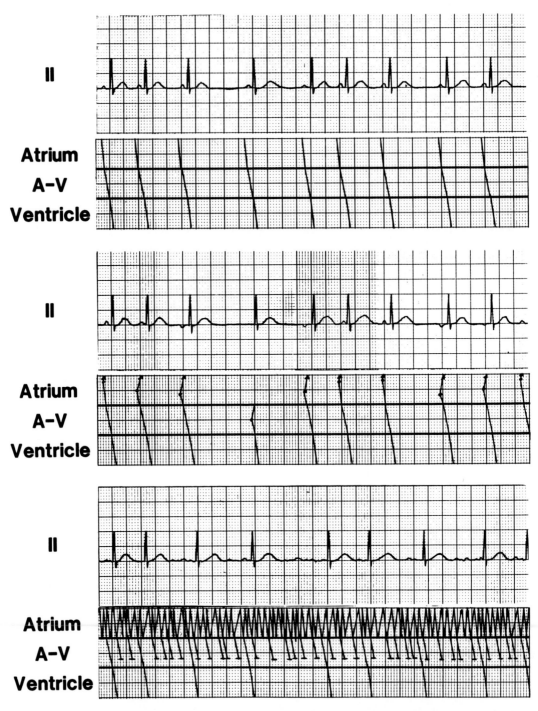

FIG. 12-92.　Category 7: RR interval—irregular; RR interval—varies continuously; PP interval—irregular; QRS duration—normal. *Top tracing*, Sinus arrhythmia. Ventricular rate—variable (RR interval = .48–.92 sec); atrial rate—variable (PP interval = .50–.88 sec); P mean vector—slight variation (+45° to +90°); PR interval—slight variation (.10–.12 sec). Inspiration began at the left side of the tracing and the patient breathed approximately every 3 seconds (20/min). *Middle tracing*, Wandering pacemaker. Ventricular rate—variable (RR interval = .48–.92 sec); atrial rate—variable (PP interval = .45–1.72 sec); P mean vector—variable, when P wave present; PR interval—slight variation, when P wave present (.10–.12 sec). *Bottom tracing*, Atrial fibrillation. Ventricular rate—variable (RR interval = .44–1.06 sec). No two RR intervals are the same. Atrial rate—fibrillation.

8. RR   INTERVAL —IRREGULAR
    RR   INTERVAL —VARIES CONTINUOUSLY
    PP   INTERVAL —IRREGULAR
    QRS DURATION—PROLONGED

(See Fig. 12-93)

a. SINUS ARRHYTHMIA WITH ABERRATION.

(1) P wave mean vector may vary between 0 and +90°.
(2) P wave precedes each QRS complex with variation in PR interval <0.02 sec.
(3) RR interval prolongs and shortens cyclically with respiration. (Sinus, atrial, and junctional pacemakers are all under vagal influence, so the rate of rhythms originating from all these sites can vary cyclically. Therefore, sinus, atrial, and junctional rhythm can all have "sinus arrhythmia".)

b. WANDERING PACEMAKER WITH ABERRATION.

(1) P wave mean vector continually changes—sinus, atrial, and junctional.
(2) QRS complexes related to all P waves—P wave either precedes QRS (sinus or atrial origin of P wave) or follows QRS (junctional origin of P wave).

c. ATRIAL FIBRILLATION WITH ABERRATION.

(1) Atrial depolarizations have fibrillation morphology.
(2) "Irregularly irregular"—RR intervals are all usually different.

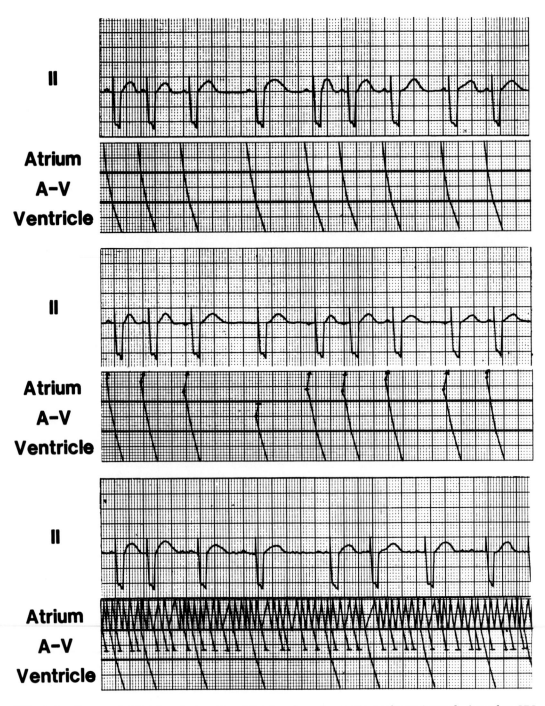

FIG. 12-93. Category 8: RR interval—irregular; RR interval—varies continuously; PP interval—irregular; QRS duration—prolonged. *Top tracing*, Sinus arrhythmia with complete right bundle branch block. Ventricular rate—variable (RR interval = .48–.92 sec); atrial rate—variable (PP interval = .50–.88 sec); P mean vector—slight variation (+45° to +90°); PR interval—slight variation (.10–.12 sec). Inspiration began at the left side of the tracing and the patient breathed approximately every 3 sec (20/min). *Middle tracing*, Wandering pacemaker with complete right bundle branch block. Ventricular rate—variable (RR interval = .48–.92 sec); atrial rate—variable (PP interval = .45–1.72 sec); P mean vector—variable, when P wave present; PR interval—slight variation, when P wave present (.10–.12 sec). *Bottom tracing*, Atrial fibrillation with complete right bundle branch block. Ventricular rate—variable (RR interval = .44–1.06 sec). No two RR intervals are the same. Atrial rate—fibrillation.

9. RR   INTERVAL —IRREGULAR
   RR   INTERVAL —VARIES CONTINUOUSLY
   PP   INTERVAL —REGULAR
   QRS DURATION—NORMAL

(See Fig. 12-94)

a. SUPRAVENTRICULAR RHYTHM (SEE CATEGORY 1D) WITH VARYING TYPE II SECOND-DEGREE AV BLOCK.

(1) RR interval varying multiple of PP interval.
(2) All R waves preceded by P wave with same PR interval.

b. SUPRAVENTRICULAR RHYTHM (SEE 1D) WITH TYPE I SECOND-DEGREE AV BLOCK (WENCKEBACH).

(1) RR interval progressively shortens.
(2) PR interval progressively lengthens until single P wave is not followed by QRS complex.

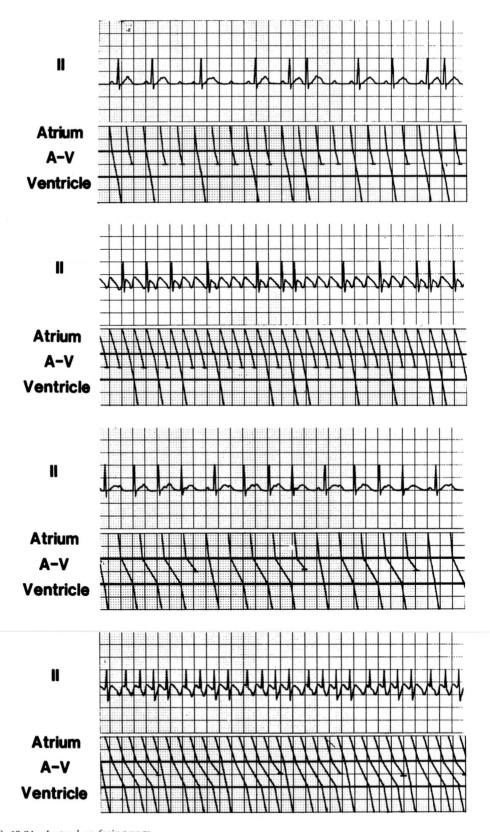

FIG. 12-94.   Legend on facing page.

10. RR   INTERVAL —IRREGULAR
     RR   INTERVAL —VARIES CONTINUOUSLY
     PP   INTERVAL —REGULAR
     QRS DURATION—PROLONGED

(See Fig. 12-95)

a. SUPRAVENTRICULAR RHYTHM (SEE CATEGORY 1D) WITH ABERRATION AND VARY-
ING TYPE II SECOND-DEGREE AV BLOCK.

(1) RR interval varying multiple of PP interval.
(2) All R waves preceded by P wave with same PR interval.

b. SUPRAVENTRICULAR RHYTHM (SEE 1D) WITH ABBERATION AND TYPE I SEC-
OND-DEGREE AV BLOCK (WENCKEBACH).

(1) RR interval progressively shortens.
(2) PR interval progressively lengthens until single P wave not followed by QRS complex.

FIG. 12-94. Category 9: RR interval—irregular; RR interval—varies continuously; PP interval—regular; QRS duration—normal. *Top tracing*, Sinus tachycardia with varying type II second-degree AV block (3:1, 2:1, 1:1 conduction).
Ventricular rate—variable (RR interval = .28–.88 sec); atrial rate = 214/min; P mean vector 0° to +90°; PR interval =
.12 sec on conducted beats. *Second tracing*, Atrial flutter with varying type II second-degree AV block (3:1, 2:1, 1:1
conduction). Ventricular rate—variable (RR interval = .20–.80 sec); atrial rate = 300/min. *Third tracing*, Sinus tachycardia with type I second-degree AV block (5:4 Wenckebach). Ventricular rate—variable. (RR intervals progressively
shorten within a group of four QRS complexes; from the beginning of the tracing, the intervals are .48, .40, .38 sec;
then the blocked P wave causes a pause of .74 sec and then the cycle begins again.) Atrial rate = 167/min; P mean
vector 0° to +90°; PR interval—variable. (PR intervals progressively lengthen within a group of four QRS complexes;
from the beginning of the tracing the intervals are .12, .24, .28, .30 sec; then a P wave without a following QRS
complex and the cycle begins again.) *Bottom tracing*, Atrial flutter with type I second-degree AV block (5:4 Wenckebach). Ventricular rate—variable. (RR intervals progressively shorten within a group of four QRS complexes; from
beginning of tracing—.32, .24, .22 sec. The blocked flutter wave causes a pause of 0.22 sec and the cycle begins
again.) Atrial rate = 300/min; Flutter-R interval—variable. (Flutter-R intervals progressively lengthen within a group
of four QRS complexes; from beginning of tracing—.12, .24, .28, .30 sec—then a flutter wave without a following QRS
complex and the cycle begins again. Flutter waves begin on each dark line every .20 sec.)
    Note: All supraventricular rhythms can have second-degree AV block (see Category 1d. on page 304), although
only sinus tachycardia and atrial flutter are shown here.

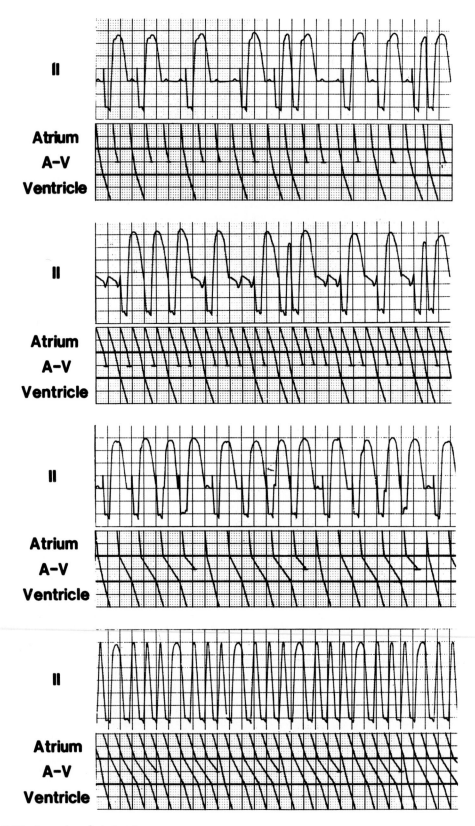

FIG. 12-95. Legend on facing page.

11. BASIC RR INTERVAL—REGULAR, BUT
    INTERRUPTED INTERMITTENTLY
    IRREGULAR RR INTERVAL—SHORT
    (PREMATURE QRS)
    QRS DURATION OF EARLY COMPLEX—NORMAL

(See Fig. 12-96)

a. ATRIAL OR JUNCTIONAL RHYTHM (SEE CATEGORY 1D) WITH SINUS CAPTURE.
   Early QRS preceded by P wave with normal P mean vector.

b. SINUS, ATRIAL, OR JUNCTIONAL RHYTHM (SEE 1D) WITH PREMATURE ATRIAL
   CONTRACTION. Early QRS preceded by P wave with abnormal P mean
   vector.

c. SINUS, ATRIAL, OR JUNCTIONAL RHYTHM (SEE 1D) WITH PREMATURE JUNC-
   TIONAL CONTRACTION. Early QRS not preceded by P wave.

FIG. 12-95.   Category 10: RR interval—irregular; RR interval—varies continuously; PP interval—regular; QRS
duration—prolonged. *Top tracing*, Sinus tachycardia with varying type II second-degree AV block (3:1, 2:1, 1:1
conduction) and complete right bundle branch block. Ventricular rate—variable (RR interval = .28–.88 sec); atrial
rate = 214/min; P mean vector 0° to +90°; PR interval = .12 sec on conducted beats (P waves are on the upstroke of
all T waves). *Second tracing*, Atrial flutter with varying type II second-degree AV block (3:1, 2:1, 1:1 conduction) and
complete right bundle branch block. Ventricular rate—variable (R-R interval = .20–.80 sec); atrial rate = 300/min.
Third tracing; Sinus tachycardia with type I second-degree AV block (5:4 Wenckebach) and complete right bundle
branch block. Ventricular rate—variable. (RR intervals progressively shorten within a group of four QRS complexes;
from the beginning of the tracing, the intervals are .48, .40, .38 sec; then the blocked P wave causes a pause of .74 sec
and then the cycle begins again.) Atrial rate = 167/min; P mean vector 0° to +90°; PR interval—variable. (PR intervals
progressively lengthen within a group of four QRS complexes; from the beginning of the tracing, the intervals are .12,
.24, .28, .30 sec; then a P wave without a following QRS complex and the cycle begins again.) The P waves cause the
various irregularities in the QRS complexes and T waves. *Bottom tracing*, Atrial flutter with type I second-degree AV
block (5:4 Wenckebach) and complete right bundle branch block. Ventricular rate—variable. (RR intervals progressively shorten within a group of four QRS complexes; from the beginning of the tracing, the intervals are .32, .24,
.22 sec. The blocked flutter wave causes a pause of .22 sec and the cycle begins again.) Flutter waves are not visible,
but the diagnosis may be inferred from the rate and pattern of the QRS complexes. The atrial rate is inferred to be
300/min.
   Note: All supraventricular rhythms can have second-degree AV block (see Category 1d), although only sinus
tachycardia and atrial flutter are shown here.

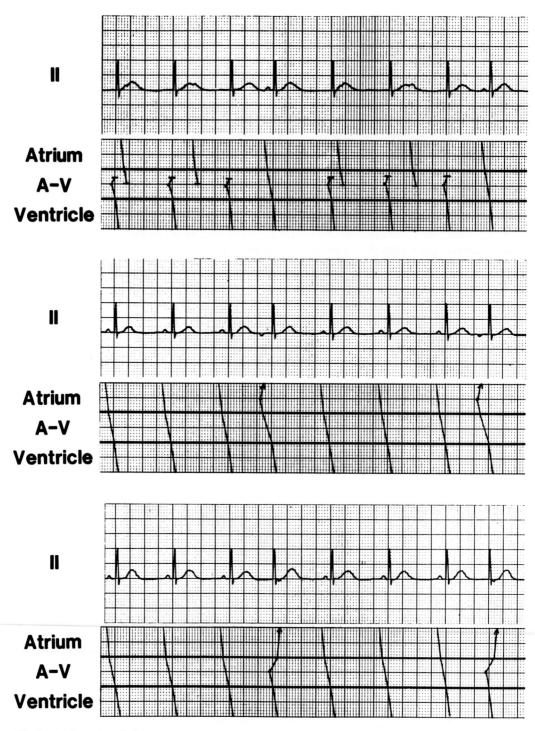

FIG. 12-96.   Legend on facing page.

12. BASIC RR INTERVAL—REGULAR, BUT INTERRUPTED INTERMITTENTLY
IRREGULAR RR INTERVAL—SHORT
(PREMATURE QRS)
QRS DURATION OF EARLY COMPLEX—PROLONGED

(See Fig. 12-97)

a. ECTOPIC ATRIAL OR JUNCTIONAL RHYTHM (SEE CATEGORY 1D) WITH SINUS CAPTURE AND ABERRATION. QRS preceded by P wave with normal P mean vector.

b. SINUS, ECTOPIC ATRIAL, OR JUNCTIONAL RHYTHM (SEE 1D) WITH PREMATURE ATRIAL CONTRACTION AND ABERRATION. QRS preceded by ectopic P wave with abnormal P mean vector.

c. SINUS, ATRIAL, OR JUNCTIONAL RHYTHM (SEE 1D) WITH PREMATURE VENTRICULAR CONTRACTION. QRS not preceded by P wave.

FIG. 12-96. Category 11: Basic RR interval—regular, but interrupted intermittently; irregular RR interval—short (premature QRS); QRS duration of early complex—normal. *Top tracing,* Junctional rhythm with intermittent sinus capture beats. Atrial rate = 60/min (PP interval is constant at 1.0 sec.) Sinus bradycardia is present also. Basic RR interval regular at .80 sec—junctional rhythm. There are two short RR intervals (.60 sec) when the third and sixth sinus P waves in the tracing occur at an appropriate time and the AV node is not refractory. Then AV conduction occurs and the P waves are followed closely by QRS complexes. The RR interval after the fourth QRS is .80 sec because the junctional rhythm begins again from the time of the last QRS complex. *Middle tracing,* Sinus rhythm with premature atrial contractions. Basic ventricular and atrial rates = 75/min (RR and PP intervals = .80 sec). The two short RR intervals (.60 sec) occur when a premature P wave (PP interval = .60 sec) with a different P axis conducts to the ventricles. The PR interval of the premature atrial contraction is .18 sec, which is longer than the .12 sec found in sinus rhythm. The PR interval is longer because the AV node is still relatively refractory when the premature atrial contraction occurs. The RR interval after the fourth QRS is .80 sec (less than compensatory pause) because the premature P wave reset the sinus node. *Bottom tracing,* Sinus rhythm with premature junctional contractions. Basic ventricular and atrial rates = 75/min (RR and PP intervals = .80 sec). The two short RR intervals (.60 sec) are caused by identical premature QRS complexes without a preceding P wave, indicating that these are premature junctional contractions. The RR interval after the fourth QRS is .80 sec (less than compensatory pause) because the premature QRS caused the atria to be activated prematurely (retrograde P wave) and reset the sinus node.

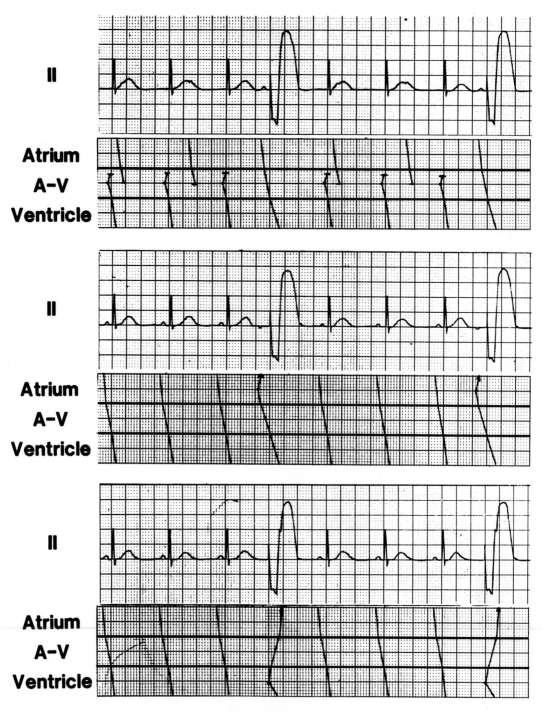

FIG. 12-97. Category 12: Basic RR interval—regular, but interrupted intermittently; irregular RR interval—short (premature QRS); QRS duration of early complex—prolonged. *Top tracing,* Junctional rhythm with intermittent sinus capture beats with complete right bundle branch block. Atrial rate = 60/min (PP interval is constant at 1.0 sec.) Sinus bradycardia is present also. Basic RR interval regular at .80 sec—junctional rhythm. There are two short RR intervals (.60 sec) when the third and sixth sinus P waves in the tracing occur at an appropriate time and the AV node is not refractory. Then AV conduction occurs and the P waves are followed closely by QRS complexes. The RR interval after the fourth QRS is .80 sec because the junctional rhythm begins again from the time of the last QRS complex. (Continued on p. 341)

13. BASIC RR INTERVAL—REGULAR, BUT INTERRUPTED INTERMITTENTLY IRREGULAR RR INTERVAL—LONG (DELAYED QRS) QRS DURATION OF DELAYED COMPLEX—NORMAL

(See Fig. 12-98)

a. SUPRAVENTRICULAR RHYTHM (SEE CATEGORY 1D) WITH INTERMITTENT TYPE II SECOND-DEGREE AV BLOCK.

(1) Supraventricular P wave occurs at regular PP interval.
(2) "Delayed" QRS occurs at twice preceding RR interval.
(3) "Delayed" QRS preceded by supraventricular P wave.

b. SUPRAVENTRICULAR RHYTHM (SEE 1D) WITH NONCONDUCTED PREMATURE ATRIAL CONTRACTION.

(1) P wave with different mean vector or morphology than supraventricular P wave occurs prematurely.
(2) "Delayed" QRS complex occurs at less than twice preceding RR interval.
(3) "Delayed" QRS preceded by supraventricular P wave.

c. PAUSE IN SUPRAVENTRICULAR RHYTHM WITH ECTOPIC ATRIAL ESCAPE.

(1) No supraventricular P wave occurs.
(2) "Delayed" QRS occurs at more than regular RR interval.
(3) "Delayed" QRS preceded by P wave with different mean vector or morphology than supraventricular P wave.

d. PAUSE IN SUPRAVENTRICULAR RHYTHM WITH JUNCTIONAL ESCAPE.

(1) No supraventricular P wave occurs.
(2) "Delayed" QRS occurs at more than regular RR interval.
(3) "Delayed" QRS not preceded by P wave.

FIG. 12-97. Cont'd *Middle tracing,* Sinus rhythm with premature atrial contractions and complete right bundle branch block. Basic ventricular and atrial rates = 75/min (RR and PP intervals = .80 sec). The two short RR intervals (.60 sec) occur when a premature P wave (PP interval = .60 sec) with a different P axis conducts to the ventricles. The PR interval of the premature atrial contraction is .18 sec, which is .06 sec longer than that of sinus rhythm. The PR interval is longer because the AV node is still relatively refractory when the premature atrial contraction occurs. The RR interval after the fourth QRS is .80 sec (less than compensatory pause) because the premature P wave reset the sinus node. *Bottom tracing,* Sinus rhythm with premature ventricular contractions. Basic ventricular and atrial rates = 75/min (RR and PP intervals = .80/sec). The two short RR intervals (.6 sec) are caused by premature QRS complexes with prolonged duration without a preceding P wave, indicating that these are premature ventricular contractions. There are retrograde P waves on the upstroke of the T waves. The RR interval after the fourth QRS is .80 sec (less than compensatory pause) because the premature QRS caused the atria to be activated prematurely (retrograde P wave) and reset the sinus node.

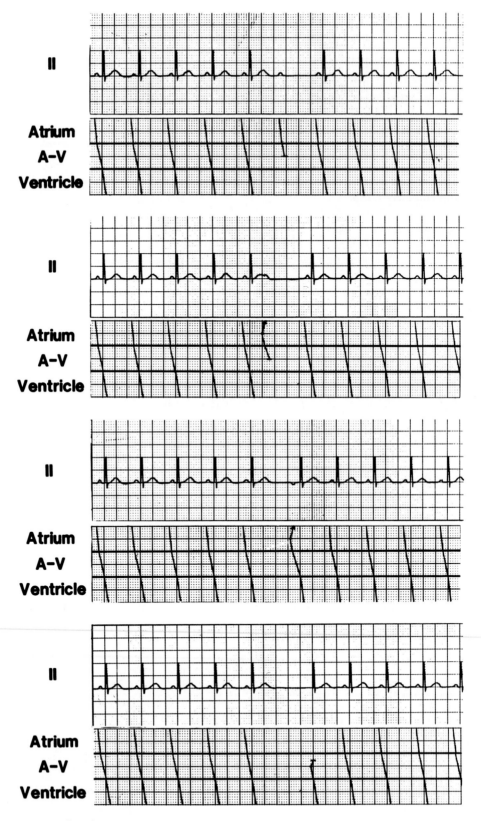

FIG. 12-98. Legend on facing page.

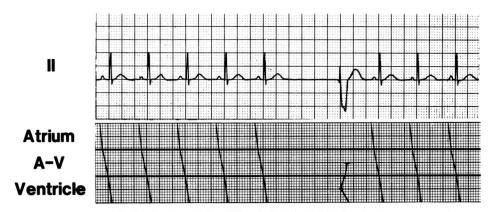

II

Atrium

A–V

Ventricle

FIG. 12-99. Category 14: Basic RR interval—regular, but interrupted intermittently; irregular RR interval—long (delayed QRS); QRS duration of delayed complex—prolonged. Sinus rhythm with sinus pause and ventricular escape beat. Basic ventricular and atrial rates = 100/min (RR and PP intervals = .60 sec). The long RR interval is 1.20 sec, which is longer than the basic RR interval. The pause is longest with a ventricular escape beat because idioventricular rhythm is the slowest in the heart. This is actually an "accelerated ventricular escape beat" because for a 4-year-old a normal ventricular escape beat would occur at a cycle length over 1.5 sec. The QRS complex preceding the delayed QRS is not followed by a sinus P wave ("pause" in sinus rhythm). The pause is ended by a QRS complex with prolonged duration without a preceding P wave—a ventricular escape beat.

---

14. BASIC RR INTERVAL—REGULAR, BUT
    INTERRUPTED INTERMITTENTLY
    IRREGULAR RR INTERVAL—LONG (DELAYED QRS)
    QRS DURATION OF DELAYED COMPLEX—PROLONGED

(See Fig. 12-99)

a. PAUSE IN SUPRAVENTRICULAR RHYTHM WITH VENTRICULAR ESCAPE.

(1) No supraventricular P wave follows preceding R wave.
(2) "Delayed" QRS occurs at more than regular RR interval.
(3) "Delayed" QRS not preceded by P wave.

←———

FIG. 12-98. Category 13: Basic RR interval—regular, but interrupted intermittently; irregular RR interval—long (delayed QRS); QRS duration of delayed complex—normal. *Top tracing*, Sinus rhythm with intermittent type II second-degree AV block. Basic ventricular and atrial rates = 100/min (RR and PP intervals = .60 sec). The long RR interval is 1.20 sec—exactly twice the basic RR interval—because sinus rhythm continues uninterrupted, despite the blocked P wave. *Second tracing*, Sinus rhythm with nonconducted premature atrial contraction. Basic ventricular and atrial rates = 100/min (RR and PP intervals = .60 sec). The long RR interval is 1.0 sec—less than twice the basic RR interval. The QRS complex preceding the pause is followed by a P wave which occurs at a time when the AV node is refractory and is not conducted to the ventricles. This premature atrial contraction resets the sinus node and sinus rhythm begins again. There is a less than fully compensatory pause following the premature atrial contraction. *Third tracing*, Sinus rhythm with sinus pause and low atrial escape beat. Basic ventricular and atrial rates = 100/min (RR and PP intervals = .60 sec). The long RR interval is 0.80 sec, which is longer than the basic RR interval. The QRS complex preceding the delayed QRS is not followed by a sinus P wave ("pause" in sinus rhythm). The pause is ended by an identical QRS complex which is preceded by a P wave with an axis of $-1°$ to $-90°$—a low atrial escape beat. *Bottom tracing*, Sinus rhythm with sinus pause and junctional escape beat. Basic ventricular and atrial rates = 100/min (RR and PP intervals = .60 sec). The long RR interval is 1.0 sec, which is longer than the basic RR interval. The pause is longer with a junctional escape beat than with an atrial escape beat because basic junctional rhythm (which determines the escape interval) is slower than atrial rhythm. The QRS complex preceding the delayed QRS is not followed by a sinus P wave ("pause" in sinus rhythm). The pause is ended by an identical QRS complex without a preceding P wave—a junctional escape beat.

Self-Assessment
Questions

As part of the self assessment, draw a ladder diagram for each arrhythmia. The answer for each question includes the correct ladder diagram.

Part or all of each tracing should be classified according to the "schema for interpretation of arrhythmias" shown in Figure 12-60. The categories are listed numerically below.

1. RR interval regular, QRS rate decreased, QRS duration normal
2. RR interval regular, QRS rate decreased, QRS duration prolonged
3. RR interval regular, QRS rate normal, QRS duration normal
4. RR interval regular, QRS rate normal, QRS duration prolonged
5. RR interval regular, QRS rate increased, QRS duration normal
6. RR interval regular, QRS rate increased, QRS duration prolonged
7. RR interval continuously irregular, PP interval irregular, QRS duration normal
8. RR interval continuously irregular, PP interval irregular, QRS duration prolonged
9. RR interval continuously irregular, PP interval regular, QRS duration normal
10. RR interval continuously irregular, PP interval regular, QRS duration prolonged
11. RR interval regular, interrupted by premature QRS of normal duration
12. RR interval regular, interrupted by premature QRS of prolonged duration
13. RR interval regular, interrupted by delayed QRS of normal duration
14. RR interval regular, interrupted by delayed QRS of prolonged duration

Question 1 (Fig. 12-100): This tracing was taken from a 16-year-old. After the two sinus beats, the next three beats can be placed into which category? (Answer with a number: 1–14.)

Question 2 (Fig. 12-100): After the two sinus beats, what is the rhythm?

A. two sinus beats (sinus rhythm) followed by three sinus beats (sinus rhythm) followed by three junctional escape beats (junctional rhythm)
B. two sinus beats (sinus rhythm) followed by three junctional escape beats (junctional rhythm) followed by three ventricular escape beats (idioventricular rhythm)
C. two sinus beats (sinus rhythm) followed by three ventricular escape beats (idioventricular rhythm) followed by three ventricular escape beats (idioventricular rhythm) from a different site
D. two sinus beats (sinus rhythm) followed by three sinus beats (sinus rhythm) followed by three ventricular escape beats (idioventricular rhythm)
E. none of the above

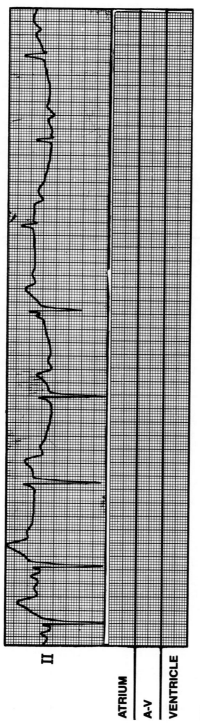

FIG. 12-100. Questions 1 and 2.

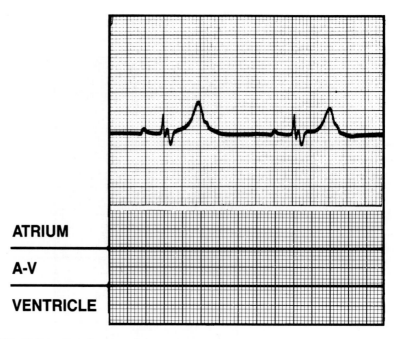

FIG. 12-101.   Questions 3 and 4.

Question 3 (Fig. 12-101): This tracing was taken from a 7-year-old. Categorize the rhythm.

Question 4 (Fig. 12-101): What is the rhythm?

A. sinus bradycardia
B. sinus bradycardia with complete right bundle branch block
C. sinus rhythm with blocked premature atrial contraction
D. sinus rhythm with complete right bundle branch block and blocked premature atrial contraction
E. sinus rhythm with complete right bundle branch block and 2:1 AV block

Question 5 (Fig. 12-102): This tracing was taken from a 4-month-old. Characterize the rhythm.

Question 6 (Fig. 12-102): Is there AV dissociation?

A. yes
B. no

Question 7 (Fig. 12-102): What is the rhythm?

A. sinus bradycardia with complete right bundle branch block and first-degree AV block
B. sinus rhythm with complete right bundle branch block and first-degree AV block

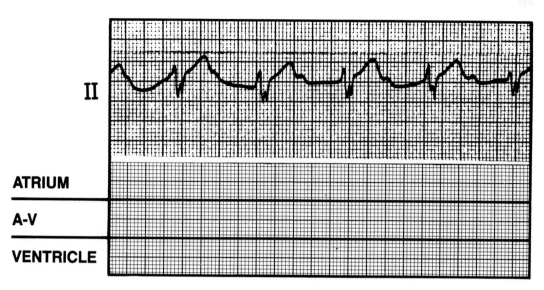

FIG. 12-102. Questions 5, 6, and 7.

C. sinus rhythm with complete right bundle branch block and second-degree AV block
D. sinus bradycardia with third-degree AV block and junctional escape rhythm
E. sinus rhythm with third-degree AV block and junctional escape rhythm

Question 8 (Fig. 12-103): This tracing was taken from a 6-month-old. Characterize the last seven beats.

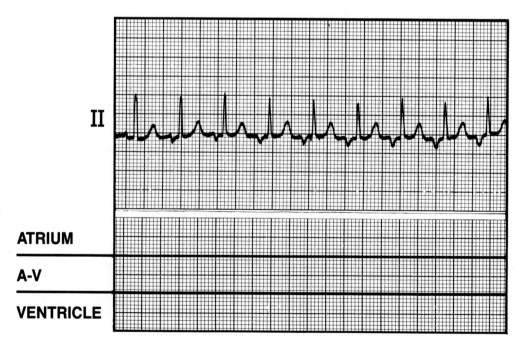

FIG. 12-103. Questions 8, 9, and 10.

Question 9 (Fig. 12-103): Is there AV dissociation?

A. yes
B. no

Question 10 (Fig. 12-103): What is the rhythm in the last seven beats?

A. junctional escape rhythm
B. accelerated junctional rhythm
C. atrial escape rhythm
D. accelerated atrial rhythm
E. sinus rhythm

Question 11 (Fig. 12-104): This tracing was taken from a 6-year-old. Characterize the rhythm.

Question 12 (Fig. 12-104): Is there AV dissociation?

A. yes
B. no

Question 13 (Fig. 12-104): What is the rhythm?

A. accelerated atrial rhythm with accelerated junctional rhythm and probable AV block
B. sinus rhythm with supraventricular tachycardia and AV block
C. sinus rhythm with junctional escape rhythm and probable AV block
D. atrial flutter with 2:1 AV block

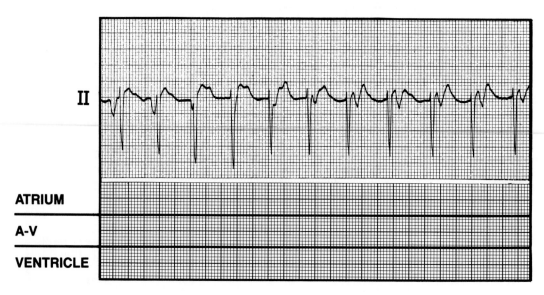

FIG. 12-104. Questions 11, 12, and 13.

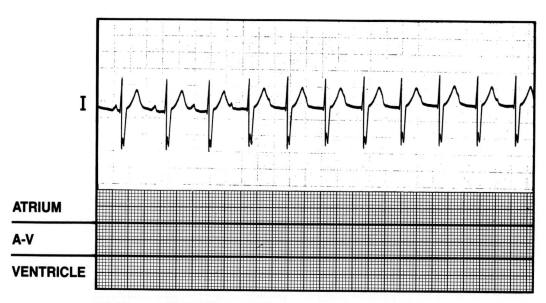

FIG. 12-105. Questions 14 and 15.

Question 14 (Fig. 12-105): This tracing was taken from a 2-year-old. Characterize the rhythm in the last six beats.

Question 15 (Fig. 12-105): What is the rhythm?

A. sinus rhythm with complete right bundle branch block and type I second-degree AV block
B. sinus rhythm and complete AV block with accelerated junctional rhythm
C. accelerated junctional rhythm with complete right bundle branch block followed by sinus rhythm with complete right bundle branch block and first-degree AV block
D. sinus rhythm and complete AV block with accelerated ventricular rhythm
E. none of the above

Question 16 (Fig. 12-106): This tracing was taken from a 2-week-old. Characterize the rhythm.

Question 17 (Fig. 12-106): Is there AV dissociation?

A. yes
B. no

Question 18 (Fig. 12-106): What is the rhythm?

A. sinus tachycardia
B. atrial flutter with 1:1 conduction
C. atrial flutter with 2:1 conduction
D. supraventricular tachycardia with 1:1 conduction
E. supraventricular tachycardia with 2:1 conduction

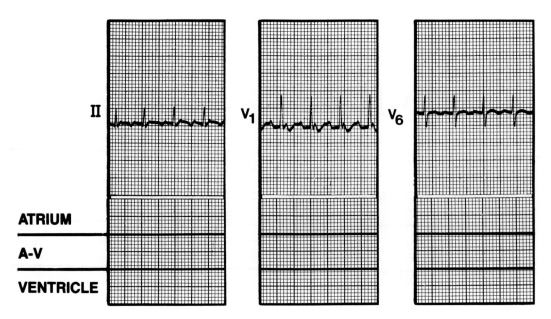

FIG. 12-106. Questions 16, 17, and 18.

Question 19 (Fig. 12-107): This tracing was taken from a 2-day-old. Characterize the rhythm involving the last three QRS complexes.

Question 20 (Fig. 12-107): What is the rhythm?

A. sinus tachycardia followed by sinus bradycardia followed by atrial fibrillation

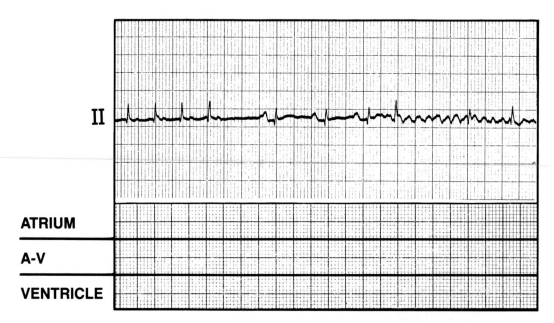

FIG. 12-107. Questions 19 and 20.

B. sinus tachycardia followed by sinus rhythm followed by atrial flutter
C. supraventricular tachycardia followed by sinus rhythm followed by atrial flutter
D. supraventricular tachycardia followed by sinus rhythm followed by atrial fibrillation
E. sinus tachycardia with 1:1 conduction followed by sinus tachycardia with 2:1 conduction followed by atrial flutter

Question 21 (Fig. 12-108): This tracing was taken from a 13-year-old. Characterize the rhythm.

Question 22 (Fig. 12-108): Is there AV dissociation?

A. yes
B. no

Question 23 (Fig. 12-108): What is the rhythm?

A. sinus bradycardia with complete left bundle branch block and junctional escape beats with complete left bundle branch block
B. atrial fibrillation with complete left bundle branch block
C. sinus rhythm with advanced second-degree AV block and intermittent junctional escape rhythm with capture beats; all beats have complete left bundle branch block
D. sinus tachycardia with type I second-degree AV block and complete left bundle branch block
E. sinus rhythm with complete AV block and ventricular escape rhythm

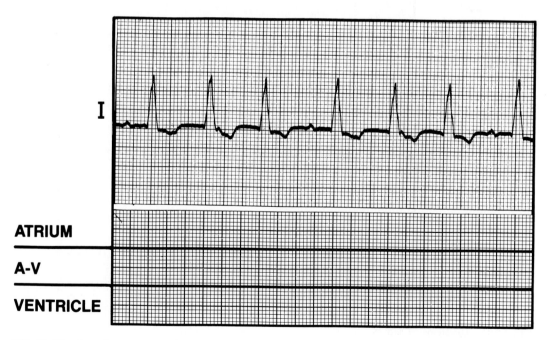

FIG. 12-108. Questions 21, 22, and 23.

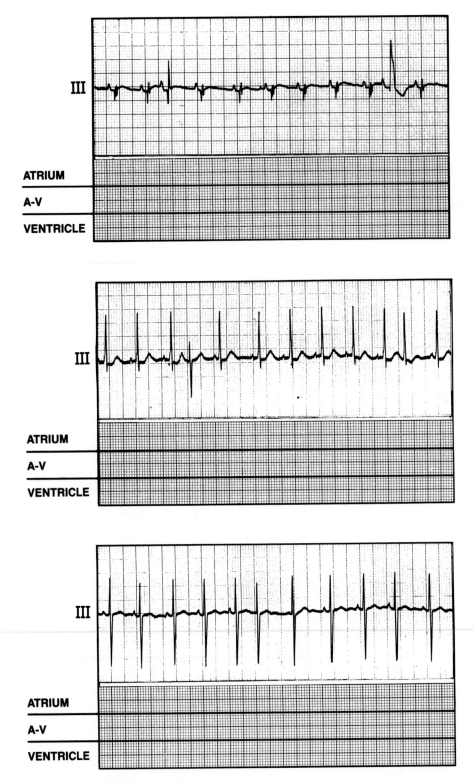

FIG. 12-109.   Questions 24 and 25.

Question 24 (Fig. 12-109): These tracings were taken from infants between 12 and 24 months old. Characterize tracings A, B, and C.

Question 25 (Fig. 12-109): Identify each of the premature beats as either:

A. premature atrial contraction
B. premature junctional contraction
C. premature ventricular contraction
D. capture beat
E. none of the above

Question 26 (Fig. 12-110): This tracing was taken from a 14-year-old. Characterize the rhythm in the first six beats.

Question 27 (Fig. 12-110): Is there AV dissociation in the first six beats?

A. yes
B. no

Question 28 (Fig. 12-110): What is the rhythm?

A. sinus bradycardia with junctional escape rhythm (and intermittent sinus capture) followed by sinus rhythm with complete left bundle branch block
B. high-grade AV block with intermittent sinus capture followed by sinus rhythm with complete left bundle branch block
C. sinus rhythm with accelerated junctional rhythm followed by sinus rhythm with complete left bundle branch block
D. sinus bradycardia with ventricular escape rhythm (and intermittent sinus capture) followed by sinus rhythm with complete left bundle branch block
E. none of the above

Question 29 (Fig. 12-111): This tracing was taken from a 7-year-old. Classify the rhythm.

Question 30 (Fig. 12-111): What is the rhythm?

A. sinus followed by premature ventricular contraction followed by accelerated junctional rhythm followed by sinus
B. sinus followed by premature atrial contraction followed by junctional rhythm followed by sinus
C. sinus followed by premature ventricular contraction followed by low atrial rhythm followed by sinus
D. sinus followed by premature junctional contraction followed by low atrial rhythm followed by sinus
E. none of the above

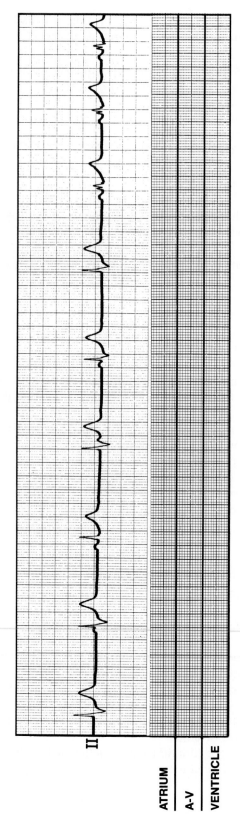

FIG. 12-110. Questions 26, 27, and 28.

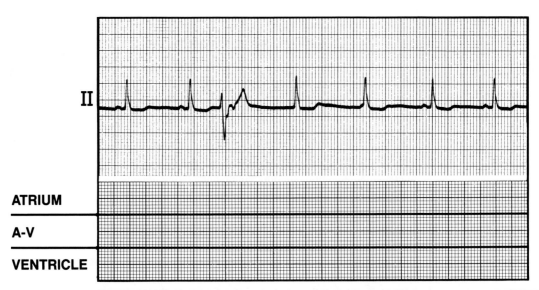

FIG. 12-111. Questions 29, 30, and 31.

Question 31 (Fig. 12-111): Which drug would be most likely to produce the tracing in this Figure?

A. imipramine
B. atropine
C. digitalis
D. quinidine
E. verapamil

Question 32 (Fig. 12-112): This tracing was taken from a 6-year-old. Characterize the rhythm.

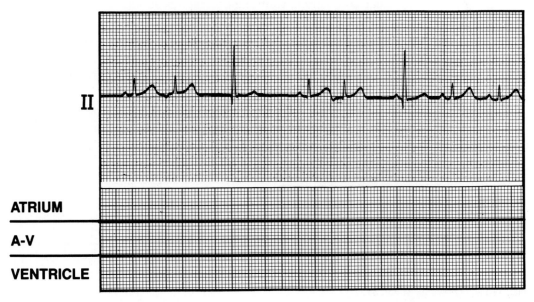

FIG. 12-112. Questions 32 and 33.

Question 33 (Fig. 12-112): What are the first three beats?

A. sinus, atrial escape beat, premature ventricular contraction
B. sinus, atrial escape beat, ventricular escape beat
C. sinus, premature atrial contraction, premature ventricular contraction
D. sinus, premature atrial contraction, ventricular escape beat
E. sinus, premature atrial contraction, premature junctional contraction

Question 34 (Fig. 12-113): This tracing was taken from a 9-year-old. Characterize the rhythm.

Question 35 (Fig. 12-113): What is the rhythm?

A. premature atrial contraction, sinus, premature atrial contraction, etc.
B. premature junctional contraction, sinus, premature junctional contraction, etc.
C. premature ventricular contraction, sinus, premature ventricular contraction, etc.
D. junctional escape beat, sinus, junctional escape beat, etc.
E. none of the above

Question 36 (Fig. 12-114): This tracing was taken from a 12-year-old. Characterize the rhythm.

Question 37 (Fig. 12-114): What is the rhythm?

A. sinus with complete right bundle branch block, premature ventricular contraction, ventricular escape beat, etc.

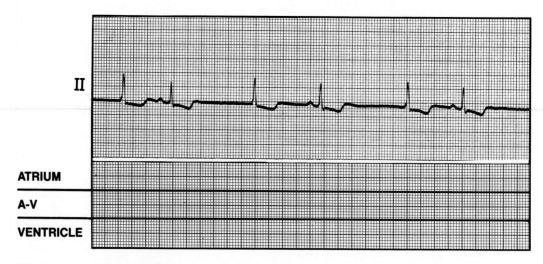

FIG. 12-113.   Questions 34 and 35.

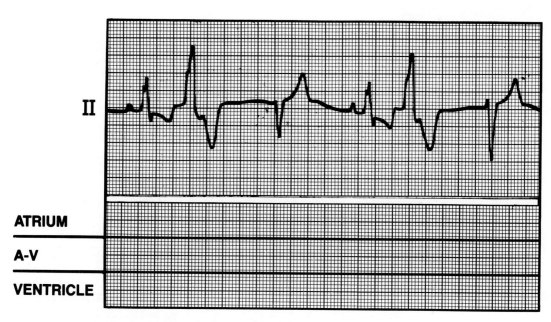

FIG. 12-114. Questions 36 and 37.

B. junctional escape beat with complete right bundle branch block, premature junctional contraction, ventricular escape beat, etc.
C. sinus with complete right bundle branch block, premature ventricular contraction, junctional escape beat, etc.
D. junctional escape beat with complete right bundle branch block, premature atrial contraction, junctional escape beat, etc.
E. sinus with complete right bundle branch block, premature junctional contraction, junctional escape beat, etc.

Question 38 (Fig. 12-115): This tracing was taken from a 17-year-old. Characterize the rhythm.

Question 39 (Fig. 12-115): Is there AV dissociation?

A. yes
B. no

Question 40 (Fig. 12-115): What is the rhythm?

A. sinus tachycardia with complete right bundle branch block
B. supraventricular tachycardia with complete right bundle block
C. atrial flutter with 2:1 AV block and complete right bundle branch block
D. ventricular tachycardia
E. none of the above

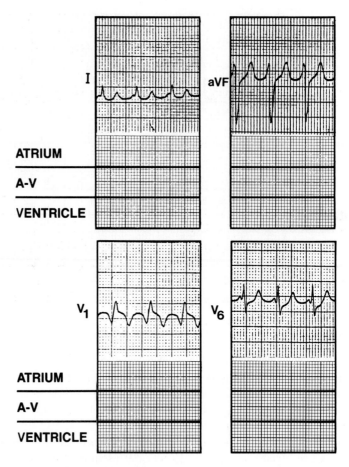

FIG. 12-115. Questions 38, 39, and 40.

Answers to Self-Assessment Questions

Answer 1 (Fig. 12-116): Category 1 (RR interval regular, QRS rate decreased, QRS duration normal). The QRS duration is .10 sec, which is normal for a 16-year-old.

Answer 2 (Fig. 12-116): B
Following the two sinus beats, there are three beats of junctional rhythm at a cycle length of 1.28 sec (47/min). The QRS complex is identical to that found in sinus rhythm. There is a sinus P wave preceding each junctional beat but the PR interval is too short to conduct. The last three beats are ventricular escape beats at a cycle length of 1.30 sec (46/min). The QRS complex is different from the sinus QRS. This might be called an "accelerated ventricular escape rhythm" since the rate is over 40/min, but 46/min is probably within the range of variability for an idioventricular rhythm. Atrial activity is not seen during the idioventricular rhythm, and therefore it is not indicated on the ladder diagram.

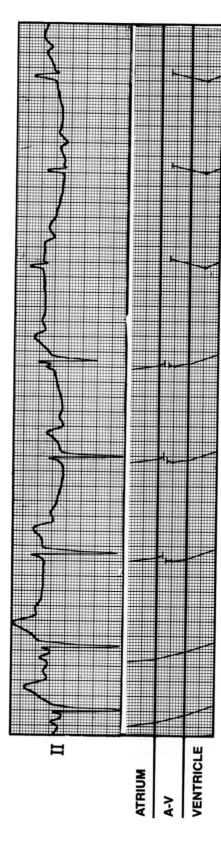

FIG. 12-116. Answers 1 and 2.

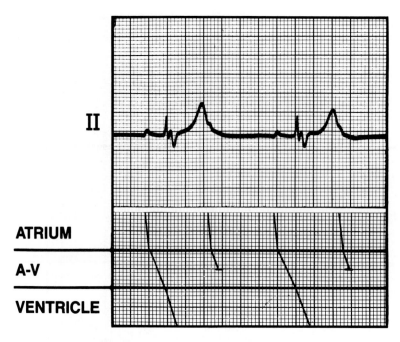

FIG. 12-117. Answers 3 and 4.

Answer 3 (Fig. 12-117): Category 2 (RR interval regular, QRS rate decreased, QRS duration prolonged).

Answer 4 (Fig. 12-117): E

There is a sinus P wave on the downslope of each T wave. All four P waves have the same morphology. Since this is positive in lead II, this suggests a sinus origin. The PP interval is regular, suggesting that this is regular sinus rhythm rather than blocked premature atrial contractions.

Answer 5 (Fig. 12-118): Category 2 (RR interval regular, QRS rate decreased, QRS duration prolonged).

Answer 6 (Fig. 12-118): A

There is AV dissociation.

Answer 7 (Fig. 12-118): E

There is an obvious P wave approximately .40 sec before each QRS complex. The intervals from the P waves to the subsequent QRS complexes are: .52, .48, .47, .44, and .45 sec. There are actually twice as many P waves as are immediately apparent. There is a notch preceding the upstroke of the first QRS complex. If the PP interval preceding this P wave is measured (.47 sec) and then "marched out," it can be seen that there is a second P wave buried within each subsequent QRS complex. The key to this tracing is in the varying, prolonged PR interval which suggests AV dissociation. In this case, there is actually complete AV dissociation with the P waves completely unrelated to the

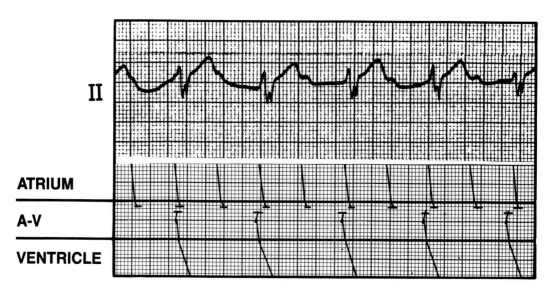

FIG. 12-118. Answers 5, 6, and 7.

QRS complexes. There is complete AV block. The site of origin of the QRS complex could either be junctional with aberrancy or ventricular in that the QRS duration is prolonged. Since the rate of 68/min is appropriate for a junctional escape rhythm, this is the answer provided. This also could have been complete AV block with an accelerated ventricular rhythm.

Answer 8 (Fig. 12-119): Category 3 (RR interval regular, QRS rate normal, QRS duration normal).

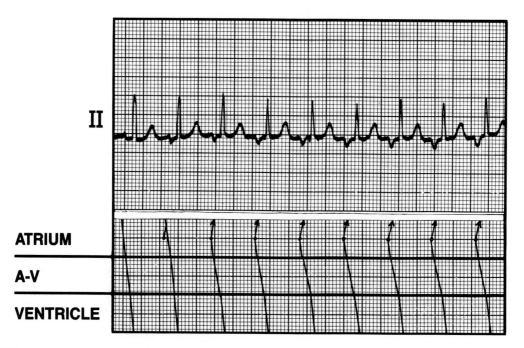

FIG. 12-119. Answers 8, 9, and 10.

Answer 9 (Fig. 12-119): B
No, there is not AV dissociation.

Answer 10 (Fig. 12-119): D
In the last seven beats there is an inverted P wave in lead II preceding each normal QRS complex at a rate of 130/min. This is an accelerated atrial rhythm. The first beat of the tracing is a sinus beat. This is followed by a fusion P wave. Note that this P wave has characteristics of both the sinus P wave and the P wave due to the accelerated atrial rhythm. The abnormal rhythm therefore begins with the second P wave of the tracing.

Answer 11 (Fig. 12-120): Category 3 (RR interval regular, QRS rate normal, QRS duration normal).

Answer 12 (Fig. 12-120): A
Yes, there is AV dissociation.

Answer 13 (Fig. 12-120): A
The P waves are negative in lead II, indicating a low atrial origin. The atrial rate (115/min) is abnormally rapid for an atrial escape rhythm in a 6-year-old. Therefore, this is an accelerated atrial rhythm. The ventricles are controlled by a rapid junctional rate (125/min). The P waves and QRS complexes are completely dissociated. There are no short RR intervals indicating a capture beat of the ventricles by the atria, although the first two P waves should probably have changed the RR interval if they had conducted. Therefore, there may also be AV block, since these first two P waves should have shortened the RR interval. AV block cannot be diagnosed with certainty, however, since there are not enough P waves on the tracing that should conduct to the ventricles (i.e., those that occur just beyond the end of the T wave).

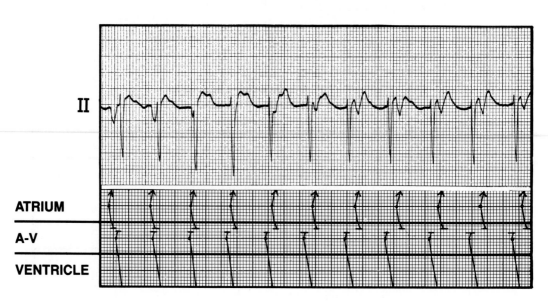

FIG. 12-120. Answers 11, 12, and 13.

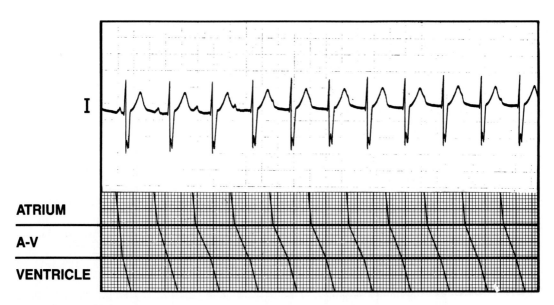

FIG. 12-121. Answers 14 and 15.

Answer 14 (Fig. 12-121): Category 9 (RR interval continuously irregular, PP interval regular, QRS duration normal). At first glance, this appears to be category 4 with a normal, regular RR interval. This is not the case, however.

Answer 15 (Fig. 12-121): A
The first three RR intervals are slightly longer than the rest. These measure .56, .52, and .50 sec. Then the RR intervals stabilize at .48 sec. The PP interval is constant throughout at .48 sec. The PR intervals are .10, .16, .21, and .22 sec. They stabilize at approximately .22 to .23 sec. This is the onset of type I second-degree AV block. While at the beginning of the tracing, there appears to be AV dissociation, the P waves are related to the QRS complexes, and therefore there is not AV dissociation.

Answer 16 (Fig. 12-122): Category 5 (RR interval regular, QRS rate increased, QRS duration normal).

Answer 17 (Fig. 12-122): B
No, there is not AV dissociation. There are twice as many atrial impulses as ventricular impulses, but the atrial and ventricular impulses are related.

Answer 18 (Fig. 12-122): C
The atrial impulses (cycle length .18 sec) are seen best in lead V_1. There is one atrial impulse immediately following each QRS complex and one preceding the QRS by .14 sec. In both lead II and V_1, the atrial impulses have the characteristics of flutter waves. There is 2:1 AV conduction. This demonstrates that atrial flutter may have a regular ventricular rate even though in small children the rate is usually irregular.

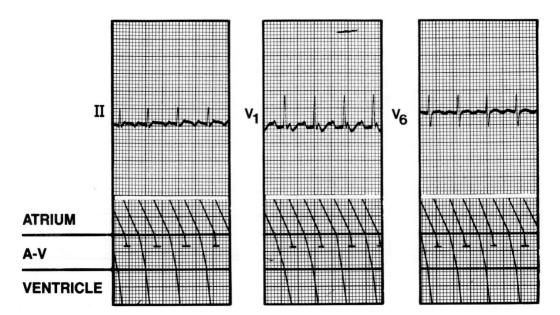

FIG. 12-122.   Answers 16, 17, and 18.

Answer 19 (Fig. 12-123): Category 9 (RR interval continuously irregular, PP interval regular, QRS duration normal).

Answer 20 (Fig. 12-123): C

There are three different rhythms on this tracing. The first is supraventricular tachycardia at a rate of 230/min. When the supraventricular tachycardia stops spontaneously, there are three beats of sinus

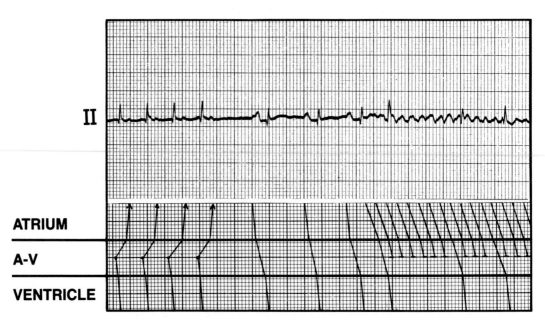

FIG. 12-123.   Answers 19 and 20.

rhythm. Atrial flutter begins spontaneously after the third sinus QRS complex. The flutter waves have a distinct morphology with a regular "PP" interval of .12 sec. In newborn infants with coexistent supraventricular tachycardia and atrial flutter, usually the supraventricular tachycardia is regular and the atrial flutter is irregular.

Answer 21 (Fig. 12-124): Category 10 (RR interval continuously irregular, PP interval regular, QRS duration prolonged).

Answer 22 (Fig. 12-124): B
No, there is not AV dissociation despite the appearance of the tracing.

Answer 23 (Fig. 12-124): D
The QRS complexes occur in groups of three. The RR intervals shorten in each group. Both of these suggest 4:3 Wenckebach (type I second-degree AV block). Most of the P waves occur on T waves or within the QRS complexes (see the ladder diagram).

Answer 24 (Fig. 12-125):
Tracings A and B are both categories 11 (RR interval regular, interrupted by premature QRS of normal duration) and 12 (RR interval regular, interrupted by premature QRS of prolonged duration). Tracing C is category 11.

Answer 25 (Fig. 12-125): All A
All five premature beats are premature atrial contractions. In tracing A, the premature P waves are clearly visible. The QRS complex following

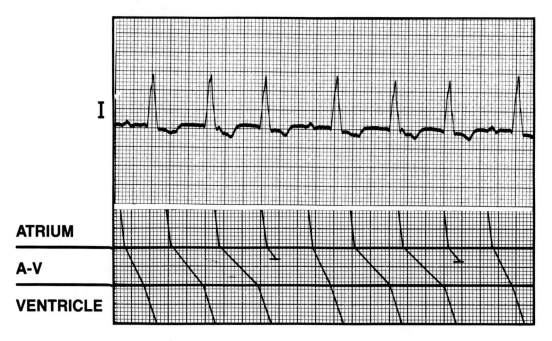

FIG. 12-124. Answers 21, 22, and 23.

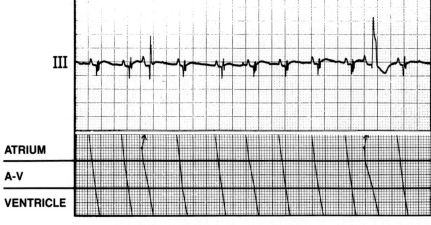

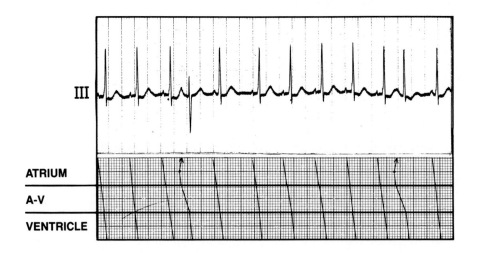

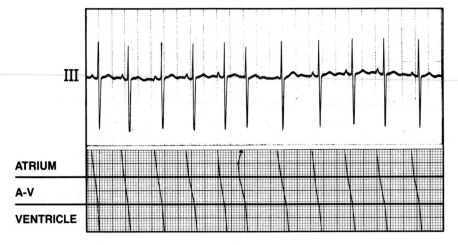

FIG. 12-125. Answers 24 and 25.

the first premature P wave is slightly aberrant and the QRS following the second premature P wave is more aberrant. In tracing B, the first premature P wave causes the T wave to be more peaked than the other T waves. The accompanying QRS is aberrant although it is not wide. The second premature atrial contraction causes a slight flattening of the T wave. It occurs slightly later, and so the following QRS is not aberrant. In tracing C, the T wave is flattened by the premature P wave. These tracings demonstrate that any variation in an otherwise uniform group of T waves is likely to be due to a P wave.

Answer 26 (Fig. 12-126): Category 11 (RR interval regular, interrupted by premature QRS of normal duration). The third QRS complex occurs slightly prematurely.

Answer 27 (Fig. 12-126): A
Yes, there is AV dissociation.

Answer 28 (Fig. 12-126): D
The first, second, fourth, fifth, and sixth QRS complexes are identical. They have a prolonged duration and occur at a cycle length of 1.32 sec (equivalent to a rate of 45/min). This is a ventricular escape rhythm. There is AV dissociation due to sinus bradycardia and the ventricular escape rhythm. Although it is tempting to call this a junctional rhythm, there are several points proving that this is a ventricular rhythm. Firstly, the QRS complexes are prolonged. Secondly, the final three QRS complexes in the tracing are conducted from the atria. These QRS complexes are completely different from those of the escape rhythm. Finally, the third QRS complex in the rhythm is narrower than the others and is preceded by a P wave; this is a fusion complex, between the QRS complex caused by the conducted P wave and the QRS complex caused by the ventricular escape rhythm. The fusion beat is narrower than both the conducted QRS and the escape QRS. This is because the sinus beats are conducted with complete left bundle branch block and the escape pacemaker is in the left bundle branch. If the timing is proper, and the ectopic pacemaker fires and activates the left ventricle just as the conducted impulse activates the right ventricle, the ventricles will be activated almost simultaneously and the resultant QRS will be narrow. Therefore, generally, beats that originate in the proximal left bundle branch in patients with left bundle branch block produce narrow QRS complexes; and beats that arise in the proximal right bundle branch in patients with right bundle branch block are narrow. For example, assume in a patient with left bundle branch block and sinus rhythm that the right ventricle is activated 20 msec after the His bundle and the left ventricle is activated 80 msec after the His bundle. If this patient with left bundle branch block has an ectopic beat that originates in the left bundle branch, it may take 20 msec to travel retrogradely to the His bundle and another 20 msec to travel down the right bundle branch to activate the right ventricle. Therefore, the right ventricle is activated 40 msec after the onset of the ectopic beat. However, since the ectopic impulse origi-

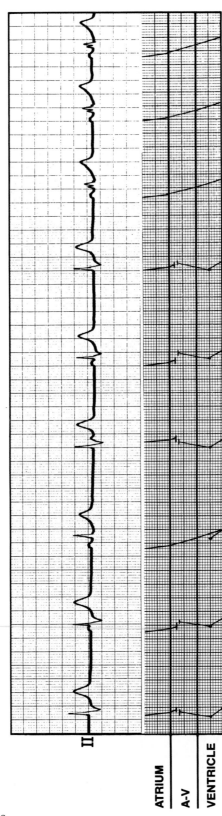

II

ATRIUM

A-V

VENTRICLE

FIG. 12-126. Answers 26, 27, and 28.

368

nates in the left bundle branch by local spread of the impulse, the time to activate the left ventricle will be shorter than in sinus rhythm (i.e., approximately 40 msec). Thus, the right ventricle and left ventricle may be activated simultaneously and the resultant QRS complex will be narrow.

Answer 29 (Fig. 12-127): Category 12 (RR interval irregular, interrupted by a premature QRS of prolonged duration).

Answer 30 (Fig. 12-127): A
The first two beats are sinus followed by a premature ventricular contraction. There is a retrograde P wave following the premature ventricular contraction. Then there are three junctional beats at a rate of 68/min. This is slightly more rapid than the usual junctional escape rhythm and may be called an accelerated junctional escape rhythm. The third QRS following the premature ventricular contraction has a shorter PR interval (.12 sec) and those beats before the premature ventricular contraction (.13 sec) and therefore the P wave on this beat may not have conducted. The final P wave conducts with the same PR interval (.13 sec) as those preceding the premature ventricular contraction. Atrial activity is not seen until just before the second QRS of the junctional rhythm. The ladder diagram has been drawn assuming a P wave is buried in the first QRS complex after the premature ventricular contraction. Alternatively, the atrial depolarization caused by the retrograde conduction from the premature ventricular contraction may have transiently suppressed the sinus node until just before the second QRS complex of the junctional rhythm.

Answer 31 (Fig. 12-127): C
Digitalis intoxication may be manifest by premature ventricular contractions and accelerated junctional rhythm or "nonparoxysmal junctional tachycardia."

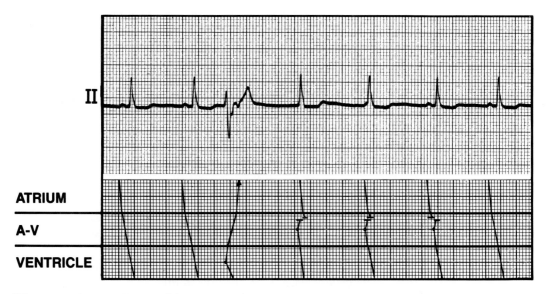

FIG. 12-127. Answers 29, 30, and 31.

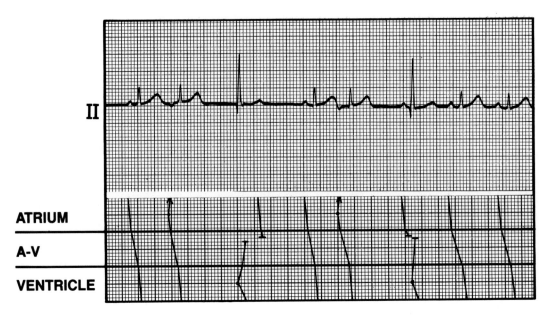

FIG. 12-128.   Answers 32 and 33.

Answer 32 (Fig. 12-128):
Category 11 (RR interval regular, interrupted by premature QRS at normal duration) and 14 (RR interval regular, interrupted by a delayed QRS of prolonged duration).

Answer 33 (Fig. 12-128): C
The first beat is sinus. The second is a premature atrial contraction. The coupling interval between the sinus and abnormal P waves is .50 sec (equivalent to a rate of 120/min). This is definitely a premature beat and not an atrial escape beat. The third beat originates from the ventricles. The coupling interval is .70 sec (equivalent to a rate of 86/min) from the previous QRS complex. This is not a ventricular escape beat because the coupling interval is too short. It could be classified as either a premature ventricular contraction or an accelerated ventricular escape beat.

Answer 34 (Fig. 12-129): Category 13 (RR interval regular, interrupted by delayed QRS of normal duration).

Answer 35 (Fig. 12-129): D
The underlying problem is sinus bradycardia. Whenever the sinus node fails to depolarize, there is a junctional escape beat with a coupling interval of 1.2 sec from the preceding QRS. The "premature" beats are actually the normal sinus capture beats. These are followed by pauses which are terminated by junctional escape beats. This rhythm is called "escape-capture bigeminy."

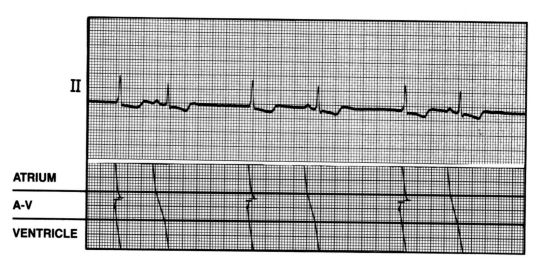

FIG. 12-129. Answers 34 and 35.

Answer 36 (Fig. 12-130):
Category 12 (RR interval regular, interrupted by premature QRS of normal duration) and 14 (RR interval regular, interrupted by delayed QRS of prolonged duration).

Answer 37 (Fig. 12-130): A
The first beat is a sinus beat conducted with complete right bundle branch block. The second QRS is premature, aberrant, and not preceded by a P wave. It occurs at a coupling interval of .52 sec. It is a premature ventricular contraction. This premature ventricular contraction is followed by a sinus P wave. Then there is a pause of 1.08 sec.

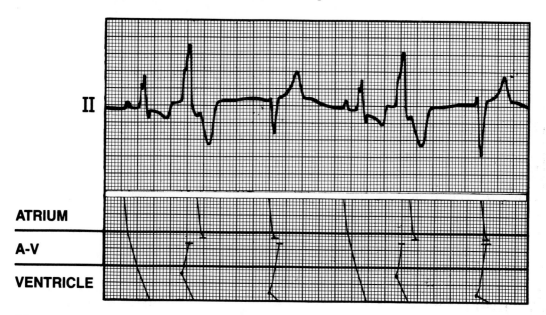

FIG. 12-130. Answers 36 and 37.

The pause is ended by a wide QRS beat. This QRS is not preceded by a P wave. It has a different morphology from the conducted sinus QRS. Therefore it is a ventricular escape beat from a different site than the premature ventricular contraction. This tracing demonstrates an example of abnormal ectopic activity (the premature ventricular contraction) immediately followed by normal ectopic activity (the escape beat).

Answer 38 (Fig. 12-131): Category 5 (RR interval regular, QRS rate increased, QRS duration normal).

Answer 39 (Fig. 12-131): B
No, there is not AV dissociation.

Answer 40 (Fig. 12-131): C
Atrial flutter may result in an irregular or a regular RR interval. In this case, it resulted in a regular RR interval. In this record, two features suggest the possibility of atrial flutter: (1) The rapid regular RR interval

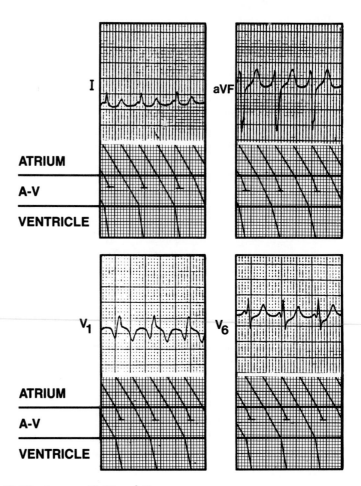

FIG. 12-131. Answers 38, 39, and 40.

without obvious P waves at a normal PR interval suggests that multiple leads should be examined for the presence of flutter waves. In this record, flutter waves are seen well only in lead V_1. (2) The ventricular rate is close to 150/min. Since the most common atrial rate for atrial flutter in a child is 300/min and since the most common type of AV block to occur with atrial flutter in an older child is 2:1, the most common rate for atrial flutter in an older child is approximately 150/min. Therefore, in a child who has a ventricular rate of approximately 150/min without an obvious cause for sinus tachycardia, there may be an extra buried P wave and atrial flutter with 2:1 block should be suspected. Any rhythm that defies interpretation is likely to be atrial flutter.

References

1. Michaelsson M., and Engle M. A.: Congenital complete heart block: an international study of the natural history. *In* Cardiovascular Clinics. Edited by A. N. Brest and M. A. Engle. Philadelphia, F. A. Davis, 1972, p. 85.
2. Pinsky W. W., Gillette P. C., Garson A., and McNamara D. G.: Diagnosis, management, and long-term results of patients with congenital complete atrioventricular block. Pediatrics *69:*728–733, 1982.
3. Southall D. P., Richards J., Mitchell P., et al.: Study of cardiac rhythm in healthy newborn infants. Br Heart J *43:*14–20, 1979.
4. Scott O., Williams G. J., and Fiddler G. I.: Results of 24 hour ambulatory monitoring of electrocardiogram in 131 healthy boys aged 10 to 13 years. Br Heart J *44:*304–308, 1980.
5. Southall D. P., Johnston F., Shinebourne E. A., et al.: A 24-hour ECG study of heart rate and rhythm patterns in a population of healthy children (unpublished data).
6. Pick A., and Langendorf R.: Interpretation of Complex Arrhythmias. Philadelphia, Lea & Febiger, 1979, pp 8–26.
7. Garson A., Gillette P. C., and McNamara D. G.: A Guide to Cardiac Dysrhythmias in Children. New York, Grune & Stratton, 1980.
8. Kugler J. D.: Sinoatrial node dysfunction. *In* Pediatric Cardiac Dysrhythmias. Edited by P. C. Gillette and A. Garson. New York, Grune & Stratton, 1981, pp 265–293.
9. Gillette P. C., and Rose A. P.: Sinus arrhythmia, wandering pacemaker, and premature atrial contractions. *In* Pediatric Cardiac Dysrhythmias. Edited by P. C. Gillette and A. Garson. New York, Grune & Stratton, 1981, pp 145–151.
10. Randall W. C., Rinkema L. E., and Moran J. F.: Overdrive suppression of atrial pacemaker tissues in the alert awake dog before and chronically after excision of the sinoatrial node. Am J Cardiol *49:*1666–1675, 1982.
11. Booth D. C., Popio K. A., and Gettes L. S.: Multiformity of induced unifocal ventricular premature beats in human subjects. Am J Cardiol *49:*1643–1653, 1982.
12. Josephson M. E., Horowitz L. N., Farshidi A., et al.: Recurrent sustained ventricular tachycardia. I. Mechanisms. Circulation *57:*431–440, 1978.
13. Watanabe Y., and Dreifus L. S.: Cardiac Arrhythmias: Electrophysiologic Basis for Clinical Interpretation. New York, Grune & Stratton, 1977, pp 217–267.
14. Southall D. P., Johnson A. M., Shinebourne E. A., et al.: Frequency and outcome of disorders of cardiac rhythm and conduction in a population of newborn infants. Pediatrics *68:*58–66, 1981.
15. Garson A.: Ventricular dysrhythmias. *In* Pediatric Cardiac Dysrhythmias. Edited by P. C. Gillette and A. Garson. New York, Grune & Stratton, 1981, pp 295–360.
16. Schamroth L.: The Disorders of Cardiac Rhythm. Oxford, Blackwell, 1970, pp 85–94.
17. Langendorf R., Pick A., and Winternitz M.: Mechanisms of intermittent ventricular bigeminy. I. Appearance of ectopic beats, dependent upon length of the ventricular cycle, the "rule of bigeminy." Circulation *11:*422–430, 1955.

18. Talbot S., and Dreifus L. S.: Characteristics of ventricular extrasystoles and their prognostic importance. Chest 67:665–674, 1975.

19. Gillette P. C., and Garson A.: Intracardiac electrophysiologic studies: use in determining the site and mechanisms of dysrhythmias. *In* Pediatric Cardiac Dysrhythmias. Edited by P. C. Gillette and A. Garson. New York, Grune & Stratton, 1981, pp 77–120.

20. Fisher D. J., Gross D. M., and Garson A.: Rapid sinus tachycardia—differentiation from supraventricular tachycardia. Am J Dis Child 137:164–166, 1983.

21. Garson A.: Supraventricular tachycardia. *In* Pediatric Cardiac Dysrhythmias. Edited by P. C. Gillette and A. Garson. New York, Grune & Stratton, 1981, pp 177–253.

22. Garson A., Gillette P. C., and McNamara D. G.: Supraventricular tachycardia in children: clinical features, response to treatment and long-term follow-up in 217 patients. J Pediatr 98:875–882, 1981.

23. Garson A., and Gillette P. C.: Junctional ectopic tachycardia in children: electrocardiography, electrophysiology and pharmacologic response. Am J Cardiol 44:298–302, 1979.

24. Gillette P. C., and Garson A.: Electrophysiologic and pharmacologic characteristics of automatic ectopic atrial tachycardia. Circulation 56:571–575, 1977.

25. Rosen M. R., Fisch C., Hoffman B. F., et al.: Can accelerated atrioventricular junctional escape rhythms be explained by delayed afterdepolarizations? Am J Cardiol 45:1272–1284, 1980.

26. Shih J. Y., Gillette P. C., and Garson A.: Atrial flutter and fibrillation. *In* Pediatric Cardiac Dysrhythmias. Edited by P. C. Gillette and A. Garson. New York, Grune & Stratton, 1981, pp 255–263.

27. Shih J. Y., Gillette P. C., Garson A., et al.: The prognosis of atrial flutter in children. Pediatr Res 14:450, 1980 (Abstr).

28. Gillette P. C., Garson A., and Kugler J. D.: Wolff-Parkinson-White syndrome in children: electrophysiologic and pharmacologic characteristics. Circulation 60:1487–1495, 1979.

29. Radford D. J., and Izukawa T.: Atrial fibrillation in children. Pediatrics 59:250–256, 1977.

30. Pedersen D., Zipes D. P., Foster P. R., et al.: Ventricular tachycardia and ventricular fibrillation in a young population. Circulation 60:988–997, 1979.

31. Videbaek J., Andersen E., Jacobsen J., et al.: Paroxysmal tachycardia in infancy and childhood. II. Paroxysmal ventricular tachycardia and fibrillation. Acta Paediatr Scand 62:349–357, 1973.

32. Garson A., Gillette P. C., Hawkins E., et al.: Epicardial tumors undetected by angiography as a cause of ventricular tachycardia in infants: electrophysiology and surgical cure. Pediatr Cardiol (in press).

33. Kossmann C. E.: Torsade de pointes: an addition to the nosography of ventricular tachycardia. Am J Cardiol 42:1054–1956, 1978.

34. Morris S. N., and Zipes D. P.: His bundle electrocardiography during bidirectional ventricular tachycardia. Circulation 48:32–38, 1973.

35. Garson A., Porter C. J., and Gillette P. C.: Ventricular tachycardia in children with a normal heart. Circulation 66; Supp II: 170, 1982.

36. Davidson R. M.: Chronic accelerated ventricular rhythm. J Electrocardiol 9:249–254, 1976.

37. Gaum W., Biancaniello T., and Kaplan S.: Accelerated ventricular rhythm in childhood. Am J Cardiol 43:162–164, 1979.

38. Benson D. W., Smith W. M., Sterba R., et al.: Mechanisms of regular, wide QRS tachycardia in infants and children. Am J Cardiol 49:1778–1788, 1982.

39. Vetter V. L., Horowitz L. N., and Josephson M. E.: Recurrent sustained ventricular tachycardia in pediatric patients. Circulation 57/58:II–196, 1978 (Abstr).

40. Gillette P., Reitman M., Gutgesell H., et al.: Intracardiac electrophysiology in children and young adults. Am Heart J 89:36–44, 1975.

41. Alimurung M., and Massell B.: The normal PR interval in infants and children. Circulation 13:257–261, 1956.

42. Bellet S.: Clinical Disorders of the Heart Beat. 3rd Ed. Philadelphia, Lea & Febiger, 1971, pp 1–36.

43. Jacobsen J., Gillette P., Corbett B., et al.: Intracardiac electrography in endocardial cushion defects. Circulation *54*:599–603, 1976.

44. Mirowski M., Arevalo F., Medrano G., et al.: Conduction disturbances in patients with patent ductus arteriosus: a study of 200 cases before and after surgery with determination of the PR interval. Circulation *25*:807–813, 1962.

45. Wenckebach K.: Zur analyse des unregelmassigen pulses. Z Klin Med *37*:475–488, 1889.

46. Mobitz W.: Über die unvollstandinge storung der errugungsuberleitung zeischen vorhof und kammer des menschichen herzens. Z Ges Exp Med *41*:180–237, 1924.

47. Denes P., Levy K., Pick A., et al.: The incidence of typical and atypical A-V Wenckebach periodicity. Am Heart J *89*:26–31, 1975.

48. Narula O., Runge M., and Samet P.: Second degree Wenckebach type AV block due to block within the atrium. Br Heart J *34*:1127–1136, 1972.

49. Young D., Eisenberg R., Fish B., et al.: Wenckebach atrioventricular block (Mobitz type I) in children and adolescents. Am J Cardiol *40*:393–399, 1977.

50. Steeg C., and Krongrad E.: Disorders of conduction. *In* Cardiac Arrhythmias in the Neonate, Infant and Child. Edited by N. Roberts and H. Gelband. New York, Appleton-Century-Crofts, 1977, pp 211–230.

51. Karpawich P. P.: First and second degree atrioventricular block. *In* Pediatric Cardiac Dysrhythmias. Edited by P. C. Gillette and A. Garson. New York, Grune & Stratton, 1981, pp 361–381.

52. Watanabe Y., and Dreifus L.: Second degree atrioventricular block. Cardiovasc Res *1*:150–158, 1967.

53. Zipes D.: Second degree atrioventricular block. Circulation *60*:465–472, 1979.

54. Langendorf R., and Pick A.: Atrioventricular block, type II (Mobitz)—its nature and clinical significance. Circulation *38*:819–821, 1968.

55. Kelly D., Brodsky S., and Krovetz L.: Mobitz type II atrioventricular block in children. J Pediatr *79*:972–976, 1971.

56. Gochberg S. H.: Congenital heart block. Am J Obstet Gynecol *88*:238–241, 1964.

57. McCue C. M., Mantakas M. E., Tingstad J. B., et al.: Congenital heart block in newborns of mothers with connective tissue disease. Circulation *56*:82–89, 1977.

58. Lev M.: Pathogenesis of congenital atrioventricular block. Prog Cardiovasc Dis *15*:145–157, 1972.

59. Pinsky W. W.: Diagnosis and management of congenital complete atrioventricular block. *In* Pediatric Cardiac Dysrhythmias. Edited by P. C. Gillette and A. Garson. New York, Grune & Stratton, 1981, pp 265–293.

60. Driscoll D. J.: Surgical complete atrioventricular block. *In* Pediatric Cardiac Dysrhythmias. Edited by P. C. Gillette and A. Garson. New York, Grune & Stratton, 1981, pp 397–404.

13

Artifacts

Recognition of artifacts is both important and satisfying:—it is an exercise in mind over matter. Causes of artifacts can be classified into six major categories.[1]

Causes of Artifacts

INCORRECT POSITIONING OF THE ELECTROCARDIOGRAM LEADS. (1) Artifacts are most commonly caused by reversing the right arm with the left arm or the right leg with the left leg. Only the limb leads on the electrocardiographic tracing are affected. If the arm leads are reversed, the P wave, QRS complex, and T wave are inverted in lead I. This can be checked by examining lead V_6, since V_6 has approximately the same vector as lead I. If the complexes in lead I and V_6 are completely different and the P waves are inverted in lead I, the limb leads are reversed (Fig. 13-1A and B). If the right leg and the left leg leads are switched, there is practically no change in the electrocardiogram (Fig. 13-1C). If the right leg and the right arm leads are switched, lead II is entirely isoelectric; in addition, the complexes in aV_R and aV_F are completely positive. It is not possible to calculate a mean vector that is entirely positive in aV_R and aV_F at the same time. Finally, lead I is entirely different from lead V_6. These leads should record similar complexes (Fig. 13-1D). If the left leg and left arm leads are switched, unlike the other errors, the resultant electrocardiogram is not obviously faulty. Instead, this error in position results in abnormal left axis deviation (Fig. 13-1E).

(2) If the chest leads are positioned in an incorrect interspace a change will result in the ECG (Fig. 13-2). If all the leads are placed one interspace too high (e.g., third instead of fourth interspace), the R waves are diminished and the S waves are augmented in leads V_4 to V_7. If the leads are placed one interspace too low, the R waves are augmented and the S waves are diminished.

(3) If electrode paste is not cleaned between chest lead placement, the entire anterior chest will become a conductor and the same "average" QRS complex will be recorded from each lead. This is a common

376

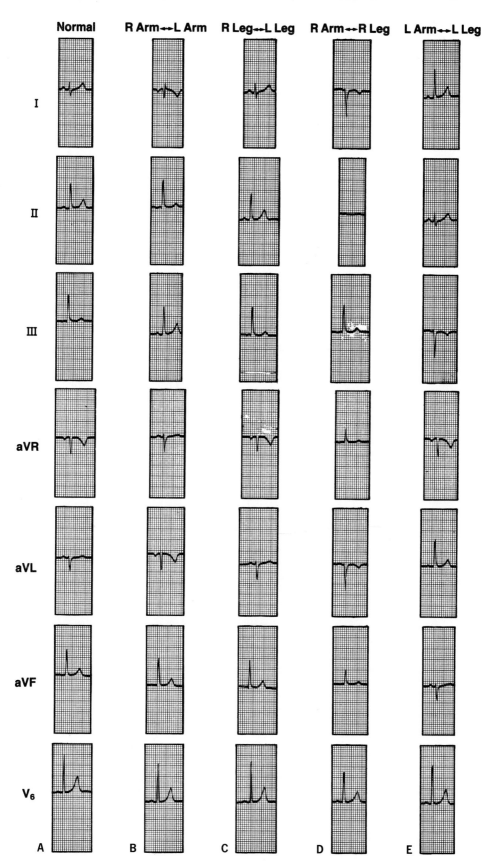

FIG. 13-1. Artifacts due to incorrect limb lead placement. *A,* Limb leads in the normal positions; *B,* right arm and left arm reversed; *C,* right leg and left leg reversed; *D,* right arm and right leg reversed; *E,* left arm and left leg reversed.

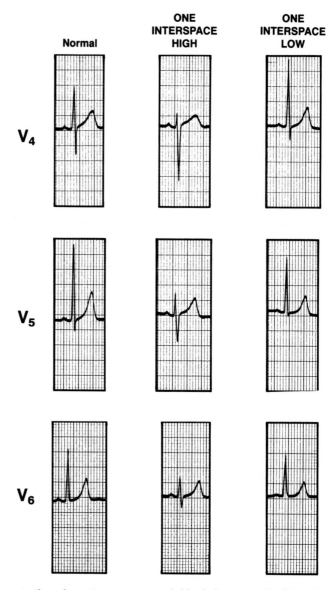

FIG. 13-2. Artifacts due to incorrect precordial lead placement. The *first* column is with the leads in the normal position. The *second* column is with the leads placed one interspace too high. The *third* column is with the leads placed one interspace too low.

problem in infants. This should be suspected if every chest lead appears similar (Fig. 13-3).

PATIENT INITIATED MOVEMENT. (1) Hiccoughs. These are monophasic or biphasic deflections which occur randomly throughout the cardiac cycle. They are usually midway in size between a P wave and QRS complex. There is no alteration in the basic rhythm (Fig. 13-4). (2) Purposeful movement. Any random depolarization on the electrocardiogram that does not affect the basic rhythm should be suspected as an

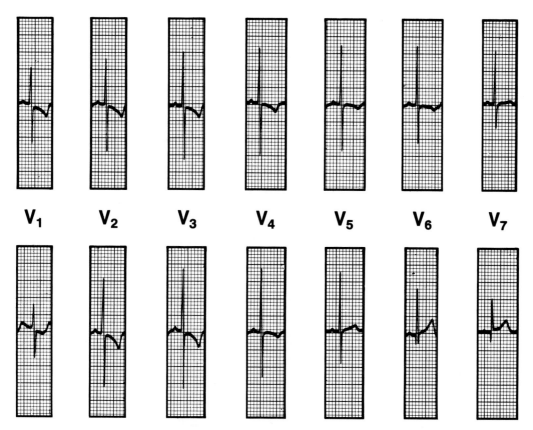

FIG. 13-3. Electrode paste improperly removed between applications of the chest electrodes. *Top* row, Paste smeared on the anterior chest wall causing all complexes to appear the same. *Bottom* row, Proper application of the paste showing a difference between complexes.

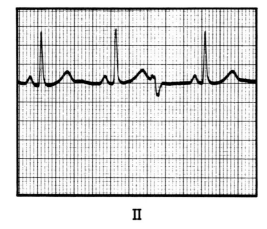

II

FIG. 13-4. Hiccough. This artifact can best be described as being midway in size between a P wave and a QRS complex. It is too large for a P wave. If it were a QRS complex, it should be followed by a T wave.

artifact. If the movement is repetitive (e.g., waving of the hand), it may simulate ventricular tachycardia. (3) Nonpurposeful movement. Convulsions, "jittery" newborns, and somatic tremors may simulate tachyarrhythmias (Fig. 13-5). (4) Respirations. The size of the QRS complex may change with normal deep inspiration (Fig. 13-6).

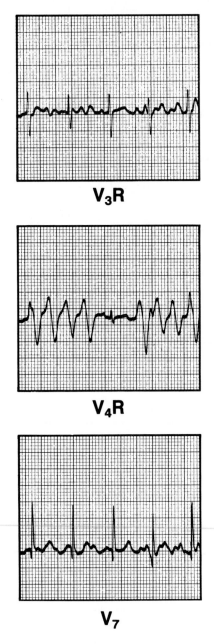

FIG. 13-5. Simultaneous tracings taken during a seizure. In lead V₄R, the tracing appears to be ventricular tachycardia, but in the other two tracings it is apparent that this is an artifact and that there is a regular supraventricular rhythm at a rate of 120/min. This demonstrates the value of having three simultaneous leads to aid in the identification of artifacts.

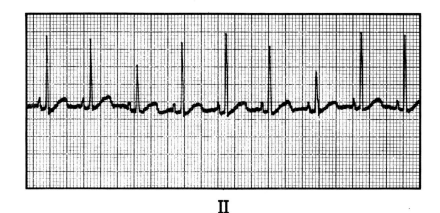

II

FIG. 13-6. Respiration. The QRS amplitude changes cyclically with approximately 2 sec between the smallest QRS complexes. This corresponds to a respiratory rate of 30/min.

THERAPEUTIC MANIPULATION OF THE PATIENT. (1) Chest percussion can occur at a rate of approximately 5/sec, which results in an artifact at a rate of 300/min (Fig. 13-7). (2) Open or closed chest massage adds artifactual complexes with each depression of the chest.

PROPERLY FUNCTIONING ELECTROCARDIOGRAPHIC SYSTEM WITH "BUILT-IN" ARTIFACT. In certain electrocardiographic recording machines, the calibration signal is provided automatically without stopping the paper. Thus, the calibration spike may be confused with parts of the true electrocardiogram and form an artifact (Fig. 13-8).

MALFUNCTIONING ELECTROCARDIOGRAPHIC SYSTEM. (1) Loss of electrode contact. Usually this is marked by an abrupt change in the baseline with an absence of cardiac depolarizations. In true asystole the base-

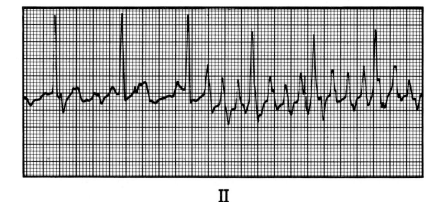

II

FIG. 13-7. Chest percussion. This is recorded from a 24-hour electrocardiogram, and the artifact occurs at a rate of approximately 300/min. Note that the RR interval is unchanged before and during the artifact.

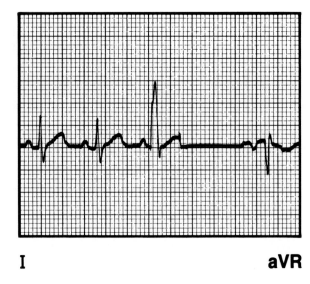

I   aVR

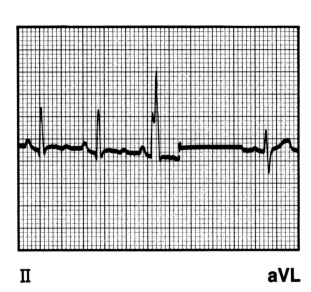

II   aVL

FIG. 13-8. Calibration fusion. These leads were recorded simultaneously. Most apparent in lead II is the onset of a normal QRS complex, and then a further spike is introduced on top of the QRS complex. This is followed by an isoelectric segment when the electrocardiograph is not recording. This simulates a premature ventricular contraction.

line usually does not change (Fig. 13-9). (2) Faulty cable shielding. Movement artifact on the electrocardiogram is seen when the cable is moved. (3) Faulty cable attachment. A repetitive artifact may be produced by low-amplitude vibration in the environment (Fig. 13-10). (4) Interference from 60-cycle leakage. (5) Faulty paper drive. Uneven stylus marks may be present, causing the paper to appear "burned." As the paper speed varies, all parts of the P wave, QRS complex, and T wave shorten and prolong with the apparent increase or decrease in

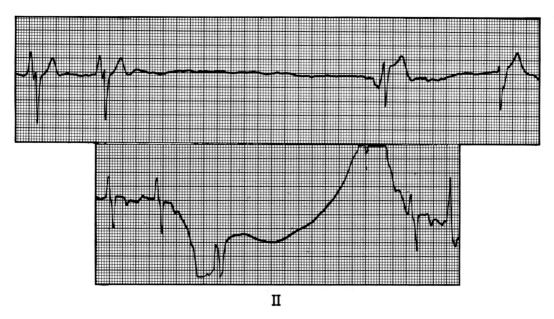

II

FIG. 13-9. Asystole versus loss of electrode contact. In the *top* tracing, there is asystole and in the *bottom* tracing, there is loss of electrode contact. Note the change in the baseline with the loss of electrode contact.

heart rate respectively (Fig. 13-11). At the slowest abnormal paper speeds, the heart rate may appear to be faster than physiologically possible, giving a hint that this may be an artifact (Fig. 13-12). (6) Faulty stylus. An arc rather than a straight line is drawn for the R wave. (7) Incorrect stylus position or improper gain. The "isoelectric" line may be unusually flat, indicating that the stylus is at the limit of its excursion

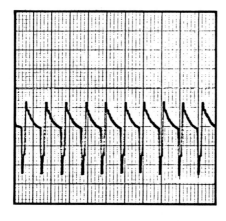

II

FIG. 13-10. Faulty cable attachment. This artifact was eliminated when the connector between the patient cable and the electrocardiograph was secured. This presumably resulted from repetitive vibrations in the pins, which were placed loosely in the slots of the connector.

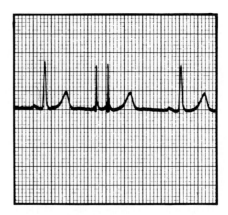

II

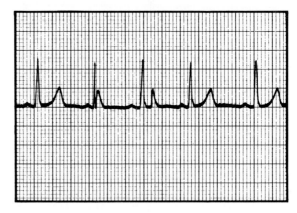

FIG. 13-11. Paper drag due to faulty paper drive. In the *top* tracing, the middle two QRS complexes are too narrow compared to the others and indicate that the paper is dragging. Also, there is an uneven stylus mark causing the paper to appear burned in the third complex. In the *bottom* tracing, in the middle three complexes, the PR, QRS, and QT intervals are all shortened to varying degrees.

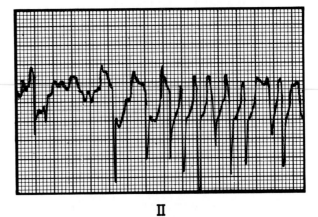

II

FIG. 13-12. Tape drag causing rapid and irregular rate. In this tracing from a 24-hour electrocardiogram, the rhythm is irregular, indicating an artifact, and the rate of 428/min is physiologically impossible for a 14-year-old child.

or "pegged" (Fig. 13-13A). This can be suspected by the lack of any deflection on one side of the isoelectric line or a heavy mark at the peak of the QRS complex (Fig. 13-13B).

CURRENT PRODUCED FROM EXTERNAL SOURCES. Overhead warmer or respirator. Either may cause cyclic production of 60-cycle current, which may be printed on the electrocardiogram. The source of the current or electrical interference may not be identified. (2) The "infusion pump artifact." This was originally described as a biphasic spike of 30 msec duration with a repetitive rate of 135/min.[2] This artifact is similar to, but wider than, a normal bipolar cardiac pacemaker artifact. The control plunger in a defective infusion pump was the source of current leak, which was transmitted through the IV tubing and scalp vein to the patient and detected on the electrocardiogram. We have recently found an artifact that even more closely resembled P waves. This was again due to current leakage from an infusion pump down a nasogastric tube and through the patient which was recorded on the electrocardiogram at a rate of 56/min (Fig. 13-14).

Systematic Approach to the Recognition of Artifacts

A systematic approach is necessary for the recognition of artifacts. The following eight points are helpful in their identification.

(1) The shape, amplitude, or duration of the wave is atypical for a P wave or a QRS complex. The normal limits for P waves and QRS com-

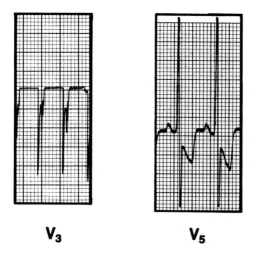

V₃   **V₅**

FIG. 13-13.   Improper stylus position. *A,* The isoelectric line is unusually flat and there are no complexes above this line. This indicates that the upper limit for the stylus was being reached at this point. The patient had ventricular tachycardia. *B,* An improper gain setting has been applied so that the QRS complexes are clipped at both the top and the bottom of the tracing. In such cases, it is impossible to tell how much larger the QRS complexes would have been without changing the gain setting.

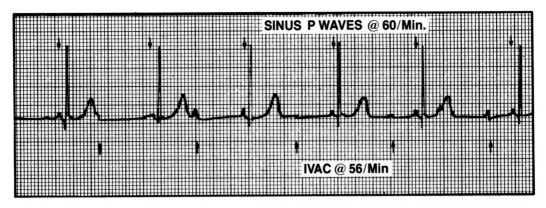

FIG. 13-14.   The infusion pump artifact. The arrows on top of the tracing demonstrate the sinus P waves occurring at a rate of 60/min. The arrows on the bottom of the tracing indicate an artifact occurring at a constant rate of 56/min due to current leak from an infusion pump with faulty shielding.

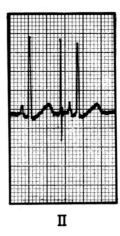

II

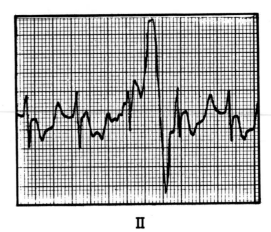

II

FIG. 13-15.   Improper duration for QRS complex. *Top*, The artifact between the two QRS complexes is too narrow to be a QRS complex and it is also not followed by a T wave. *Bottom*, The artifact in the middle of the tracing is too wide to be a premature ventricular contraction in a 1-month-old child. It is also accompanied by a baseline shift.

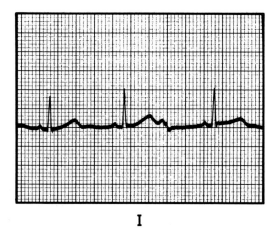

I

FIG. 13-16. Absence of a T wave following a "QRS complex." This artifact has the appearance of a QRS complex but is not followed by a T wave.

plexes are defined in Chapter 6 on the normal electrocardiogram. For example, many artifacts are "narrower" than a normal QRS and some artifacts last longer than even the most prolonged bundle branch block pattern (Figs. 13-10 and 13-15).

(2) If a wave has the appearance of a "QRS complex" but is not followed by a T wave, an artifact should be suspected (Fig. 13-16).

(3) Artifacts may be accompanied by a shift in the baseline (Fig. 13-17).

(4) An artifact that repeats itself must be differentiated from tachycardia. In a repetitive artifact the rate may be too rapid to be physiologically possible. The maximum regular atrial or ventricular rate is approximately 450/min in an infant (130 msec between waves) and 300/min in a child (200 msec between waves). Therefore, if there is less than 130 msec between successive regular waves in an infant, or less

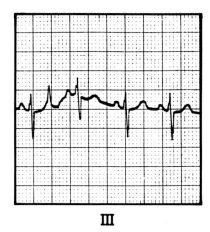

III

FIG. 13-17. Baseline shift. This hiccough is suspected as an artifact because it is too large for a P wave, is not followed by a T wave, and results in a baseline shift.

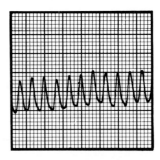

FIG. 13-18. Rapid rate that is physiologically impossible. This tracing was recorded on a 24-hour electrocardiogram from a 6-year-old child. Although these artifacts may appear similar to QRS complexes, the rate of 480/min is not physiologically possible for any rhythm in a child of this age.

than 200 msec in a child, an artifact should be suspected (Fig. 13-18).

A single artifact must be distinguished from a premature beat. Some artifacts occur "too early" to be physiologically possible. The normal atrial or ventricular effective refractory period is approximately 200 msec in an infant and 250 msec in a child. Thus, at least this amount of time is necessary before the atrium or ventricle can depolarize again. Therefore, for example, if a wave follows a QRS complex by 180 msec in a 14-year-old child, this second wave is unlikely to be a QRS complex (Fig. 13-19).

(5) Repetitive artifacts may simulate parasystole. The artifact will usually occur at a variable interval from the preceding P wave or QRS complex, but there may be a constant interval between the artifacts (Fig. 13-20).

(6) The basic rhythm is unaffected by the artifact. An artifact may only affect part of the QRS, in which case the QRS may be "seen through" the artifact (Fig. 13-21). Alternatively, the basic RR interval

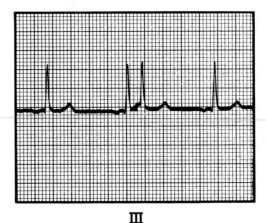

III

FIG. 13-19. Unphysiologically premature. This tracing was recorded from a normal 14-year-old. The third QRS complex occurs 180 msec after the last QRS. This is too premature in an adolescent. The cause of the artifact can be established by the shift in the baseline and the burned appearance to the paper. The electrocardiograph was stopped and started at this time.

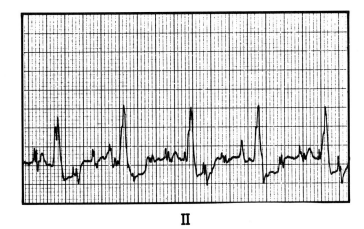

II

FIG. 13-20. Artifact parasystole. This tracing was recorded on a telemetry unit while a patient was brushing her teeth. The QRS complexes are regular and the artifact is somewhat irregular and occurs at approximately 300 times per minute. The artifact, which simulates P waves, has a fairly regular interval between spikes, but is unrelated to the QRS complexes. Also, preceding the first, third, and fifth QRS complexes, the true P waves can be seen in the tracing.

may be entirely unaffected by the artifact and the QRS "marches through" with the artifact present or absent (Fig. 13-22). In general, following an episode of supraventricular or ventricular tachycardia, the sinus node is suppressed and takes a few beats to regain its normal regular rate. Following a repetitive artifact, the sinus rate does not change, making preceding tachycardia less likely (Fig. 13-23). Finally, if a T wave is the first complex to follow a pause, the pause must have been an artifact since a T wave is unlikely without a preceding QRS complex (Fig. 13-24).

(7) Artifacts may be phasic with external influences. Knowledge of the rate of the artifact may help to predict the external source. The

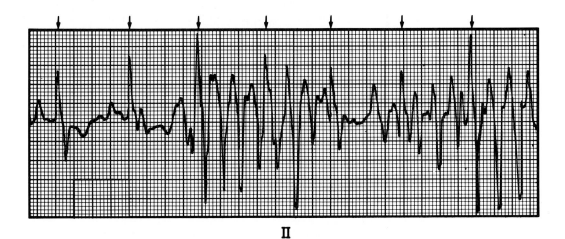

II

FIG. 13-21. QRS "seen through" the artifact. The arrows mark the QRS complexes which continue undisturbed through the movement artifact.

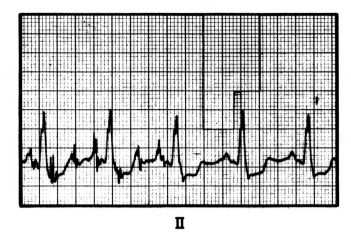

II

FIG. 13-22.   QRS "marches through" the artifact. In the patient who was brushing her teeth during the recording in Figure 13-20, the toothbrushing stopped in this recording and the basic rhythm continued unaffected.

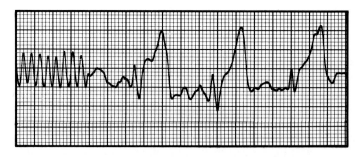

FIG. 13-23.   Lack of "sinus pause." The absence of a pause in the rhythm following a rapid rate may indicate that the rapid rate was an artifact. In this tracing, the rapid artifact stops and there is no pause in the QRS rate.

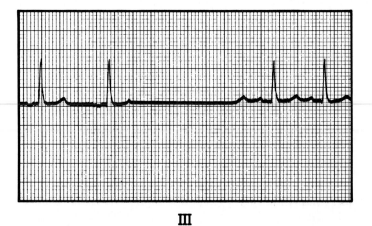

III

FIG. 13-24.   Pause ends with a T wave. The pause in this tracing might have been real except for the undue evenness of the baseline and the fact that the pause ends with a T wave, implying that there must have been a QRS complex preceding the T wave which was not recorded.

infusion pump artifact shown in Figure 13-14 occurred at the same rate as the infusion: 56 times/min (interval of 1.07 sec between artifacts). Muscle movement related to respiration should occur between 15 and 60 times/min (interval every 1 to 4 sec) (Fig. 13-6); or toothbrushing occurs at approximately a rate of 300/min (interval of 200 msec) (Fig. 13-20).

(8) Artifacts usually occur more than once. Therefore, even if a wave on the electrocardiogram cannot be positively identified as either due to depolarization of the heart or due to an artifact, further observation of the remainder of the tracing or a subsequent tracing (perhaps under different circumstances with a more rapid or slower heart rate) will usually reveal the true identity (Fig. 13-25).

Despite all the guidelines, occasionally it is impossible to distinguish artifact from arrhythmia (Fig. 13-26). In these cases, clinical correlation is mandatory. A faulty interpretation of an artifact may cause an "electrocardiographic casualty." Sometimes these casualties are fatal.

A

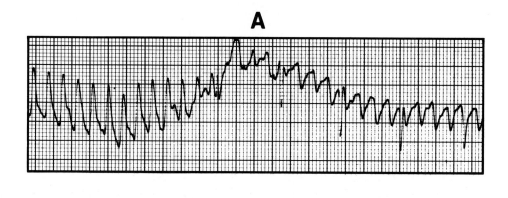

B   **C**

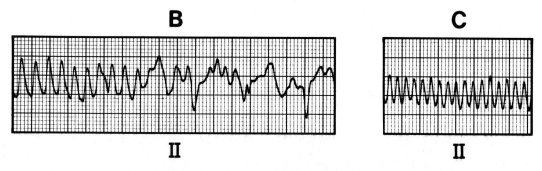

II   **II**

FIG. 13-25. Identification of an artifact at a different point in time. These tracings all were recorded from a 24-hour electrocardiogram. *A*, It is not possible to identify the rhythm. It appears that there is a rapid, wide QRS rhythm that inexplicably changes to a rhythm simulating atrial flutter with block. *B*, Four hours later, the artifact has a similar morphology but actually disappears before the last QRS complex in the tracing. *C*, The artifact has become even smaller and now has a physiologically impossible rate, identifying the entire process as an artifact.

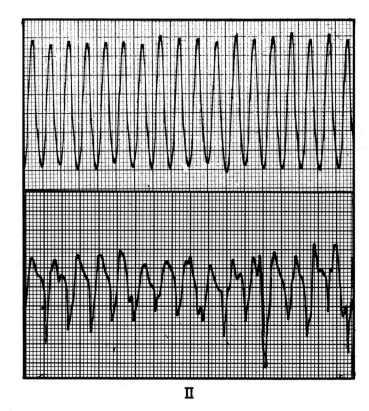

II

FIG. 13-26. Which is the artifact? The *top* tracing is ventricular tachycardia; the *bottom* tracing is the artifact.

Self-Assessment Questions

Question 1: Interpret the following electrocardiogram taken from a 7-year-old child (Fig. 13-27).

A. ventricular tachycardia
B. artifact
C. both
D. neither

Question 2: Interpret the following electrocardiogram taken from a 4-year-old child (Fig. 13-28).

A. ventricular bigeminy
B. artifact
C. both
D. neither

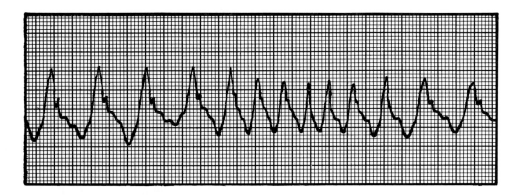

II

FIG. 13-27. Question 1.

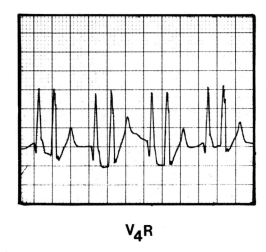

V₄R

FIG. 13-28. Question 2.

Question 3: Interpret the following tracing taken from an 8-year-old child (Fig. 13-29).

A. accelerated junctional rhythm
B. artifact
C. both
D. neither

Answers to Self-Assessment Questions

Answer 1: B
This could be a 7-beat run of supraventricular tachycardia. Ventricular tachycardia would be unlikely with the same QRS morphology. This

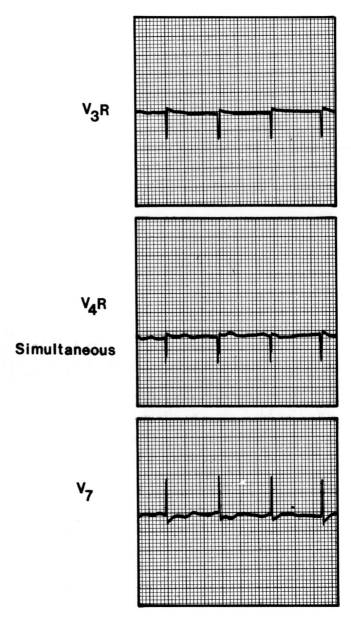

FIG. 13-29.   Question 3.

was taken from a 24-hour electrocardiographic monitor with tape drag. At the beginning and end, it is sinus rhythm with bundle branch block. The QRS is .20 sec. In the middle, the same QRS morphology shortens duration progressively to a QRS duration of .07 sec. This is much more likely to be tape drag.

Answer 2: D

In analyzing this record, note: (1) Each complex has a reasonable morphology for a QRS complex; (2) there could be a "T wave" after each

QRS; (3) but the "QRS complexes" fall too close together for a 4-year-old. (4) Therefore, either one of the pair of complexes is an artifact, or (5) the first complex is a P wave and the second is an R wave. This is the case. The patient had severe right atrial enlargement and this was recorded in a right chest lead.

Answer 3: B

The "spikes" are too narrow to be QRS complexes. The "T waves" are random, low frequency occurrences. This was recorded from a patient in asystole with a temporary pacemaker which was not capturing. These are only pacemaker artifacts with no QRS complexes. If a heart rate monitor had been attached, it would have registered "105/minute" without any QRS complexes: a potential electrocardiographic casualty.

References

1. Stanger P., Lister G., Silverman N. H., et al.: Electrocardiograph monitor artifacts in a neonatal intensive care unit. Pediatrics *60*:689–695, 1977.
2. Sahn D. J., and Vaucher Y. E.: Electrical current leakage transmitted to an infant via an IV controller: an unusual ECG artifact. J Pediatr *89*:301–302, 1976.

Appendix

TABLE A-1.

| AGE | FRONTAL PLANE QRS MEAN VECTOR (degrees) | | | | | |
	Min*	2%*	Mean	98%	Max	No. Subjects
Less than 1 day	38	59	137	−167	−160	189
1–2 days	27	64	134	−161	−160	179
3–6 days	−8	77	132	−167	−162	180
1–3 weeks	−43	65	110	161	−176	117
1–2 months	−77	31	74	113	113	114
3–5 months	−7	1	60	104	112	108
6–11 months	−3	1	56	99	118	136
1–2 years	−2	1	55	101	115	191
3–4 years	−10	1	55	104	145	209
5–7 years	−48	1	65	143	200	224
8–11 years	−35	1	61	119	145	232
12–15 years	−13	1	59	130	198	245

*The limits of "normal" include the 2nd and 98th percentile. The "Min" and "Max" are the minimum and maximum values in the sample of normal children. Statistically, these would be considered "abnormal."

TABLE A-2.

| AGE | HEART RATE (beats/min) | | | | | |
	Min	2%	Mean	98%	Max	No. Subjects
Less than 1 day	88	93	123	154	168	189
1–2 days	57	91	123	159	170	179
3–6 days	87	91	129	166	166	181
1–3 weeks	96	107	148	182	188	119
1–2 months	114	121	149	179	204	112
3–5 months	101	106	141	186	188	109
6–11 months	100	109	134	169	176	138
1–2 years	68	89	119	151	165	191
3–4 years	68	73	108	137	145	210
5–7 years	60	65	100	133	139	226
8–11 years	51	62	91	130	145	233
12–15 years	51	60	85	119	133	247

TABLE A-3.

	PR Interval (sec) in Lead II					
Age	Min	2%	Mean	98%	Max	No. Subjects
Less than 1 day	.07	.08	.11	.16	.17	188
1–2 days	.07	.08	.11	.14	.15	176
3–6 days	.07	.07	.10	.14	.14	181
1–3 weeks	.06	.07	.10	.14	.14	115
1–2 months	.06	.07	.10	.13	.13	106
3–5 months	.06	.07	.11	.15	.15	104
6–11 months	.04	.07	.11	.16	.18	127
1–2 years	.08	.08	.11	.15	.15	192
3–4 years	.08	.09	.12	.16	.20	210
5–7 years	.08	.09	.12	.16	.18	219
8–11 years	.08	.09	.13	.17	.21	227
12–15 years	.08	.09	.14	.18	.22	237

TABLE A-4.

	QRS Duration (sec) in V_5					
Age	Min	2%	Mean	98%	Max	No. Subjects
Less than 1 day	.018	.031	.051	.075	.078	187
1–2 days	.030	.032	.048	.066	.069	176
3–6 days	.027	.031	.049	.068	.072	180
1–3 weeks	.036	.036	.053	.080	.084	117
1–2 months	.033	.033	.053	.076	.084	115
3–5 months	.027	.032	.054	.080	.081	108
6–11 months	.030	.034	.054	.076	.081	135
1–2 years	.033	.038	.056	.076	.078	192
3–4 years	.039	.041	.057	.072	.078	210
5–7 years	.042	.042	.059	.079	.090	223
8–11 years	.039	.041	.062	.085	.087	229
12–15 years	.027	.044	.065	.087	.099	224

TABLE A-5.

| AGE | Q AMPLITUDE IN LEAD III (mm at normal standardization) | | | | | |
	Min	2%	Mean	98%	Max	No. Subjects
Less than 1 day	0.0	0.0	1.4	4.5	4.5	189
1–2 days	0.0	0.0	1.4	5.1	6.6	179
3–6 days	0.0	0.0	1.6	4.8	5.4	181
1–3 weeks	0.0	0.0	1.5	5.6	5.8	119
1–2 months	0.0	0.0	1.5	5.4	7.5	113
3–5 months	0.0	0.0	1.8	6.6	6.6	109
6–11 months	0.0	0.0	2.1	6.3	8.5	133
1–2 years	0.0	0.0	1.5	5.3	5.8	192
3–4 years	0.0	0.0	1.0	4.2	5.0	212
5–7 years	0.0	0.0	0.9	3.2	4.3	214
8–11 years	0.0	0.0	0.6	2.6	3.0	222
12–15 years	0.0	0.0	0.5	3.0	3.3	244

TABLE A-6.

| AGE | Q AMPLITUDE IN V_6 (mm at normal standardization) | | | | | |
	Min	2%	Mean	98%	Max	No. Subjects
Less than 1 day	0.0	0.0	0.3	2.0	2.6	189
1–2 days	0.0	0.0	0.4	2.4	3.4	179
3–6 days	0.0	0.0	0.6	3.1	4.0	181
1–3 weeks	0.0	0.0	0.8	3.1	3.1	119
1–2 months	0.0	0.0	0.7	2.9	4.0	115
3–5 months	0.0	0.0	0.8	2.9	4.0	109
6–11 months	0.0	0.0	0.8	3.2	3.6	138
1–2 years	0.0	0.0	1.0	3.1	4.6	192
3–4 years	0.0	0.0	1.2	3.5	4.6	210
5–7 years	0.0	0.0	1.2	4.7	6.0	222
8–11 years	0.0	0.0	1.0	3.0	3.2	221
12–15 years	0.0	0.0	0.8	3.1	5.0	243

TABLE A-7.

	R Amplitude in V_1 (mm at normal standardization)					
Age	Min	2%	Mean	98%	Max	No. Subjects
Less than 1 day	3.6	5.2	13.8	26.1	29.2	189
1–2 days	0.9	5.3	14.4	26.9	38.0	177
3–6 days	1.0	2.8	12.9	24.2	27.2	181
1–3 weeks	2.5	3.2	10.6	20.8	23.0	119
1–2 months	2.8	3.3	9.5	18.4	20.6	115
3–5 months	0.7	2.7	9.8	19.8	25.2	109
6–11 months	1.4	1.4	9.4	20.3	24.0	138
1–2 years	2.0	2.6	8.9	17.7	34.4	192
3–4 years	0.4	1.0	8.1	18.2	20.6	211
5–7 years	0.0	0.5	6.7	13.9	14.8	219
8–11 years	0.0	0.0	5.4	12.1	15.4	230
12–15 years	0.0	0.0	4.1	9.9	12.6	244

TABLE A-8.

	S Amplitude in V_1 (mm at normal standardization)					
Age	Min	2%	Mean	98%	Max	No. Subjects
Less than 1 day	0.0	0.0	8.5	22.7	28.4	189
1–2 days	0.0	0.0	9.1	20.7	30.0	178
3–6 days	0.0	0.0	6.6	16.8	21.4	181
1–3 weeks	0.0	0.0	4.2	10.8	14.2	119
1–2 months	0.0	0.0	5.0	12.4	13.4	115
3–5 months	0.0	0.0	5.7	17.1	26.6	109
6–11 months	0.0	0.4	6.4	18.1	24.4	138
1–2 years	0.0	0.7	8.4	21.0	33.0	191
3–4 years	0.6	1.8	10.2	21.4	26.2	212
5–7 years	0.8	2.9	12.0	23.8	29.4	219
8–11 years	1.8	2.7	11.9	25.4	28.8	226
12–15 years	1.4	2.8	10.8	21.2	23.0	235

TABLE A-9.

AGE	R AMPLITUDE IN V_6 (mm at normal standardization)					
	Min	2%	Mean	98%	Max	No. Subjects
Less than 1 day	0.0	0.0	4.2	11.1	22.8	189
1–2 days	0.0	0.0	4.5	12.2	17.0	179
3–6 days	0.0	0.3	5.2	12.1	14.5	181
1–3 weeks	1.2	2.6	7.6	16.4	24.0	119
1–2 months	3.1	5.2	11.6	21.4	24.2	115
3–5 months	5.0	6.4	13.1	22.4	25.0	109
6–11 months	5.8	5.8	12.6	22.7	24.6	138
1–2 years	3.7	5.9	13.3	22.6	24.6	192
3–4 years	7.6	8.1	14.8	24.4	36.0	209
5–7 years	6.4	8.4	16.3	26.5	28.4	223
8–11 years	7.0	9.2	16.3	25.4	33.0	233
12–15 years	5.5	6.5	14.3	23.0	32.2	246

TABLE A-10.

AGE	S AMPLITUDE IN V_6 (mm at normal standardization)					
	Min	2%	Mean	98%	Max	No. Subjects
Less than 1 day	0.0	0.0	3.2	9.6	16.3	189
1–2 days	0.0	0.0	3.0	9.4	12.4	179
3–6 days	0.0	0.0	3.5	9.8	10.4	181
1–3 weeks	0.0	0.0	3.4	9.8	13.0	119
1–2 months	0.0	0.0	2.7	6.4	6.4	115
3–5 months	0.0	0.0	2.9	9.9	12.8	109
6–11 months	0.0	0.0	2.1	7.2	14.2	138
1–2 years	0.0	0.0	1.9	6.6	10.4	192
3–4 years	0.0	0.0	1.5	5.2	5.4	210
5–7 years	0.0	0.0	1.2	4.0	4.3	217
8–11 years	0.0	0.0	1.0	3.9	4.6	232
12–15 years	0.0	0.0	0.8	3.7	4.4	241

TABLE A-11.

AGE	R/S RATIO IN V_1					
	Min	2%	Mean	98%	Max	No. Subjects
Less than 1 day	.04	.1	2.2	U	U	178
1–2 days	.03	.1	2.0	U	U	171
3–6 days	.06	.2	2.7	U	U	174
1–3 weeks	.9	1.0	2.9	U	U	103
1–2 months	.2	.3	2.3	U	U	104
3–5 months	.03	.1	2.3	U	U	97
6–11 months	.02	.1	1.6	3.9	5.2	130
1–2 years	.01	.05	1.4	4.3	5.2	185
3–4 years	.01	.03	.9	2.8	4.6	209
5–7 years	0.0	.02	.7	2.0	4.4	212
8–11 years	0.0	0	.5	1.8	2.2	225
12–15 years	0.0	0	.5	1.7	3.0	234

Note: U = undefined (S wave may equal zero)

TABLE A-12.

AGE	R/S RATIO IN V_6					
	Min	2%	Mean	98%	Max	No. Subjects
Less than 1 day	0.0	0	2.0	U	U	174
1–2 days	0.0	0	2.5	U	U	168
3–6 days	0.0	.1	2.2	U	U	177
1–3 weeks	0.0	.1	3.3	U	U	118
1–2 months	.08	.2	4.8	U	U	113
3–5 months	.1	.2	6.2	U	U	106
6–11 months	.1	.2	7.6	U	U	132
1–2 years	.2	.3	9.3	U	U	187
3–4 years	.3	.6	10.8	U	U	207
5–7 years	.3	.9	11.5	U	U	205
8–11 years	.9	1.5	14.3	U	U	208
12–15 years	.8	1.4	14.7	U	U	209

Note: U = undefined (S wave may equal zero)

TABLE A-13.

	R Amplitude in V_6 + S Amplitude in V_1 (mm at normal standardization)					
Age	Min	2%	Mean	98%	Max	No. Subjects
Less than 1 day	1.4	1.4	12.6	28.0	40.8	189
1–2 days	1.6	1.6	13.7	28.7	32.8	179
3–6 days	2.8	2.8	11.7	24.7	27.2	181
1–3 weeks	2.7	3.0	11.7	21.0	24.0	119
1–2 months	6.8	6.8	16.5	29.1	30.2	115
3–5 months	6.6	7.2	18.6	34.9	42.2	109
6–11 months	6.1	7.3	19.0	32.2	34.4	138
1–2 years	5.8	7.7	21.7	39.0	51.8	192
3–4 years	10.4	13.0	25.1	41.8	45.4	210
5–7 years	12.4	13.6	28.2	47.1	52.4	217
8–11 years	14.1	15.3	28.1	45.5	57.4	225
12–15 years	6.9	11.4	25.1	41.1	43.6	235

TABLE A-14.

	R + S Amplitude in V_4 (mm at normal standardization)					
Age	Min	2%	Mean	98%	Max	No. Subjects
Less than 1 day	5.0	9.2	31.9	52.5	55.6	189
1–2 days	14.8	16.0	32.6	52.2	54.2	179
3–6 days	6.7	10.2	31.4	49.0	52.5	181
1–3 weeks	12.3	15.1	30.5	49.1	51.2	119
1–2 months	19.0	19.6	36.4	53.5	54.2	115
3–5 months	14.2	18.0	37.8	61.4	63.0	109
6–11 months	18.0	18.0	33.6	52.8	58.0	138
1–2 years	10.7	15.9	33.6	49.5	53.0	192
3–4 years	16.8	17.8	35.1	53.5	73.4	209
5–7 years	9.8	16.6	35.8	54.1	57.4	211
8–11 years	14.6	16.9	34.9	53.1	54.2	214
12–15 years	7.7	8.9	29.0	50.3	53.6	233

TABLE A-15. *Sex Differences in R Wave Amplitudes in Age Group 12 to 15 Years*

Lead	Sex	R Wave Amplitude (mm at normal standardization)		
		2%	Mean	98%
V_1	Girls	.1	3.5	9.6
	Boys	.2	4.2	10.3
V_5	Girls	6.3	16.3	29.9
	Boys	10.9	24.1	34.7
V_6	Girls	5.9	12.2	19.1
	Boys	8.0	15.9	24.1

Notes: Based upon 105 boys and 142 girls; difference between boys and girls highly significant ($p < 0.0001$) for each lead

TABLE A-16.

Heart Rate	QT Duration (sec) According to Heart Rate in Lead V_5					
	Min	2%	Mean	98%	Max	No. Subjects
80 to 90/min	.222	.293	.343	.380	.396	168
90 to 95/min	.273	.280	.329	.372	.378	101
95 to 100/min	.270	.290	.325	.361	.432	111
100 to 105/min	.267	.274	.318	.364	.423	143
105 to 110/min	.255	.264	.307	.355	.417	139
110 to 115/min	.228	.247	.300	.367	.372	168
115 to 120/min	.207	.245	.293	.344	.360	159
120 to 125/min	.222	.233	.289	.351	.363	137
125 to 130/min	.198	.228	.280	.334	.345	175
130 to 135/min	.204	.212	.273	.331	.336	121
135 to 140/min	.210	.228	.272	.325	.330	139
140 to 150/min	.195	.218	.263	.308	.318	164

TABLE A-17. *Summary of Normal Values*

Age Group	*Heart Rate (BPM)	Frontal Plane QRS Vector (degrees)	PR Interval (sec)	**Q III (mm)§	**Q V6 (mm)	RV1 (mm)	SV1 (mm)	R/S V1	RV6 (mm)	SV6 (mm)	R/S V6	**SV1 + RV6 (mm)	**R + S V4 (mm)
Less than 1 day	93–154 (123)	+59 to –163 (137)	.08–.16 (.11)	4.5	2	5–26 (14)	0–23 (8)	.1–U (2.2)	0–11 (4)	0–9.5 (3)	.1–U (2.0)	28	52.5
1–2 days	91–159 (123)	+64 to –161 (134)	.08–.14 (.11)	6.5	2.5	5–27 (14)	0–21 (9)	.1–U (2.0)	0–12 (4.5)	0–9.5 (3)	.1–U (2.5)	29	52
3–6 days	91–166 (129)	+77 to –163 (132)	.07–.14 (.10)	5.5	3	3–24 (13)	0–17 (7)	.2–U (2.7)	.5–12 (5)	0–10 (3.5)	.1–U (2.2)	24.5	49
1–3 weeks	107–182 (148)	+65 to +161 (110)	.07–.14 (.10)	6	3	3–21 (11)	0–11 (4)	1.0–U (2.9)	2.5–16.5 (7.5)	0–10 (3.5)	.1–U (3.3)	21	49
1–2 months	121–179 (149)	+31 to +113 (74)	.07–.13 (.10)	7.5	3	3–18 (10)	0–12 (5)	.3–U (2.3)	5–21.5 (11.5)	0–6.5 (3)	.2–U (4.8)	29	53.5
3–5 months	106–186 (141)	+7 to +104 (60)	.07–.15 (.11)	6.5	3	3–20 (10)	0–17 (6)	.1–U (2.3)	6.5–22.5 (13)	0–10 (3)	.2–U (6.2)	32	61.5
6–11 months	109–169 (134)	+6 to +99 (56)	.07–.16 (.11)	8.5	3	1.5–20 (9.5)	.5–18 (4)	.1–3.9 (1.6)	6–22.5 (12.5)	0–7 (2)	.2–U (7.6)	32	53
1–2 years	89–151 (119)	+7 to +101 (55)	.08–.15 (.11)	6	3	2.5–17 (9)	.5–21 (8)	.05–4.3 (1.4)	6–22.5 (13)	0–6.5 (2)	.3–U (9.3)	39	49.5
3–4 years	73–137 (108)	+6 to +104 (55)	.09–.16 (.12)	5	3.5	1–18 (8)	.2–21 (10)	.03–2.8 (.9)	8–24.5 (15)	0–5 (1.5)	.6–U (10.8)	42	53.5
5–7 years	65–133 (100)	+11 to +143 (65)	.09–.16 (.12)	4	4.5	.5–14 (7)	.3–24 (12)	.02–2.0 (.7)	8.5–26.5 (16)	0–4 (1)	.9–U (11.5)	47	54
8–11 years	62–130 (91)	+9 to +114 (61)	.09–.17 (.13)	3	3	0–12 (5.5)	.3–25 (12)	0–1.8 (.5)	9–25.5 (16)	0–4 (1)	1.5–U (14.3)	45.5	53
12–15 years	60–119 (85)	+11 to +130 (59)	.09–.18 (.14)	3	3	0–10 (4)	.3–21 (11)	0–1.7 (.5)	6.5–23 (14)	0–4 (1)	1.4–U (14.7)	41	50

*2%–98% (mean)
**98th percentile

§mm at normal standardization
U undefined (S wave may equal zero)

Index

Page numbers in *italics* indicate figures; page numbers followed by "t" indicate tables; page numbers followed by "Q" indicate material in "Questions."

Abdominal distention, AV block and, 264t
escape beats and escape rhythms and, 205t
Aberration. See also *Bundle branch block; Interventricular conduction delay; Wolff-Parkinson-White*
in escape rhythms, 201, *203*
in sinus tachycardia, 231, *235*, 351Q, *351*
in supraventricular tachycardia, 124, 237
differential diagnosis of, 261
premature beats vs., atrial flutter/fibrillation, 215, *218, 219*, 220
Absence of cardiac activity, 393Q, *394*
Accelerated atrial rhythm, causes of, 241
electrocardiographic criteria for, 239, 241, *242, 243*, 347, 348Q, *348*
Accelerated junctional rhythm, category 3, in morphology schema, 302t, 312, *313*
causes of, 241
electrocardiographic criteria for, 239, 241, *242, 244*, *245*, 348Q, *348*
with aberration, category 4, in morphology schema, 302t, 316, *317*
and complete AV block, category 4, in morphology schema, 302t, *319*
with AV dissociation, in morphology schema, 285, *288*
with complete AV block, 269, *274*
Accelerated ventricular rhythm, electrocardiographic criteria, *242*, 259, *260*
with AV dissociation, in morphology schema, 285, *288*
Accessory AV connection. See *Wolff-Parkinson-White*
Acidosis, 172t, 178, 241t
supraventricular tachycardia and, 241t
Action potential, atrial and ventricular, 9, 25, *25, 26*, 44
AV node and, 12, *25, 26*
changes with injury, *152*, 152, 154, *154*
changes with ischemia, 151, *152, 153*
drug effects on, 170, *171*. See also specific drugs
duration of, dependency on preceding cycle length, 215, *218, 219*, 220
"fast response," 9, 10, *10*, 16Q

His bundle and, 9, *25, 26*
phases of, 10–11, *10*
sinus node and, 12, 25, *25*
"slow response," 9, *10*, 12, 16Q
systemic effects on, 170, *171*. See also specific effects
Activation, left ventricular, anatomy of, 5, *6*
right ventricular, anatomy of, 6
sequence of, 25–27, *25*
ventricular endocardial, 39, *41*, 46Q
ventricular epicardial, 42, *42*
Acute rheumatic fever. See *Rheumatic fever*
Adrenal insufficiency, 172t, 188
Adrenogenital syndrome, and hyperkalemia, 173
"Advanced" AV block. See *AV block, "Advanced"*
Amines, sympathetic. See *Sympathetic amines*
Amyloid, low-voltage QRS and, 70
Analysis of electrocardiograms, introduction to, 274–276, *275*
Anatomy, conduction system, 3–6, *4*
left atrial, *4*, 4, 6Q
right atrial, *4*, 4–6, 6Q
Anemia, sinus tachycardia, 236t
Anesthetic drugs, 172t, 183
premature ventricular contractions and, 214t
Aneurysm, ventricular, 164–165
Anomalous left coronary artery, 161–162, *161, 163*, 164–165
ischemic changes and, 151
left axis deviation and, 131
Anomalous pulmonary venous return, *total*, papillary muscle infarction and, 162
Antiarrhythmic drugs, 178–183
Antidepressants. See *Tricyclic antidepressants*
Antidromic supraventricular tachycardia. See *Wolff-Parkinson-White*
Anxiety, sinus tachycardia and, 236t
T wave changes and, 149
Aortic insufficiency, 107
left axis deviation and, 131
Aortic stenosis, 103, 106, 107
ischemic changes and, 151
left axis deviation and, 131

Aortic stenosis *(Continued)*
  papillary muscle infarction and, 162
  postoperative AV block and, 274
Aortic valve surgery, left anterior hemiblock and,
      133
  left bundle branch block and, 127
Appendicitis, 189
Arrhythmia(s), 195–375. See also specific
      arrhythmias
  continuously irregular, in morphology schema,
      303t, 329–337
  electrophysiologic approach, 197–274
  intermittently irregular, in morphology schema,
      303t, 327–343
  morphologic approach to, 274–344
  regular RR interval in, in morphology schema,
      302t, 304–328
Arrhythmia category(ies), criteria for, 301, 304
  1, 304, *305, 306, 307,* 344Q
  2, 302t, 308, *309, 310, 311,* 346Q
  3, 302t, 312, *313, 314, 315,* 347Q, 348Q
  4, 302t, 316, *317, 318, 319*
  5, 302t, 320, *321, 322, 323,* 349Q, 357Q
  6, 302t 324, *325, 326, 327, 328*
  7, 303t, 329, *330*
  8, 303t, 331, *332*
  9, 303t, 333, *334,* 349Q, 350Q
  10, 303t, 335, *336,* 351Q
  11, 303t, 337, *338,* 353Q, 355Q
  12, 303t, 339, *340,* 353Q, 356Q
  13, 341, *342,* 303t, 356Q
  14, 303t, 343, *343*
  summary of, 302t, 303t, 344
Arrhythmogenic right ventricular dysplasia,
      ventricular tachycardia and, 258t
Artery, AV nodal, 5
  of Haas, 5
  sinus node, 3
Artifacts, 376–395
  arc for straight line, 383
  baseline shift, 387, *387*
  "burned" paper, 382, *384*
  calibration spike, 381, *382*
  causes of, 376–385
  chest massage during cardiac arrest, 381
  chest percussion, 381, *381*
  current from external sources, 385, *386*
  faulty cable attachment, 382, *383*
  faulty cable shielding, 382
  faulty paper drive, 382, *384*
  faulty stylus, 383
  hiccough, 378, *379*
  impossible to distinguish, 391, *392*
  improper calibration, 383, *385*
  improper gain, 383, *385*
  incorrect positioning of leads, 376, *377, 378, 378,
      379*
  incorrect stylus position, 383, *385*
  "infusion pump," 385, *386*
  lack of sinus suppression after "tachycardia," 389,
      390
  loss of electrode contact, 381, 382, *383*
  malfunctioning ECG system, 381–385, *383, 384,
      385*
  nonpurposeful movement, 380, *380*
  not affecting rhythm, 388, *389, 390*
  pacemaker spike, 393Q, *394*

  patient-initiated movement, 378–380, *379, 380, 381*
  pause ends with T wave, 389, *390*
  "pegged" tracing, 383, *385*
  phasic, caused by external influences, *381, 386,
      389, 389, 391*
  purposeful movement, 378
  QRS "marches through," 389, *390*
  QRS "seen through," 388, *389*
  recognition of, systematic, 385–392
  repetitive, 391, *391*
    "parasystole," 388, *389*
  respirations, 380, *381*
  reversed limb leads, 96Q, *96,* 376, *377*
  simulating right atrial enlargement, 392Q, *393*
  simulating ventricular tachycardia, *392,* 392Q, *393*
  60 cycle interference, *382, 385*
  smeared electrode paste, 376, 378, *379*
  T wave before QRS, 389, *390*
  therapeutic manipulation of patient, 381, *381*
Ashman phenomenon, 215, *218, 219,* 220
Asplenia, P wave, 83, 84, *85*
Asystole, 257
  loss of electrode contact vs., 383
Athletes, escape beats and escape rhythms in, 205t
Atrial activity, in morphology schema. See
      Morphology schema
Atrial bigeminy, 220, 222, *222*
  blocked, 209, 210 *211*
Atrial bradycardia. See *Ectopic atrial bradycardia*
Atrial couplets, 223
Atrial dilation, atrial flutter and, 243, 248t
Atrial ectopic tachycardia. See *Ectopic atrial
      tachycardia*
Atrial enlargement, biatrial, *112,* 113
  left, 63, 65
    P-terminal forces, *111,* 111, 112, 115Q, *115*
    P wave duration, *111,* 112, *115,* 115Q
  premature atrial/junctional contractions, 211t
  right, 63, 65
    P wave amplitude and, 110–111, *110,* 113Q, *114*
    simulating artifact, 392Q, *393*
  with nonsinus P wave, 110, 112
Atrial escape beat(s), ectopic, in morphology
      schema, 303t, 341, *342*
  escape rhythm and, electrocardiographic criteria
      for, 196, 199t, *199,* 199, 200, *206,* 242
  in morphology schema, *300*
  premature atrial contraction confused with, 209
Atrial fibrillation, aberration vs. premature beats
      and, 215, *218, 219,* 220
  causes of, 251t
  differential diagnosis of, 259, 261
  electrocardiographic criteria for, 249–251, *249, 250*
  hypothermia and, 186
  in morphology schema, 281, *282, 283,* 290, 303t,
      329, *330*
  in myotonic dystrophy, 187
  with aberration, in morphology schema, 303t, 330,
      332
  with complete AV block, 273
  Wolff-Parkinson-White, 250, *250*
    in morphology schema. See *Arrhythmia
        category(ies),* 8
Atrial fibrosis, prolonged P wave and, 112
Atrial flutter, aberration vs. premature beats and,
      215, 218, 219, 220
  advanced AV block and, *270*

Atrial flutter *(Continued)*
  causes of, 243, 248t
  confusion with supraventricular tachycardia, 237
  differential diagnosis of, 259, 261
  electrocardiographic criteria for, 241, 243, *246, 247,*
      248, *248,* 350Q, *350,* 357Q, *358*
  in morphology schema, 281, *282, 283,* 302t, 320,
      323
  intrauterine, 243
  systemic effects causing, 172t
  with aberration, 302t, 324, *328*
    type I block and, 303t, 335, *336*
    with type II AV block, 302t, *311*
      category 6, 302t, *319* 324, *328*
      varying, 303t, 335, *336*
  with complete AV block, *273*
  with 2:1 block, 349Q, *350,* 357Q, *358*
  with type I block, 303t, 334, *335*
  with type II AV block, 302t, *315,* 320, *323*
  with type II block varying, 303t, 334, *335*
Atrial fusion, *253*
Atrial ischemia, prolonged P wave and, 112
Atrial parasystole, 225, *228*
Atrial premature beat. See *Premature beat(s)*
Atrial premature contractions. See *Premature atrial*
      contractions
Atrial rate, normal conduction to ventricles, 263
Atrial repolarization, ST segment shift and, 158
Atrial rhythm, accelerated. See *Accelerated atrial*
      rhythm
  ectopic. See *Ectopic atrial rhythm*
  with AV block in morphology schema, 302t, 304,
      306
Atrial septal defect, first-degree AV block and, 263
  primum, left axis deviation and, 54, 131
  secundum, 124, 125, *125*
Atrial stretch, first-degree AV block and, 263
Atrial trigeminy, 221, *223*
Atrio-His fiber. See *Lown-Ganong-Levine*
Atrioventricular block. See *AV block*
Atrioventricular node. See *AV node*
Atrium, activation time in, 26, 66
  conduction in, 4, 5, 6Q
  depolarization. See *Depolarization, atrial*
  repolarization. See *Repolarization, atrial*
Atropine, central nervous system injury and, 185
Atypical bundle branch block, in supraventricular
      tachycardia, 261, *262*
"Atypical" Wenckebach, 266
Automaticity, atrial, digitalis and, 179
    normal, 198
  defined, 11
  hierarchy of, 198
  increased, digitalis and, 179
    in accelerated rhythms, 241
  junctional, normal, 198
  sinus nodal, 12, 198
  ventricular, 198
Autonomic imbalance, adrenal insufficiency and,
      188
AV block, "advanced," 269, *270, 271*
    in morphology schema, *296*
  atrial fibrillation and, 250
  capture beats and, 229, 231, *232*
  cardiac tumor and, 159
  causes of, 264t
  complete, 269, 271, 272, 273, *273,* 274, 346Q, *347*

accelerated junctional rhythm and, in
      morphology schema, 302t, *319*
  acquired, 274
  causes of, 264t, 271
  congenital, 271, 272, 273
  lupus erythematosus and, 272
  progression from bundle branch block, 124
  site of escape rhythm, 272, 274
  ventricular tachycardia and, 302t, *319*
  with accelerated junctional rhythm, 269, 274
    in morphology schema, 302t, *315*
  with atrial fibrillation, *273*
  with atrial flutter, *273*
  with junctional rhythm, 269, 346Q, *347*
    in morphology schema, 302t, 304, *307*
  with sinus bradycardia, 269, *274*
  with ventricular escape rhythm, in morphology
      schema, 302t, 308, *311*
  complete AV dissociation and, 269
  connective tissue disease and, 187
  defined, 261, 263
  digitalis intoxication and, 179
  electrocardiographic criteria for, 261, 263–274
  first-degree, causes of, 263, 264, 264t
    digitalis and, 179
    electrocardiographic criteria for, 263–264, *264*
    hypermagnesemia and, 177
  "high grade." See *AV block, "Advanced"*
  hyperkalemia and, 173
  hypocalcemia and, 177
  hypoxia/acidosis and, 178
  imipramine and, 183
  in atrial flutter, 243, *246, 247,* 248, *248,* 349Q, *350*
  in AV node, 263
  insecticides and, 184
  myocarditis and, 157
  sarcoid and, 189
  second degree, AV dissociation, 269, *271*
    electrocardiographic criteria, 265–269, *265, 266,*
        267, 268, 269, 270, 271, 357Q, *358*
    site of, 269
    2:1. See *AV block, 2:1*
    type I. See *Wenckebach*
    type II, 267–269, *267, 270,* 357Q, *358*
      causes of, 264t, 269
      His bundle block, 269
      in morphology schema, 284, *287, 290, 292,*
          295, 300
  site of Wenckebach, 267
  supraventricular tachycardia and, 237, *240*
  systemic effects causing, 172t, 189Q, 192
  third-degree. See *AV block, complete*
  tricyclic antidepressants and, 183
  2:1, 267, 268, *268, 270,* 346Q, *346,* 349Q, *350,* 357Q,
      358
    sinus rhythm with aberration and, in
        morphology schema, 302t, *318*
    with ectopic atrial rhythm and aberration, in
        morphology schema, 302t, *310, 314, 318*
    with sinus rhythm and aberration, in
        morphology schema, 302t, *310*
    with sinus rhythm, in morphology schema,
        302t, *314*
  type I, atrial flutter, and morphology schema,
      303t, 334, *335*
    atrial flutter with aberration and, in
        morphology schema, 303t, 335, *336*

AV block, type I (Continued)
  sinus tachycardia with aberration and, in
      morphology schema, 303t, 335, 336
  with sinus tachycardia, in morphology schema,
      303t, 334, 335
  type II, atrial flutter with aberration and, in
      morphology schema, 302t, 319, 324, 328
  in morphology schema, 303t, 333, 334
  intermittent, with supraventricular rhythm, in
      morphology schema, 303t, 341, 342
  sinus tachycardia with aberration and, in
      morphology schema, 302t, 318
  supraventricular rhythm with aberration and,
      in morphology schema, 302t, 316, 317, 318
  supraventricular tachycardia and, in
      morphology schema, 302t, 314, 320, 322
  varying, atrial flutter and, in morphology
      schema, 303t, 334, 335
    sinus tachycardia and, in morphology
        schema, 303t, 333, 334
      with aberration, 303t, 335, 336
    supraventricular rhythm and, in morphology
        schema, 303t, 333, 334
  with aberration, 302t, 310, 318, 327
  with atrial flutter and aberration, in
      morphology schema, 302t, 311
  with atrial flutter, in morphology schema, 302t,
      315, 320, 323
  with sinus tachycardia, in morphology schema,
      303t, 314
    aberration and, in morphology schema, 302t,
        310
  with supraventricular rhythm and aberration,
      in morphology schema, 302t, 308, 310, 311
  with supraventricular rhythm, in morphology
      schema, 304, 306
  verapamil and, 183
  Wenckebach, in morphology schema, 290, 292
  with atrial flutter, in morphology schema, 302t,
      304, 307
  with atrial rhythm, in morphology schema, 302t,
      304, 306
  with AV dissociation, in morphology schema, 285,
      288
  with sinus rhythm, in morphology schema, 302t,
      304, 306
  with sinus tachycardia, in morphology schema,
      302t, 304, 306
  with supraventricular rhythms, in morphology
      schema, 291
  with supraventricular tachycardia, in morphology
      schema, 302t, 304, 306
AV canal, left axis deviation and, 54, 131
  postoperative AV block and, 274
AV conduction, intermittent, in AV dissociation, 229
  normal, conducted P waves and, 269
  normal rate of, 263
  rapid, bypass tract, 243, 250, 250
AV dissociation, accelerated junctional rhythm and,
      239, 244, 245, 348Q, 348
  accelerated ventricular rhythm and, 259, 260
  capture beats and, 229, 230, 231, 232, 233
  causes of, in morphology schema, 284–286, 287,
      288
  combination of causes, 269, 271, 274, 348Q, 348
  complete AV block and, 269
  definition of, 201

differential diagnosis of tachyarrhythmias, and
    261
  in morphology schema, 282, 284–286, 286, 287,
      288
  junctional rhythm and, 196, 200, 201, 345
  junctional tachycardia and, 236–237, 239, 240
  second-degree AV block and, 269, 271
  ventricular escape rhythm and, 353Q, 354
  ventricular tachycardia and, 251, 253, 254, 255,
      256, 257
AV node, abnormal, in ventricular inversion, 273
  activation time for, 26
  anatomy of, 4, 5, 4, 6Q, 7Q
  block, Wenckebach, 267
  bypass tract, rapid conduction in, 243, 250, 250
  normal conduction through, 263
  refractory period of, 263
"Axis." See Mean vector
"Axis deviation," 52–55, 54, 58Q, 58

Band, moderator, 6
Barbiturates, action potential and, 170, 171
Baseline shift. See Artifacts
Beat(s), premature, See Premature beats
  capture, 229, 230, 231, 232, 233
Biatrial enlargement. See Atrial enlargement
Bidirectional tachycardia, 179, 180, 252, 257
Bifocal tachycardia, 179, 180, 252, 257
Bigeminy, 220, 221, 222, 224
  atrial, blocked, 209, 210, 211
  "escape-capture," 356Q, 356, 370
  multiform, 224, 225
Biventricular hypertrophy. See Ventricular
    hypertrophy
Block, bifascicular, 134–135, 135, 144Q, 144
  familial, 134
  bundle branch. See Bundle branch block
  entrance, sinoatrial, 3
  exit, sinoatrial, 3
  fascicular, 130–134
  right bundle branch, with left axis deviation. See
      also Block, bifascicular.
    with left axis deviation, causes of, 134–135
  trifascicular, 135
Blocked atrial bigeminy, 209, 210, 211
Blood pressure, AV block and, 264t
  escape beats and escape rhythms and, 205t
Body chemistry, effects of, 173–178
Bradycardia, central nervous system injury and, 185
  halothane and, 183
  sinus. See Sinus bradycardia
  U wave, 45, 173
Bundle, AV. See His bundle
Bundle branch(es), anatomy of, 4, 5
  left, anatomy of, 4, 5
  lesion, 5
  refractory period of, 263
Bundle branch block, alternating, in tachycardia,
      179, 180
  Ashman phenomenon, 215, 218, 219, 220
  atypical, in supraventricular tachycardia, 261, 262
  bilateral, type II, second degree, 269
  hyperkalemia and, 177
  hypermagnesemia and, 177
  hyperthyroidism and, 187
  in morphology schema, 279, 280, 280, 281
  in myotonic dystrophy, 187

Bundle branch block *(Continued)*
  left, 126–130, *127, 128,* 145Q, *145*
    calculation of mean vector in, 127, *129*
    causes of, 127
    complete, 126–129, *127, 128,* 145Q, *145*
    functional, during supraventricular tachycardia, 124
    Mahaim confused with, 141
    in morphology schema, 279, *280,* 280, *281*
    incomplete, 130
    pseudoinfarction Q wave, 164
    T wave, 127
    vectors, 126–127, *128*
    with left axis deviation, 127, *129*
    Wolff-Parkinson-White confused with, 138
  myocarditis and, 157
  quinidine and, 181
  right, calculation of mean vector, *123,* 123, 124
    causes of, 124
    central vs. peripheral, 119, 124
    changes with surgery, 120, *121*
    complete, 119–125, *120, 121,* 143Q, 144Q, *144*
    congenital, 124
    from His lesion, 119
    functional, during supraventricular tachycardia, 124
    in morphology schema, 279, *280,* 280, *281*
    incomplete, *125,* 125, 126
    T waves and, 124
    vectors and, 119–122, *122*
    with left axis deviation, *123,* 123, 124, 134, 135, *135,* 144Q, *144*
    with right ventricular hypertrophy, 124
    Wolff-Parkinson-White confused with, 138
  sarcoid and, 189
  systemic effects causing, 172t, 189Q, 190Q, 192, 193
Bundle branch bypass tract, 139, 141, *142, 143,* 143Q
Bundle of His. See *His bundle*
Bundle of Kent. See *Kent bundle*
"Burned" paper, 382, *384*
Bypass tract, in AV conduction, 263

Cable attachment, faulty, 382, *383*
Cable shielding, faulty, 382
Caffeine, supraventricular tachycardia and, 241t
Calcium, 9–12, 172t, 214t
Calibration, improper, 383, *385*
Calibration spike, 381, *382*
Capture beats, 229, *230,* 231, *232, 233,* 356Q, 356
  bigeminy with, 356Q, *356,* 370
  differential diagnosis of, 214, 215, 220
  in differential diagnosis of tachyarrhythmias, 261
  in morphology schema, 293, 294, *296,* 303t, 337, *338*
  ventricular tachycardia and, 251, *254, 256*
  with aberration, morphology schema, 303t, 339, *340*
Cardiac malposition, 83–98
Cardiac output, increased, sinus tachycardia and, 236t
Cardiac tumor, 159
  low-voltage QRS and, 70
  premature ventricular contractions and, 214t
  ventricular tachycardia and, 258t
Cardiomyopathy, atrial fibrillation and, 251t
  atrial flutter and, 248t
  AV block and, 264t

bifascicular block and, 134
hypertrophic, 101, 103, *103,* 107
  left bundle branch block and, 127
  pseudoinfarction Q wave and, 164
left axis deviation and, 131
premature ventricular contractions and, 214t
supraventricular tachycardia and, 241t
ventricular tachycardia and, 258t
Categories of arrhythmias. See *Arrhythmia category(ies)*
Cells, atrial, orientation of, 4
  P, 3, 5
  Purkinje, anatomy of, 6
  transitional, 3
Central nervous system effects, 184–185
Central nervous system injury, 172t, 184–185
  pseudoinfarction Q wave and, 164
  ST elevation and, 158
Central venous pressure line, premature atrial junctional contractions, 211t
Cerebrovascular accident, U wave and, 174
Chagas disease, myocarditis and, 157
Chemistry body, effects of, 173–178
Chest leads, incorrect positioning of, 376, *378*
Chest massage, during cardiac arrest, 381
Chest percussion, 381, *381*
Chest trauma, supraventricular tachycardia and, 241t
Chloride, 10, 12
Chloroform, 183
Chronic tachycardia, ectopic focus and, 237
Clockwise rotation, pseudoinfarction Q wave and, 164
Coarctation of aorta, first-degree AV block and, 263
  left ventricular hypertrophy and, 103
Coarse atrial fibrillation, 249, *249*
Cola, supraventricular tachycardia and, 241t
Compensatory pause, 215, *216*
  in morphology schema, 291
Complete AV block. See *AV block, complete*
Conduction, AV, phenytoin/lidocaine and, 182
  cell-to-body surface, 16
  cell-to-cell, 16
  digitalis and, 179
  intraatrial, 3, 6Q, 7Q
    digitalis and, 179
  preferential atrial, 4, 5, 6Q
  sinoventricular, in hyperkalemia, 173
Conduction delay, interatrial, P wave duration and, *111,* 112
  intraatrial, hyperkalemia and, 173
Conduction disturbance, interventricular, 119–148
Conduction system, anatomy of, 3–6, *4*
Conduction time, internodal, 5, 7Q
Congenital heart disease, atrial fibrillation in, 251t
  atrial flutter in, 248t
  AV block in, 264t
  bidirectional tachycardia in, 252, *257*
  premature ventricular contractions in, 214t
  supraventricular tachycardia in, 241t
  ventricular tachycardia in, 258t
Congestive heart failure,
  sinus tachycardia in, 236t
Connective tissue disease, 172t, 187
Contractions, premature. See *Premature atrial/junctional/ventricular contractions*
Cor pulmonale, ST elevation and, 158

Coronary artery, anomalous. See *Anomalous left coronary artery*
Corrected transposition. See *Inversion, ventricular*
Cortisone, hypokalemia and, 173
Couplets, 223, *223, 224*
Coupling interval, 225, *226, 227, 228*
  shortest observed, 388, *388*
Current, ionic, 10–18
Current flow, 13, *13, 14, 15*
Cushing's disease, hypokalemia and, 174
Cyclopropane, 172t, 183

Decongestants, sinus tachycardia and, 236t
Delayed QRS. See *QRS complex*
Delta wave, Mahaim conduction and, 141
  Wolff-Parkinson-White and, *137,* 138
Depolarization, atrial, derivation of, 36–39, *37, 44*
    direction of, 56, *57, 59Q, 59*
  basic principles of, 9–18
  diastolic, 11
  ionic flow during, 12–14, *13, 14, 15*
  ventricular, derivation of, 39–43, *40, 41, 42, 44, 46Q*
Dextrocardia, 84–88, *86, 87, 89, 90, 95Q*
Dextrorotation, *86, 87, 88, 89, 91, 95Q*
Diagrams, ladder, 195, *197*
Diarrhea, hypokalemia and, 173
Diethyl ether, 183
Differential diagnosis, premature beats in, 214–215, 220
  tachyarrhythmias in, 259, 261
Digitalis, 172t, 178–181, *179, 180,* 190Q, *191*
  action potential and, *170,* 171
  AV block and, 264t
  bidirectional tachycardia and, 252, *257*
  escape beats and escape rhythms and, 205t, 355Q, *355*
  hypercalcemia and, 175
  hypokalemia and, 174
  premature atrial/junctional contractions and, 211t
  premature ventricular contractions and, 214t
  ST segment changes and, 158
Digitalis toxicity, 172t, 179–181, *180*
Diphtheria, complete AV block and, 274
Dipole, 12–16, *13*
"Dipole vector," 15, *15,* 16, 17Q
Discs, intercalated, 16
Disease, right atrial, escape beats and escape rhythms and, 205
Disopyramide, 172t, 181, *181,* 182
"Dispersion of refractoriness," 45, 47Q
Dissociation, AV. See *AV dissociation*
Dissociation, "isorhythmic," 286, *288,* 304
Diuretics, hypokalemia and, 173
"Dome and dart." See *P wave*
Double outlet right ventricle, first-degree AV block and, 263
  left axis deviation and, 131
Drugs, anesthetic. See *Anesthetic drugs*
  antiarrhythmic, 178–183
  AV block and, 264t
  psychotropic, 183
  premature ventricular contractions and, 214t
  sinus tachycardia and, 236t, 259
  supraventricular tachycardia and, 241t
Duchenne's muscular dystrophy. See *Muscular dystrophy*

Ductus arteriosus, first-degree AV block and, 263
  ischemia and injury and, 155, 156, *156*
Dysplasia, arrhythmogenic right ventricular, ventricular tachycardia and, 258t
Dysrhythmias. See *Arrhythmias*
Dystrophy, muscular. See *Muscular dystrophy*

"Early repolarization," 70, 150, *150,* 151
  ST segment shift and, 158, 165Q, *166*
Eating, T wave changes and, 150
Ebstein's anomaly, first-degree AV block and, 263
Ectopic atrial bradycardia, in morphology schema, 302t, 304, *305*
  with aberration, in morphology schema, 302t, 308, *309*
Ectopic atrial escape beat, in morphology schema, 303t, 341, *342*
Ectopic atrial rhythm, in morphology schema, 302t, 312, *313*
  with aberration, in morphology schema, 302t, 316, *317*
    with 2:1 block, in morphology schema, 302t, *310, 318*
  with 2:1 block, in morphology schema, 302t, *314*
Ectopic atrial tachycardia, in morphology schema, 302t, 320, *321*
  with aberration, in morphology schema, 302t, 324, *325*
Ectopic focus mechanism, in tachyarrhythmias, 237, 239
Edema, low-voltage QRS and, 69
  myocardial, hypothyroidism and, 187
Effusion, pericardial, low-voltage QRS and, 70
  pleural, low-voltage QRS and, 70, 80Q, *80*
Electrical interference, ventricular fibrillation confused with, 254, 257, *258*
Electrocardiogram, calibration and paper speed of, 22–23, *22, 23,* 33Q
  computer analysis of, 23–25, *24*
  explanation of hypothetical recording, 13, 14, *14,* 17Q
  leads. See *Leads*
  normal, 61–82
    adolescent, 61, *62*
    neonatal, 61, *62*
  normal values. See *Normal values*
  predictive value in hypertrophy, 99
  standardization and measurement, 22–23, 33Q, 80Q
  waves and intervals, 25–27
Electrocardiograph, American Heart Association standards, 21
  direct writing, 19–22, *21*
  frequency response, 20–22, 34Q
  operation of, 19–25
  signal distortion in, 20
Electrode contact, loss of, 381, 382, *383*
Electrode paste, smeared, 376, 378, *379*
Electrolytes, 173–178
Electrophysiologic approach to arrhythmias, 197–274
Electrophysiology, cellular, 9–18
Emetine intoxication, ST segment changes and, 158
Encephalitis, supraventricular tachycardia and, 241t
Endocardial activation. See *Activation*
Endocarditis, AV block and, 264t
  bifascicular block and, 134

Endocarditis *(Continued)*
  left bundle branch block and, 127
  left posterior hemiblock and, 134
  right bundle branch block and, 124
Endocrine disease, hypokalemia and, 174
Entrance block, parasystole, 225, *227, 228*
Epicardial activation. See *Activation*
Epinephrine, action potential and, *170,* 171
  sinus tachycardia and, 259
Escape, atrial. See *Atrial escape beat(s)*
  junctional. See *Junctional escape beat(s)*
  ventricular. See *Ventricular escape beat(s)*
Escape beat(s), 198–205
  causes of, 205t, 205
  in morphology schema, 303t, 341, *342, 343, 343*
  premature beat vs. 206–208, *207,* 356Q, 357
Escape rates, normal, 198, 199t
Escape rhythm, 198–205
  causes of, 205t, 205
  in complete AV block, 272
  with aberrancy, 201, *203*
"Escape-capture" bigeminy, 356Q, *356,* 370
Ether, diethyl, 183
Ethyl chloride, 183
Exchange transfusion, supraventricular tachycardia
    and, 241t
Exercise, sinus tachycardia and, 236t
Exit block, parasystole and, 225, *227, 228*
External influences, phasic cause of artifacts, *381,*
    386, 389, 389, 391

Fabry's disease, short PR interval and, 139
Fascicle, left anterior, anatomy of, *4, 5,* 7Q
  left posterior, anatomy of, *4, 5,* 7Q
"Fast response." See *Action potential*
Fear, T wave changes and, 149
Fever, sinus tachycardia and, 236t, 259
  supraventricular tachycardia and, 241t
Fibrillation, atrial. See *Atrial fibrillation*
  ventricular. See *Ventricular fibrillation*
Fine atrial fibrillation, 249, *249*
Fixed coupling, 225, *226, 227, 228*
Flutter, atrial. See *Atrial flutter*
Flutter waves, absence of, in supraventricular
    tachycardia, 237
  in atrial flutter, 241, *246, 247, 248, 248*
  in morphology schema, 281, *282, 283*
Focus, ectopic, parasystolic, 225, *227, 228*
Frequency response, 20–22, 34Q
Friedreich's ataxia, 172t, 187
  pseudoinfarction Q wave, 164
Frontal plane, 27, *28*
Fusion, atrial, *253*
  due to Wolff-Parkinson-White, *137,* 138
  premature ventricular contractions and, 212, *214*
  ventricular tachycardia and, 251, *253, 254, 255, 256*
Fusion beats, differential diagnosis of
    tachyarrhythmias, 261

Gain, improper, 383, *385*
Galvanometer, explanation of hypothetical
    recording, 13, 14, *14,* 17Q
  string, 19, *20, 21*
"Grouped beating," Wenckebach, 266

Halothane, 172t, 183
  action potential and, *170,* 171
  premature ventricular contractions and, 214t

Head injury. See *Central nervous system injury*
Heart failure, congestive, low-voltage QRS and, 70
Heart rate, accelerated atrial rhythm and, 239, 241,
    242
  accelerated junctional rhythm and, 239, 241, *242*
  accelerated ventricular rhythm and, *242,* 259, *260*
  escape, normal, 198, 199t
  impossibly rapid, 383, *384, 388*
  in differential diagnosis of tachyarrhythmias, 259,
    261
  in morphology schema. See *Morphology schema*
  maximum observed, 387, 388
  method of determination, 62, 63, *63, 64,* 79Q, 396t
  normal, AV block and, 263
  ventricular tachycardia and, *242,* 251
Hemiblock, left anterior, 130–133, *132, 133,* 143Q. See
    also *Left axis deviation*
  causes of, 131–133
  familial, 133
  genesis of, 130–131, *132*
  pseudoinfarction Q wave and, 164
  S wave in V_6 and, 103, *104*
  left posterior, *132, 133,* 133, 134
  right axis deviation and, 105
Hexaxial system, 30, 31, *31,* 34Q
Hiccough, 378, *379*
"High-grade" AV block. See *AV block, "Advanced"*
His bundle, abnormal, in ventricular inversion, 273
  anatomy of, 4, *4, 5,* 6Q, 7Q
  block, type II second-degree, 269
  refractory period and, 263
Horizontal plane, 27, *28*
H-V interval, trifascicular block and, 135
Hyperaldosteronism, hypokalemia and, 173
Hypercalcemia, 172t, 174–175, *176,* 214t
  action potential and, 170, *171*
  AV block and, 264t
  digitalis and, 175
  escape beats and escape rhythms and, 205t
  premature atrial/junctional contractions and, 211t
Hyperkalemia, 172t, 173, 174, 214t
  action potential and, 170, *171*
  AV block and, 264t
  conduction delay and, 135, *136*
  hypoglycemia and, 178
  ST segment changes and, 158
Hypermagnesemia, 172t, 177
Hypernatremia, 172t, 178
Hyperparathyroidism, hypercalcemia and, 174
Hypertension, U waves and, 46
Hyperthyroidism, supraventricular tachycardia and,
    241t
Hypertrophy, biventricular, 69
  ventricular, 99–110
    predictive value of ECG in, 99
Hyperventilation, T wave changes and, 150
Hypervitaminosis D, hypercalcemia and, 174
Hypocalcemia, 172t, 175–177, *177*
  action potential and, 170, *171*
  AV block and, 264t
  Q-OT interval and, 77, *78, 81,* 81Q
  sinus tachycardia and, 236t
Hypoglycemia, 172t, 178
  AV block and, 264t
  diffuse conduction delay and, 135, *136*
  escape beats and escape rhythms and, 205t
  premature atrial/junctional contractions and, 211t

Hypoglycemia *(Continued)*
  premature ventricular contractions and, 214t
  supraventricular tachycardia and, 241t
Hypokalemia, 172t, 173–174, *175*, 214t
  action potential and, 170, *171*
  AV block and, 264t
  bidirectional tachycardia and, 252, *257*
  digitalis and, 174
  hypomagnesemia and, similarities, 177–178
  plus hypocalcemia, 178
  premature atrial/junctional contractions and, 211t
  U waves and, 45
Hypomagnesemia, 172t, 177–178
Hyponatremia, 172t, 178
Hypoparathyroidism, hypocalcemia and, 175
Hypophosphatasia, hypercalcemia and, 174
Hypotension, supraventricular tachycardia and, 241t
Hypothermia, 186, *186*
  AV block and, 264t
  escape beats and escape rhythms and, 205t
  U waves and, 45
Hypothyroidism, 172t, 187, *188*
  AV block and, 264t
Hypovolemia, sinus tachycardia and, 236t, 259
Hypoxia, 172t, 178
  action potential and, 170, *171*
  AV block and, 264t
  escape beats and escape rhythms and, 205t
  premature atrial/junctional contractions and, 211t
  premature ventricular contractions and, 214t

Idioventricular rhythm. See *Ventricular escape rhythm*
Ileus, 189
Imipramine, 183
  premature atrial/junctional contractions and, 211t
  premature ventricular contractions and, 214t
Increased cardiac output, sinus tachycardia and, 236t
Infarction, myocardial. See *Myocardial infarction*
  papillary muscle, 162
Infection, sinus tachycardia, 236t
"Infusion pump," 385, *386*
Injury, ischemia causing, 155, *155*, 156, *156*, *160*
  myocardial, 152–159, 165Q
  myocarditis, 156–157, *157*
  pericarditis, 157–159, *158*
  subendocardial, 154, *154*, 165Q
  subepicardial, 152, *154*, 165Q
Insecticides, organophosphorous, 184
Instrumentation, electrocardiographic, 19–25
Interference, 60 cycle, 382, 385
Interval, interectopic. See *Parasystole*
Interventricular conduction delay, diffuse, 135, *136*
  in morphology schema, 280, *280*, *282*
Intracranial pressure. See also *Central nervous system*
  AV block caused by, 264t
  escape beats and escape rhythms caused by, 205
Inversion, ventricular, 90, *92*, 95Q
  AV block and, 90
  complete AV block and, 273
  left axis deviation and, 90
  postoperative AV block and, 274
  QR pattern and, 100
Ions. See individual ions
"Irregularly irregular." See *Atrial fibrillation*

Irregular rhythm, continuously irregular, defined, 286, *289*, *290*
  intermittently irregular, 291, 293–301, *293*, *294*, *295*, *296*, *297*, *298*, *299*, *300*, *301*
  defined, 286, *289*, *290*
Ischemia, 151–152, *152*, *153*, 165Q
  causes of, 151, 152
  conduction delay and, 135, *136*
  strain vs., 152
  subendocardial, 151, *152*, *153*, 165Q
    central nervous system injury and, 185
  transmural, 151, *152*, *153*, 165Q
  U wave and, 173
"Isochronic" dissociation, 286, *288*, 304
Isoelectric line, defined, *26*, 27, 67, 77, *78*
  use of PR segment and, 38, 46Q, 67, 77, *78*
Isoproterenol, sinus tachycardia, 259

J point, defined, *26*, 27
  elevation of. See *"Early repolarization"*
"J" wave, central nervous system injury and, 185, *186*
  hypothermia and, 186, *186*
James fiber. See *Lown-Ganong-Levine*
Jervell-Lange-Nielsen, 45, 172t, 184, *185*, 192Q, *192*
"Jittery" newborn, artifacts and, 380
Junctional bigeminy, 220, 222, *222*
Junctional bradycardia, electrocardiographic criteria for, 205
Junctional contractions, premature. See *Premature junctional contractions*
Junctional couplets, 223
Junctional escape beat(s), escape rhythm and, electrocardiographic criteria, *196*, 199t, *200*, 200–201, *206*, *207*, 242, 344Q, *345*, 353Q, *355*, 356Q, *356*
  in morphology schema, *294*, *301*, 303t, *341*, *342*
  premature junctional contraction confused with, 210–211, *294*
Junctional ectopic tachycardia, 237, 239, *240*
  with Wenckebach, *266*
Junctional parasystole, 225, *228*
Junctional premature contractions. See *Premature junctional contractions*
Junctional rhythm. See also *Junctional escape rhythm*
  accelerated. See *Accelerated junctional rhythm*
  capture beats and, 229, *230*, 231
  central nervous system injury and, 185
  digitalis toxicity and, 179
  in morphology schema, 302t, 304, *305*
  with aberration, 201
in morphology schema, 302t, 308, *309*
  with AV dissociation, in morphology schema, 284, *285*, *288*
  with complete AV block, 269, 273, 274, 346Q, *347*
    in morphology schema, 302t, 304, *307*
Junctional tachycardia, AV dissociation and, 236–237, 239, *240*
  capture beats and, 231, *233*
  digitalis toxicity, 179
Junctional trigeminy, 221, 223

Katz-Wachtel criterion, in biventricular hypertrophy, 108–110, *109*, *114*, 115
Kawasaki's disease, 162, 163, *164*
  ischemic changes and, 151

Kent bundle. See also *Wolff-Parkinson-White*
operation on, 6Q
Kyphoscoliosis, 95

Ladder diagrams, 195, 197
Lancisi, muscle of, 6
Leads, 27–33
augmented, 28–31, *29, 30, 31,* 34Q
bipolar, 28, *29*
chest, incorrect positioning, 376, *377, 378, 378, 379*
right chest, left chest, precordial, 31–33, *32*
definition of planes and, 27–28, *28*
Frank, X, Y, Z, 28
frontal plane, defined, 28–31, *29, 30, 31,* 34Q
horizontal plane, 31–33, *32*
limb, 28–31, *29, 30, 31,* 34Q
magnitude of voltage, 16
reversed limb, 376, *377*
ST elevation relating to epicardial injury, 159
transition, 69
unipolar, *29, 30*
Left anterior hemiblock. See *Hemiblock*
Left atrial enlargement. See *Atrial enlargement*
Left atrium, P wave direction and, 56, *57*
Left axis deviation. See also *Hemiblock*
causes of, 54, 90, 91, 131–133
defined, 53, 54, *54,* 58Q, *58*
in myotinic dystrophy, 187
Left bundle branch block. See *Bundle branch block*
Left ventricular hypertrophy. See *Ventricular hypertrophy*
Lidocaine, 172t, 182
Limb leads, reversed, 96Q, *96,* 376, *377*
"Long-short" phenomenon, 215, *218, 219,* 220
Loss of electrode contact, 381, *382, 383*
Low right atrial pacemaker. See *Rhythm, low atrial*
Low right atrium, P wave direction and, 56, *57*
Low-voltage QRS. See *QRS complex*
Lown-Ganong-Levine, 138–139, *140, 141,* 143Q
atrial flutter and, 243
supraventricular tachycardia and, 241t
L-transposition. See *Inversion, ventricular*
Lupus erythematosus, 187
congenital complete AV block and, 272

Mahaim conduction, 139, 141, *142, 143,* 143Q
Malabsorption, hypocalcemia and, 175
Malfunctioning ECG system, 381–385, *383, 384, 385*
Malposition, 83–98
Mannosidosis, short PR interval and, 139
Massage, chest, during cardiac arrest, 381
Mean vector, amplitude method, 49, *50, 52*
area method, 49, *50, 51*
defined, 49
left bundle branch block, 127, *129*
perpendicular method, 49–51, *50,* 53, 57Q, *58*
P wave, frontal plane, 56, *57,* 59Q, *59,* 64
horizontal plane, 57
QRS, dextrocardia, *87, 88, 89,* 95Q, 96Q
dextrorotation, *86, 87, 88, 89,* 91
frontal plane, 49–52, *50, 51, 52,* 53, 57Q, *58*
normal values, 396t
horizontal plane, 55
ventricular inversion, 90, *92*
right bundle branch block, *123,* 123, 124
T wave, frontal plane, 55, *56,* 71
horizontal plane, 55, 71

Mechanical stimulation, premature ventricular
contractions, 214t
Mechanism, tachyarrhythmias, 237
Membrane, cell, 9
Metabolic diseases, 187–188
Microelectrode, 9
Mitral insufficiency, P wave changes in, 111
Mitral prolapse, 152
ventricular tachycardia and, 258t
Mobitz type 1. See *Wenckebach*
Moderator band, 6
Morphology schema, step 1, PR interval regular, 276, *276, 277*
step 2, QRS rate, 276, *278, 278, 279*
step 3, QRS duration, 279, *280,* 280, *281*
step 4, atrial activity, 280–286, *282, 283, 284, 285, 286, 287, 288*
step 4a, P wave morphology, 280–281, *282, 283*
step 4b, P wave mean vector, 282, *284, 285*
step 4c, P-QRS relationship, 282, 284–286, *286, 287, 288*
step 5, RR interval irregular, 286
step 6, continuous vs. intermittently irregular, 286, *289, 290*
step 7, continuously irregular rhythms, 286, 290, *290, 292*
step 8, intermittently irregular rhythms, 291, 293–301, *293, 294, 295, 296, 297, 298, 299, 300, 301*
step 8a, premature QRS, 291–294, *293, 294, 295, 296, 297*
step 8b, premature-narrow QRS, 293, *296*
step 8c, premature-wide QRS, 293, 294, *298*
step 9, delayed QRS, 294, *294, 295, 297, 299, 300, 301*
step 9a, delayed-narrow QRS, 294, *295, 297, 299, 300, 301*
step 9b, delayed-wide QRS, 297, *301*
Mosque sign, in hypothyroidism, 187, *188*
Movement artifacts, 378, *380, 380*
Mucocutaneous lymph node syndrome. See *Kawasaki's disease*
Multiform bigeminy, 224, *225*
Multiform premature beats, 220, *221*
Muscular dystrophy, 101, *103,* 172t, 186–187
pseudoinfarction Q wave and, 164
Mustard operation, 5
accelerated junctional rhythm and, 241, *244*
escape beats and escape rhythm and, 205
Myocardial infarction, 159–164, *160, 161, 163, 164,* 167Q, *167*
acute ischemia and injury and, 155, *155*
anterior, QR pattern and, 100
AV block and, 264t
evolution of, 159, 160, *160*
left anterior hemiblock and, 133
left bundle branch block and, 127
patterns mimicking. See *Pseudoinfarction*
pericarditis vs., 159, 165Q, *166*
Myocardial injury, 152–159, 165Q
Myocardial ischemia. See *Ischemia*
Myocarditis, 156–157, *157*
AV block and, 264t
bifascicular block and, 134
complete AV block and, 274
diffuse conduction delay and, 135, *136*
left axis deviation and, 133

Myocarditis *(Continued)*
  left bundle branch block and, 127
  left posterior hemiblock and, 134
  low voltage QRS and, 69, 80Q, *80*
  premature ventricular contractions and, 214t
  prolonged P wave and, 112
  right bundle branch block and, 124
  sinus tachycardia and, 236t
  supraventricular tachycardia and, 241t
Myotonic dystrophy, 172t, 187
Myxedema, low-voltage QRS and, 69

Neonatal stress, hypocalcemia and, 175
Neuromuscular disorders, 186–187
Neurosurgical procedures, 184–185
Nervous system, central. See *Central nervous system*
  sympathetic, T wave changes and, 149–150
Newborn, hydropic, atrial flutter, 243
  preterm, and Q-OT interval, 77
Node(s). See *AV node; Sinus node*
Nonparoxysmal junctional tachycardia. See
      Accelerated junctional rhythm
Nonparoxysmal tachycardia, and ectopic focus, 237
Normal children, atrial fibrillation in, 251t
  atrial flutter in, 243, 248t
  escape beats and escape rhythms in, 205
  first-degree AV block in, 263
  premature atrial contractions in, 210
  premature ventricular contractions in, 214t
  type II second-degree AV block in, 269
  ventricular tachycardia in, 254, 258t
  Wenckebach in, 267
Normal values, computer method of analysis, 23
  Davignon's population, 61, *61*
  definition of normal percentiles, 62
  heart rate, 62, 63, 79Q
  P wave amplitude and configuration, 63, 64, *65*
  PR interval, 65, *66*, 79Q, 81Q, 397t
  QRS amplitude, 68, 69, *80*, 81Q, 398t, 399t, 400t,
      401t, 402t, 403t, 404t
  QRS duration, 67, *80*, 81Q, 397t
  QT interval, 75, 76, 77, *81*, 81Q, 403t
"Northwest axis", 54, *54, 55*

Obesity, low-voltage QRS and, 70
Ocular pressure, AV block and, 264t
  escape beats and escape rhythms and, 205t
Organophosphorous insecticides, 184
Orthostatic T wave changes, See *Posture*
Osborne wave. See *"J" wave*

P cells, 3
P wave, amplitude of, right atrial pressure vs.
      volume, 109–111
  artifact resembling, infusion pump, 385, *386*
  asplenia and, 83, 84, *85*
  atrial activation and, 25
  atypical appearance of, artifact, *379, 385, 386*
  AV dissociation and, conduction to ventricles, 229
  axis. See *Mean vector, P wave*
  defined, 26
  derivation of, 36–39, *37, 44*
  direction of, 56, *57*, 59Q, *59*
  "dome and dart," 83, *84*
  "dropped." See *AV block, second-degree*
  duration of, measurement of, 26, *26*
    quinidine and, 181

  enlargement of, after supraventricular tachycardia,
      111
  in atrial situs inversus, 83–84, *90*, 96Q, *96*
  in myotonic dystrophy, 172t, 187
  low-voltage, hypothyroidism, 187
  mean vector. See also *Mean vector, P wave*
    in morphology schema. See *Morphology
        schema*
  morphology of, in morphology schema. See
        Morphology schema
  nonconducted. See *AV block*
    refractoriness causing, 229
  normal amplitude and configuration, 26, *26*, 63,
      64, 65
  normal AV conduction and, 269
  P terminal forces and, left atrial pressure vs.
      volume, 111
  polysplenia and, 83, 84, *86*
  premature, 208
  prolonged, *111*, 112
  retrograde, in junctional rhythm, *200, 201*
    in morphology schema, 283, 284, *285, 287*
    in ventricular rhythm, *201*
  situs ambiguous, 83, 84, *85, 86*
  supraventricular tachycardia and, 74, 75, *238*, 239t,
      240
  T wave vs., 72, 73, *74*
Pacemaker(s), subsidiary, 198
  wandering. See *Wandering pacemaker*
Pacemaker "spike" artifact, 393Q, *394*
Paper drag, *382, 384*, 392Q, *393*
Paper drive, faulty, 382, *384*
Paper speed, faulty, 382, *384*, 392Q, *393*
Papillary muscle infarction. See *Infarction*
Parasystole, 225, *226, 227, 228*
  repetitive artifact causing, *388, 389*
Paroxysmal tachycardia, reentry and, 237
Paste, smeared, 376, *378, 379*
Patent ductus arteriosus. See *Ductus arteriosus*
Pathways, atrial, specialized, 3–5, *4*, 6Q, 7Q
Pause, compensatory, 215, *216*
"Pause," in supraventricular rhythm, 295, *300, 301*
  with ectopic atrial escape beat, in morphology
      schema, 303t, 341, *342*
  with junctional escape beat, in morphology
      schema, 303t, 341, *342*
  with ventricular escape beat, in morphology
      schema, 303t, 343, *343*
Pectus excavatum, 90–93, *93, 94*, 95Q
"Pegged" tracing, 383, *385*
Percussion, chest, 381, *381*
Pericarditis, 157–159, *158*, 165Q, *166*
  connective tissue disease and, 187
  constrictive, low-voltage QRS and, 70
  differentiation from early repolarization, *150*, 151,
      165Q, *166*
  myocardial infarction vs., 159, 165Q, *166*
  myxomatous, 187
Peritoneal inflammation, 172t, 189
Pharyngeal stimulation, AV block and, 264t
  escape beats and escape rhythms and, 205t
Phase 0–4. See *Action potential, phases of*
Phenothiazines, 172t, 183
  premature ventricular contractions and, 214t
  U wave and, 174
Phenylephrine, supraventricular vs. sinus
      tachycardia, 259

Phenytoin, 172t, 182
Pheochromocytoma, 172t, 188
Plane(s), defined, 27, *28*
Pneumomediastinum, 94
Pneumonectomy, 94, 95Q
Pneumopericardium, ST segment changes and, 158
Pneumothorax, 94
  low-voltage QRS and, 70, 80Q, *80*
  pseudoinfarction Q wave and, 164
  ST segment changes and, 158
Polysplenia, P wave, 83, 84, *86*
Pompe's disease, short PR interval and, 139, *141*
Position, ventricular, 84–90
Position, leads. See *Leads*
Positional abnormalities, 83–98
Postoperative patients, premature ventricular
  contractions, 214t
Postprandial, sinus tachycardia and, 236t
Posture, T wave changes and, 150
Potassium, 9–12, 172t, 214t
Potential, direction of depolarization and, 14, 15,
  17Q
  direction of repolarization and, 15
  recording of, in hypothetical cell, 14, *14*
P-P interval, constant, in morphology schema, 290,
  290, 291, *292*
  variable, in morphology schema, 286, 290, *290*, 292
P-QRS relationship, in morphology schema. See
  Morphology schema
PR interval, defined, 26, *26*, 33Q, 65
  hyperthyroidism and, 187
  hypothermia and, 186, *186*
  normal values for, 65, 66, *66*, 397t, 79Q, 81Q
  phenytoin and, 182
  progressive lengthening. See *Wenckebach*
  prolonged. See *AV block, first-degree*
  propranolol and, 182
  quinidine and, 181
  short, causes of, 65, 66, 139
    Lown-Ganong-Levine and, 138–139
    Wolff-Parkinson-White and, 136–138
  tricyclic antidepressants and, 183
  verapamil and, 183
PR segment, defined, 26, *26*, 67
  depression of, 67, 77, *78*
  elevation and depression of, 159
Preexcitation, 135–147
  supraventricular tachycardia and, 135
Premature atrial contraction(s), aberration in, 209,
  209, 352, 353Q
  in morphology schema, 294, 303t, 339, *340*
  association with atrial flutter, 243
  blocked or nonconducted, 209, *210*, 211
  capture beat vs., 229, *230*
  causes of, 210t, 211
  compensatory pause and, 215, *216*
  differential diagnosis of, 214–215, 220
  digitalis toxicity and, 179
  electrocardiographic criteria for, 208–210, *206*,
    208, *209*, *210*, *211*, *221*, *222*, *226*, *228*, 352,
    353Q, *355*, 356Q
  in morphology schema, 293, 294, *296*, 303t, 337,
    338
  nonconducted, in morphology schema, 295, *300*,
    303t, 341, *342*
  sarcoidoisis and, 189
  uniform vs. multiform, 220, *221*

Premature beat(s), 205–231
  aberrant conduction vs., atrial flutter/fibrillation,
    215, *218*, *219*, 220
  capture beats vs., 229, *230*, 231
  defined, 205–208, *206*
  differential diagnosis of, 214–215, 220
  escape beat vs., 206–208, *207*
  "impossibly premature," artifact, 388, *388*, 392Q,
    393
  morphology of, uniform vs. multiform, 220, *221*
  patterns of, bigeminy/trigeminy/couplets, 220, 221,
    222, *223*, 223, *224*, 225
Premature junctional contraction(s), causes of, 211t,
  212
  differential diagnosis of, 214–215, 220
  electrocardiographic criteria for, *206*, *207*, 210–
    212, *222*, *226*, *228*
  in morphology schema, 293, 294, *296*, 303t, 337,
    338
  with aberration, 212
    confused with premature ventricular
      contraction, 294, *298*
    in morphology schema, 294, *298*
Premature QRS. See *QRS complex*
Premature ventricular contraction(s), aberrant
  premature junctional contraction confused
  with, 294, *298*
  causes of, 213, 214t
  in morphology schema, 294, *298*, 303t, 339, *340*
  compensatory pause and, 215, *216*
  differential diagnosis of, 214, 215, 220
  digitalis toxicity and, 179, *180*
  electrocardiographic criteria and, 206, 212, 213,
    213, *214*, *216*, *217*, *218*, *219*, *221*, *223*, *224*,
    225, *226*, *227*, 353Q, *355*, 356Q, 357Q
  junctional vs., with aberrancy, 201
  quinidine toxicity and, 181
  sarcoid and, 189
  site of origin of, 212
  uniform vs. multiform, 220, *221*
  Wolff-Parkinson-White confused with, 215, *217*
Prematurity interval, shortest observed, 388, *388*
Procainamide, 172t, 181, *181*, 182
  toxicity of, diffuse conduction delay and, 135, *136*
  U wave and, 173
Prolapse, mitral. See *Mitral prolapse*
Propranolol, 172t, 182
  AV block and, 264t
  escape beats and escape rhythms and, 205t
Prosthetic material, pseudoinfarction Q wave, 164
Protected focus. See *Parasystole*
Proximity effect, 33
Pseudoinfarction, 163, 164, *165*, 166Q, *166*, 167Q
  causes of, 91
Psychotropic drugs, 183
Pulmonary embolism, P wave changes and, 111
  U waves and, 46
Pulmonary stenosis, 100–101, *101*
  first-degree AV block, 263
  ischemic changes and, 151
Purkinje cells, 6

Q wave, absent, in left ventricular hypertrophy, *106*,
  108, 113Q
  amplitude of, normal values, 68, 69, 398t
  cardiac tumor and, 159, 164
  clockwise rotation and, 164

Q wave *(Continued)*
   deep, in left ventricular hypertrophy, *106*, *107*,
      108, 113Q, 116Q, *116*
   defined, *26*, *27*
   Friedreich's ataxia and, 164
   hypertrophic cardiomyopathy and, 164
   in right bundle branch block, 120
   in right ventricular hypertrophy, 99–100, 113Q,
      115Q, 116Q, *116*, 164
   intracranial hemorrhage and, 164
   Kawasaki's disease and, 162, 163, *164*
   left anterior hemiblock and, 164
   left bundle branch block and, 164
   left ventricular hypertrophy and, 163, 166Q, *166*
   muscular dystrophy and, 164, 186–187
   myocardial infarction and, 159, 160, *160*, *161*, 163,
      167Q, *167*
   myocarditis and, 156–157, *157*, 164
   normal characteristics of, 68, 69
   papillary muscle infarction and, 162
   pneumothorax and, 164
   prosthetic material and, 164
   pseudoinfarction and, causes of, 163, 164, *165*,
      166Q, *166*, 167Q
   scleroderma and, 164
   ventricular inversion and, 164
   Wolff-Parkinson-White and, 164, 166Q, *166*
Q-OT interval, defined, *26*, *27*
   normal values of, 77, *78*, 81, 81Q
   prolonged, hypocalcemia and, 176
      premature infants, 176
QR pattern, 99–100, *100*, 113Q, 115Q, 116Q, *116*
   confusion with RSR', 100, 115Q, 116Q, *116*
QRS complex, acidosis and, 178
   amplitude of, normal, 68, 69, *80*, 81Q, 398t, 399t,
      400t, 401t, 402t, 403t, 404t
   atypical appearance of, artifact and, *379*, 385,
      386
   axis. See *Mean vector, QRS*
   beginning in analysis of arrhythmias, 274
   bizarre, hyperkalemia and, 173
   cancellation of forces and, 39
   changes in, with age, 69
   defined, *26*, *26*, 27
   delayed, in morphology schema. See *Morphology*
      schema
   derivation of, 39–43, *40*, *41*, *42*, *44*, 46Q
   dextrocardia and, *87*, 88, 95Q, 96Q, *96*
   dextrorotation and, *86*, *87*, 88, *89*, 91, 95Q
   differences in, with race, 69
      with sex, 69, 403t
   hypoxia and, 178
   in normal ventricular position, 84–85
   low-voltage, 69, 70, 80Q, *80*
      cardiac tumor and, 159
      connective tissue disease and, 187
      hypothyroidism and, 187
      myocarditis and, 156, *157*
   mean vector. See *Mean vector, QRS*
   morphology of, normal, 68, *80*, 81Q
   muscular dystrophy and, 186–187
   normal, 67–70
   not followed by T wave, artifact and, *387*, *387*
   premature, in morphology schema. See
      Morphology schema
   prolongation of, hyperkalemia and, 173
      in morphology schema, 279, 280, *280*, *281*

QRS duration and, normal, 67, *80*, 81Q, 397t
quinidine and, 181
supraventricular tachycardia and, 237, *238*
systemic effects on, 172t
tricyclic antidepressants and, 183
ventricular inversion and, 90, 92, 95Q
QRS delayed, in morphology schema, 303t. *See also*
   Arrhythmia category(ies) 13, *14*
QRS duration. See also *QRS complex*
   in morphology schema. See *Morphology schema*
   normal, in morphology schema, 302t. See also
      Arrhythmia category(ies) 1, 3, 5, 7, 9, 11, 13
   prolonged, in morphology schema, 302t. See also
      Arrhythmia category(ies) 2, 4, 6, 8, 10, 12, 14
QRS premature, in morphology schema, 303t. See
      also *Arrhythmia category(ies) 11, 12*
QRS rate, decreased, in morphology schema, 302t.
      See also *Arrhythmia category(ies) 1, 2*
   increased, in morphology schema, 302t. See also
      Arrhythmia category(ies) 5, 6
   in morphology schema. See *Morphology schema*
   normal, in morphology schema, 302t. See also
      Arrhythmia category(ies) 3, 4
QRS-T, angle, 55, *56*, 58Q, *58*
   concordance, mechanism of, *44*, 45
   discordance, defined, 55, *56*, 58, 59Q
      mechanism of, *44*, 45
QS wave, *26*, 68
QT interval, acidosis and, 178
   adrenal insufficiency and, 188
   central nervous system injury and, 184–185
   correction for heart rate, 75, 76, 77, *81*, 81Q, 403t
   defined, *26*, *27*, 74
   digitalis and, 179, *179*, 190Q, *191*
   halothane and, 183
   hypothermia and, 186, *186*
   hypoxia and, 178
   measurement of, method of, 74, 75, 76, 80Q, *81*,
      81Q
   normal values, 75, 76, 77, *81*, 81Q, 403t
   phenytoin and, 182
   pheochromocytoma and, 188
   prolonged, congenital, 45, 172t, 184, *185*, 192Q,
      192, 214t
      hypocalcemia and, 176
      mitral prolapse and, 152
      systemic effects causing, 172t, 189, 192, *192*
      Torsade-de-Pointes and, 181, *181*
      ventricular tachycardia and, 258t
   propranolol and, 182
   short, hypercalcemia and, 174
      systemic effects causing, 172t, 190Q, *191*, 193
   tricyclic antidepressants and, 183
QTc interval. See *QT interval, correction for heart*
   rate
Quinidine, 172t, 181, *181*, 182
   action potential and, *170*, 171
   AV block and, 264t
   premature ventricular contractions and, 214t
   toxicity of, diffuse conduction delay and, 135, *136*
   U wave and, 45, 173

Race, QRS complex differences and, 69
Rate. See *Heart rate*
Reentry mechanism, in tachyarrhythmias, 237
Refractory period, absolute, 10, *11*
   atrial and ventricular, in artifact recognition, 388

Refractory period *(Continued)*
  AV node, 263
  bundle branches, 263
    capture beats, 229
  effective, 10, *11*
  His bundle, 263
  relative, 10, *11*
Renal failure, hyperkalemia and, 173, 190Q, *191*
Repolarization, atrial, derivation of, 36–39, *37, 44*
  basic principles of, 9–18
  ionic flow during, *14, 15, 15*
  ventricular, derivation of, 43–45, *43, 44*, 46Q
  ventricular Purkinje, derivation of, 45, *46*, 47Q
Respiration, as artifact, 380, *381*
Respiratory distress, supraventricular tachycardia, 241t
"Resting membrane potential," 9
Retrograde P wave. See *P wave*
Reversed limb leads, 96Q, *96*, 376, *377*
Rheumatic fever, AV block and, 264t
  sinus tachycardia and, 236t
Rhythm, accelerated atrial, electrocardiographic criteria for, 239, 241, 242, 243, 347, 348Q, *348*
Rhythm, accelerated junctional. See *Accelerated junctional rhythm*
Rhythm, accelerated ventricular. See *Accelerated ventricular rhythm*
Rhythm, atrial ectopic, in situs inversus, 83, 84, *84*
Rhythm, junctional. See *Junctional rhythm*
  left atrial, 83, *84*
Rhythm, low atrial, in polysplenia, 83, 84, *86*
  PR interval in, 66
  sinus. See *sinus rhythm*
  terminal, children, 257
  unaffected by artifact, 388, *389, 390*
Rhythm disturbances. See *Arrhythmias*
Right atrial disease, escape beats and escape rhythms, 205
Right atrial enlargement. See *Atrial enlargement*
Right axis deviation, causes of, 53
  defined, 52–53, *54*
  right ventricular hypertrophy and, 105
Right bundle branch block. See *Block, bundle branch, right*
  incomplete. See *RSR' pattern*
Right ventricular dysplasia, arrhythmogenic, 258t
Right ventricular hypertrophy. See *Ventricular hypertrophy, right*
Romano-Ward, 172t, 184, *185*, 192
Rotation, clockwise, and left axis deviation, 90–93, *93, 94*
RR interval, continuously irregular, in morphology schema, 303t. See also *Arrhythmia category(ies)* 7–10
  in morphology schema. See also *Morphology schema*
  intermittently irregular, in morphology schema, 303t. See also *Arrhythmia category(ies)* 11 to *14*
  irregular, in morphology schema, 286
  progressive shortening. See *Wenckebach*
  regular, in morphology schema, 276, *276, 277*, 302t. See also *Arrhythmia category(ies)* 1 to 6
  shortened, capture beats, 229, *230*, 231, *232, 233*
  shortest observed, 387, *388*
RSR' pattern, clockwise rotation and, 91, *93, 94*
  confusion with QR, 100, 115Q, *116*, 116Q

genesis of, 125
  in aortic stenosis and coarctation, 103, *104*
  incomplete right bundle branch block and, 104, 125, *126*
  in normals, 26, 68, 79Q, *79*, 125
  in right bundle branch block, 68, 79Q, 121, *125*
  in right ventricular hypertrophy, 68, 79Q, *79*, 104, 105, *105*, 113Q, 114Q, *114*, 125, 126
  width of components in, 121
Rubella, and left axis deviation, 133
R wave, amplitude of. See *QRS complex*
  defined, 26, *27*, 69
R' wave, defined, 26, *27*

S wave, amplitude of. See *QRS complex*
  defined, 26, *27*, 69
S' wave, defined, 26, *27*
Sagittal plane, 27, *28*
Sarcoid, 172t, 189
  AV block and, 264t
"Sawtooth" baseline. See *Flutter waves*
Schema for analysis of arrhythmias. See *Morphology schema*
Scleroderma, 187
  pseudoinfarction Q wave and, 164
Seizure, during ECG, 380, *380*
Sepsis, sinus tachycardia and, 231, 236t, 259
  supraventricular tachycardia and, 241t
Septal defect, ventricular. See *Ventricular septal defect*
Septal hypertrophy. See *Ventricular hypertrophy*
Septal myectomy, and left anterior hemiblock, 133
  left bundle branch block and, 127
Sex, QRS complex differences and, 69, 403t
Single ventricle, left axis deviation and, 54, 131
Sinoatrial block, digitalis and, 179
  hypercalcemia and, 175
  quinidine and, 181
Sinoventricular conduction, hyperkalemia, 173
Sinus arrhythmia, electrocardiographic criteria, *196*, 198–199
  in morphology schema, 277, *283*, 290, *290*, 303t, 329, *330*
  with aberration, in morphology schema, 303t, 331, *332*
  with Wenckebach, *266*
Sinus bradycardia, blocked atrial bigeminy confused with, 210, *211*
  capture beats and, 229, *230*, 231
  central nervous system injury and, 185
  digitalis and, 179
  electrocardiographic criteria for, 202, *204*, 205, 356Q, *356*
  hypercalcemia and, 175
  hypothyroidism and, 187
  in morphology schema, 279, 302t, 304, *305*
  insecticides and, 184
  propranolol and, 182
  systemic effects causing, 172t
  verapamil and, 183
  with aberration, in morphology schema, 302t, 308, *309*
  with AV dissociation, in morphology schema, 284, *285, 288*
Sinus capture beats. See *Capture beats*
Sinus node, absence of, in polysplenia, 83, 84, *86*
  anatomy of, 3, 6Q

Sinus node *(Continued)*
  P wave direction in, 56, *57*
Sinus node artery, 3
Sinus pause. See *"Pause"*
Sinus rhythm, electrocardiographic criteria for, *196,*
      198, *206, 242*
  in morphology schema, *277,* 302t, 312, *313*
  with aberration, with 2:1 block, in morphology
      schema, 302t, *310, 318*
    in morphology schema, 302t, 316, *317*
  with AV block, morphology schema, 302t, 304, *306*
  with 2:1 block, morphology schema, 302t, *314*
Sinus suppression, lack of, by artifact, 389, *390*
Sinus tachycardia, causes of, 231, 236t, 259
  central nervous system injury and, 185
  differential diagnosis of, 259, 261
  electrocardiographic criteria for, 231, *234, 235,*
      242t, 351Q, *351*
  heart rate and, 231, 242t
  hyperthyroidism and, 187
  in morphology schema, *279, 292,* 302t, *320, 321*
  in muscular dystrophy, 186
  insecticides and, 184
  response to intervention, 231, 259
  systemic effects causing, 172t
  T wave changes and, 151
  tricyclic antidepressants and, 183
  with aberration, 231, *235, 236,* 351Q, *351*
    and type I block, in morphology schema, 303t,
        335, *336*
    and type II AV block, in morphology schema,
        302t, *310, 318*
    and varying type II block, in morphology
        schema, 303t, 335, *336*
    in morphology schema, 302t, 324, *325*
  with AV block, in morphology schema, 302t, 304,
      306
  with type I block, in morphology schema, 303t,
      334, *335*
  with type II AV block, in morphology schema,
      302t, *314*
  with varying type II block, in morphology
      schema, 303t, 333, *334*
    Wolff-Parkinson-White, *236*
Site of block, type II, 269
    Wenckebach, 267
Site of origin, escape rhythm in AV block, 272, 274
Situs, atrial, 83–84, *84, 90*
Situs ambiguous, P wave, 83, 84, *85, 86*
Situs inversus, P wave, 83–84, *84, 90,* 96Q, *96*
"Slow response." See *Action potential*
Sodium, 9–12
"Specialized tracts," 5, 6Q, 7Q
ST depression, hypokalemia, 173
ST elevation, aneurysm and, 164–165
  differentiation from early repolarization, *150,* 151,
      165Q, *166*
  leads relating to area of injury, 159
  myocardial infarction and, genesis of, 160, *160,*
      161
  neonatal epicardial injury, 159
ST segment, absent, hypothyroidism and, 187, *188*
  cardiac tumor and, 159
  central nervous system injury and, 185
  connective tissue disease and, 187
  defined, *26, 27*

  depression of, caused by Ta wave, 38, *38,* 46Q, 77
    with subendocardial injury, 154, *154,* 165Q
  digitalis and, 179, *179,* 190Q, *191*
  elevation and depression of, causes of, 157–158
  elevation of, with subepicardial injury, 152, *154,*
      165Q
  hyperthyroidism and, 187
  hypothermia and, 186, *186*
  myocardial injury and, *152,* 152–153
  myocarditis and, 156–157, *157*
  normal configuration of, 70
  peritoneal inflammation and, 189
  prolonged, hypocalcemia and, 175
  right bundle branch block and, 124
  short, hypercalcemia and, 174
  systemic effects on, 172t, 190Q, 193
Stellate ganglion, 184
Straight back syndrome, 90–93, *93, 94*
Strain, left ventricular, genesis of, *106,* 106–107, *114*
    in right chest leads, 101, *102*
    ischemia vs., 152
  right ventricular, 101, *101*
Stress, neonatal, hypocalcemia and, 175
ST/T ratio, *150,* 151, 165Q, *166*
Stylus, faulty, 383
Stylus position, incorrect, 383, *385*
Subendocardial ischemia. See *Ischemia*
Subsidiary pacemakers, 198
  loss of, 205
Supernormal period, 11, *11*
Supraventricular rhythm, defined, in morphology
        schema, 304
  with aberration, type I block and, in morphology
        schema, 303t, 335, *336*
    type II AV block and, in morphology schema,
        302t, 308, *310, 311,* 316, *317, 318*
    varying type II block and, in morphology
        schema, 303t, 335, *336*
  with intermittent type II block, in morphology
        schema, 303t, 341, *342*
  with type I block, in morphology schema, 303t,
        333, *334*
  with type II AV block, in morphology schema,
        302t, 304, *306,* 312, *314, 315*
  with varying type II block, in morphology
        schema, 303t, 333, *334*
Supraventricular tachycardia. See also *Accelerated*
        atrial/junctional rhythm
  aberration causing T wave changes, 151
  AV block and, 237, *240*
    advanced, 270
  AV dissociation and, 236–237, *240*
  causes of, 241t
  confusion with atrial flutter, 237, 243
  defined, 235–236
  differential diagnosis of, 259, 261
  electrocardiographic criteria for, 235–239, *238,*
        239t, *240,* 242t, 350Q, *350*
  heart rate, 237, 242t
  in morphology schema, 302t, *320, 321, 322*
  Lown-Ganong-Levine and, 138
  Mahaim conduction and, 141
  P wave enlargement, 111
  P waves and, 74, 75, 237, *238,* 239t, *240*
  preexcitation and, 135
  QRS aberration and, 124

Supraventricular tachycardia *(Continued)*
QRS complex and, 237, *238*
response to intervention and, 259
T wave changes and, 151
with aberration, in morphology schema, 302t, *318*, *324*, *326*, *327*
with aberration, with type II AV block, in morphology schema, 302t, *310*, *327*
with AV block, in morphology schema, 302t, 304, *306*
with AV dissociation, in morphology schema, 302t, *320*, *322*
with type II AV block, in morphology schema, 302t, *314*, *320*, *322*
with Wenckebach, *266*
Wolff-Parkinson-White and, 138
antidromic, 261, *262*
Surgery, bifascicular block and, 134
complete AV block and, 274
escape beats and escape rhythms and, 205t
left bundle branch block and, 127
left posterior hemiblock and, 134
premature atrial/junctional contractions, 211t
premature ventricular contractions and, 214t
right bundle branch block and, 124
supraventricular tachycardia and, 241t
Sympathetic nervous system, T wave changes and, 149–150
Sympathetic tone, central nervous system injury and, 185
congenital prolonged QT interval and, 184
halothane and, 183
insecticides and, 184
Sympathomimetic amines, 214t
premature atrial/junctional contractions, 211t
sinus tachycardia, 236t, 259
supraventricular tachycardia, 241t
Systemic alterations, effects of, 170–194
summary table of, 172t
Systemic lupus erythematosus. See *Lupus erythematosus*

T wave, absent, artifact, 387, *387*
adrenal insufficiency and, 188
alternating, 184
axis. See *Mean vector, T wave*
before QRS, as artifact, 389, *390*
bizarre, 184, 192Q, *192*
cardiac tumor, 159
central nervous system injury and, 185
changes in, in ischemia, 151–152, *152*, *153*
changes in, in left ventricular hypertrophy, 106, 106–107, *114*
primary, 55
in right ventricular hypertrophy, 100–101, *101*, 113Q
secondary, 55
connective tissue disease and, 187
derivation of, 43–45, *43*, *44*, 46Q
duration of, prolonged in hypokalemia, 176
functional changes in, 149–151
genesis in right ventricular hypertrophy, 101
genesis in right ventricular strain, 101
halothane and, 183
"hyperacute," in myocardial infarction, 160, *160*
hyperkalemia and, 173
hyperthyroidism and, 187
hypokalemia and, 173, *175*
hypokalemia plus hypocalcemia and, 178
hypothyroidism and, 187, *188*
in congenital prolonged QT interval, 184, *185*, 192Q, 192
inverted in midprecordial lead and, 151
left bundle branch block and, 127
low-voltage, hypothyroidism and, 187
mean vector. See *Mean vector, T wave*
mitral prolapse and, 152
myocardial infarction and, genesis of, 160, *160*, 161
myocarditis and, 156–157, *157*
normal amplitude of, 70, 71, *71*, *72*, *73*
normal progression with age, 55, 71
normal shape of, 70, *70*, *71*, *72*, *73*
P wave differentiated from, 72, 73, *74*
peritoneal inflammation and, 189
phenothiazines and, 183
pheochromocytoma and, 188
primary and secondary changes in, 149
quinidine and, 181
right bundle branch block and, 124
systemic effects on, 172t, 190Q, 193
tricyclic antidepressants and, 183
U wave differentiated from, 45, 47Q, 71–73, *71*, *72*, *73*
Tachyarrythmias, 231–261. See also specific tachyarrythmias
defined, 231
central nervous system injury and, 185
differential diagnosis of, 259, 261
imipramine and, 183
in connective tissue disease, 187
in muscular dystrophy, 186
tricyclic antidepressants and, 183
Tachycardia, differential diagnosis of, 259, 261
"impossibly rapid," artifact, *384*, 388, *388*
intrauterine, 243
junctional. See *Junctional tachycardia*
sinus. See *Sinus tachycardia*
supraventricular. See *Supraventricular tachycardia*
ventricular. See *Ventricular tachycardia*
"wide QRS." See *"Wide QRS"*
Ta wave, defined, 26
derivation of, 36–39, *37*, *38*, *44*
shape of, 36, *38*, *39*
ST segment shift and, 158
"Tape drag," 382, *384*, 392Q, *393*
Terminal rhythm, in children, 257
Tetralogy of Fallot, postoperative, accelerated junctional rhythm and, 241, *245*
postoperative, right bundle branch block and, 124
postoperative AV block and, 274
postoperative bifascicular block and, 134
Theophylline, sinus tachycardia, 259
"Threshold potential," 11
Thyrotoxicosis, sinus tachycardia and, 236t
Tofranil. See *Imipramine*
Torsade-de-Pointes, insecticides and, 184
morphology of, 252, *256*
quinidine toxicity and, 181, *181*
Total anomalous pulmonary venous return, papillary muscle infarction and, 162
Toxicity, drug. See specific drugs

T-P interval, defined, *26, 27,* 67, 77, 78
Tracts, internodal, 3–5, *4,* 6Q, 7Q
Transitional cells, 3
Transmural ischemia. See *Ischemia*
Transposition of great arteries, escape beats and
     escape rhythms and, 205
Trauma, chest, supraventricular tachycardia and,
     241t
Tremor, during ECG, 380
Triangle, Burger, 29, *30*
   Einthoven, 29, *30*
Trichloroethylene, 183
Tricuspid atresia, left axis deviation and, 54, 131
Tricyclic antidepressants, 172t, 183
   premature ventricular contractions and, 214t
Trigeminy, 221, *223*
T-U wave, 45
Tumor. See *Cardiac tumor*
Type 1 antiarrhythmic drugs. See *Quinidine*
"Typical" Wenckebach, 265, *265,* 271

U wave, bradycardia and, 173
   causes of, 45, 47Q
   cerebrovascular accident and, 174
   defined, *26, 27,* 71
   derivation of, 45, 46, 47Q
   hypokalemia and, 173
   hypokalemia plus hypocalcemia and, 178
   inversion of, 45
   ischemia and, 173
   left ventricular hypertrophy and, 173
   mitral prolapse and, 152
   normal amplitude and, 71, *71, 72, 73*
   phenothiazines and, 173, 183
   procainamide and, 173
   quinidine and, 173, 181
   T wave differentiated from, 45, 47Q, 71–73, *71, 72,*
     73
Uniform premature beats, 220, *221*
"Unipolar" lead, explanation of hypothetical
     recording, 13, 14, *14*
Uremia, AV block, 264t

Vagal maneuvers, supraventricular vs. sinus
     tachycardia, 259
Vagal tone, AV block and, 264t
   AV conduction and, 263
   central nervous system injury and, 185
   digitalis and, 179
   escape beats and escape rhythms and, 205
   halothane and, 183
   quinidine and, 181
Vagus nerve, pacemaker suppression by, 12
Variable coupling. See *Coupling interval*
Vasodilators, sinus tachycardia, 236t
Vector, atrial depolarization and, 36, *37,* 46Q
   atrial repolarization and, 36, 38, 46Q
   direction of, 16, 17Q
   P wave and, 36, *37,* 46Q
   QRS, 39–43, *40, 44,* 46Q
   summation of, 16
   T wave and, 44, *44,* 45, 46Q
   Ta wave and, 36, 38, 46Q
   U wave and, 45, 46
   ventricular depolarization and, 39–43, *40, 44,* 46Q
   ventricular repolarization and, 44, *44,* 45, 46Q

Ventricle, depolarization. See *Depolarization,*
     ventricular
   position abnormalities, 84–90
   repolarization. See *Repolarization, ventricular*
   stretch and U waves, 46
Ventricular bigeminy, 220, 221, *222, 224*
Ventricular catheters, premature ventricular
     contractions, 214t
Ventricular contractions, premature. See *Premature*
     ventricular contractions
Ventricular couplets, 223, *223*
Ventricular dysplasia, arrhythmogenic right, and
     ventricular tachycardia, 258t
Ventricular escape beat(s), escape rhythm and,
     electrocardiographic criteria, *196,* 199t, 201,
     202, 206, 242, 344Q, *345,* 353Q, *354,* 356Q,
     357
   in morphology schema, 297, *301,* 303t, 343, *343*
   premature ventricular contractions confused with,
     213
Ventricular escape rhythm, digitalis toxicity and, *180*
   in complete AV block, 272
   in morphology schema, 302t, 308, *309*
   with complete AV block, in morphology schema,
     302t, 308, *311*
Ventricular fibrillation, electrocardiographic criteria
     and, 254, 257, *258*
   hyperkalemia and, 173
Ventricular hypertrophy, biventricular, 108–110, *109,*
     114, 115Q, *115*
   left, *106,* 106–108, 113Q
     adolescents, 107
     left axis deviation and, 54
     pseudoinfarction Q wave and, 163, 166Q, *166*
     R and S waves, *106,* 107
     U wave, 173
   right, 99–105, 113Q
     pseudoinfarction Q wave, 164
     R wave in V$_1$, 101, 102, 113Q
     RSR′, 68
     RSR′ in V$_1$, 104, 105, *105,* 113Q
     R/S ratio and, 103, 113Q
     right axis deviation and, 53
     S wave in V$_6$, 102–103, 113Q
     with bundle branch block, 124
   septal, 101, 103, *103,* 107
Ventricular inversion, pseudoinfarction Q wave, 164
Ventricular parasystole, 225, *227*
Ventricular premature contractions. See *Premature*
     ventricular contractions
Ventricular rhythm, accelerated. See *Accelerated*
Ventricular septal defect, 107
   first-degree AV block, 263
   postoperative, right bundle branch block and, 124
   postoperative AV block, 274
Ventricular septal hypertrophy. See *Ventricular*
     hypertrophy
Ventricular tachycardia. See also *Accelerated*
     ventricular rhythm
   anesthetics and, 183
   AV dissociation and, 251, *253,* 254, *255, 256,* 257
   bidirectional, digitalis toxicity and, 179, *180*
     tachycardia morphology and, 252, 257
   capture beats and, 231, *233,* 251, *254, 256*
   cardiac tumor and, 159
   causes of, 254, 258t

Ventricular tachycardia *(Continued)*
    complete AV block and, in morphology schema, 302t, *319*
    differential diagnosis of, 259, 261
    electrocardiographic criteria for, 251, 252, *252*, *253*, *254*, *255*, *256*, *257*
    fusion, 251, *253*, *254*, *255*, *256*
    hyperkalemia and, 173
    imipramine and, 183
    in morphology schema, 302t, 316, *317*, 324, *326*, *327*, *328*
    insecticides and, 184
    psychotrophic drugs and, 183
    QRS complex and, 251, *252*
    quinidine toxicity and, 181, *181*
    simulating artifact, *392*, 392Q, *393*
    systemic effects causing, 172t, 190Q, 193
    Torsade-de-Pointes, morphology of, 252, *256*
        quinidine toxicity and, 181, *181*
    tricyclic antidepressants and, 183
Ventricular trigeminy, 221, 223, *223*
Ventricular tumor. See *Cardiac tumor*
Ventriculotomy, right bundle branch block and, 124
Verapamil, 172t, 183
    AV block and, 264t
Vitamin D deficiency, hypocalcemia and, 175
Vmax, defined, 10
Voltage, magnitude of, *15*, 15, 16
Volume overload, U waves and, 46
Vomiting, hypokalemia and, 173

Wandering pacemaker, central nervous system injury and, 185
    electrocardiographic criteria for, 202, *203*
    in morphology schema, 209, 303t, 329, *330*
    with aberration, in morphology schema, 303t, *331*, *332*
Wavefront, depolarization, 13, 14, *13*, *14*, *15*, 17Q
    repolarization, 14, 15, *14*, *15*
Wenckebach, 265–267, *265*, *266*, *268*, *271*, 349Q, *349*, 351Q, *351*
    AV node block and, 267
    causes of, 264t, 267
    central nervous system injury and, 185
    in digitalis toxicity, 179
"Wide QRS" tachycardia, differential diagnosis of, 259, 261
    positive in all chest leads, 261, *262*
Wolff-Parkinson-White, 65, *66*, 136–138, *137*, *139*, 143Q, 144Q, *144*, 145Q, *145*
    atrial fibrillation, 250, *250*, 251t
    atrial flutter, 243
    confused with premature ventricular contractions, 215, *217*
    in morphology schema, 279, *280*, 280, *281*
    intermittent, 215, *217*, 236
    pseudoinfarction Q wave, 164, *166*, 166Q
    sinus tachycardia, 236
    supraventricular tachycardia, 241t
        antidromic, 261, *262*
    surgical change in electrocardiogram, *250*